Head and Neck Cancer:
Diagnosis and Management

Head and Neck Cancer: Diagnosis and Management

Edited by Amber Hooper

hayle
medical

New York

Hayle Medical,
750 Third Avenue, 9th Floor,
New York, NY 10017, USA

Visit us on the World Wide Web at:
www.haylemedical.com

This book contains information obtained from authentic and highly regarded sources. Copyright for all individual chapters remain with the respective authors as indicated. All chapters are published with permission under the Creative Commons Attribution License or equivalent. A wide variety of references are listed. Permission and sources are indicated; for detailed attributions, please refer to the permissions page and list of contributors. Reasonable efforts have been made to publish reliable data and information, but the authors, editors and publisher cannot assume any responsibility for the validity of all materials or the consequences of their use.

ISBN: 978-1-63241-692-6

Trademark Notice: Registered trademark of products or corporate names are used only for explanation and identification without intent to infringe.

Cataloging-in-Publication Data

Head and neck cancer : diagnosis and management / edited by Amber Hooper.
   p. cm.
Includes bibliographical references and index.
ISBN 978-1-63241-692-6
1. Head--Cancer--Diagnosis. 2. Head--Cancer--Treatment. 3. Neck--Cancer--Diagnosis.
4. Neck--Cancer--Treatment. I. Hooper, Amber.
RD661 .H43 2019
616.992 715--dc23

Table of Contents

Preface

This book aims to highlight the current researches and provides a platform to further the scope of innovations in this area. This book is a product of the combined efforts of many researchers and scientists, after going through thorough studies and analysis from different parts of the world. The objective of this book is to provide the readers with the latest information of the field.

The group of cancers that begin in the throat, mouth, nose, salivary glands, sinuses and larynx are collectively called head and neck cancer. Some of the common symptoms are neck pain, sinus congestion, mass in the neck, bad breath, enlarged lymph glands, hoarse voice, etc. The diagnosis of head and neck cancer is done ideally through a needle biopsy of the lesion and a histopathological investigation. Depending on the tumor site, health issues, previous primary tumor occurrence, relative morbidity of treatment options, etc., an appropriate treatment strategy is devised. Most head and neck cancers are treated through surgical resection and radiation therapy. Chemotherapy may also be combined with other treatment strategies for better survival and control of the cancer. The topics covered in this extensive book deal with the diagnosis and management of head and neck cancer. It elucidates new treatment techniques and their applications in a multidisciplinary manner. Researchers and students in this field will be assisted by this book.

I would like to express my sincere thanks to the authors for their dedicated efforts in the completion of this book. I acknowledge the efforts of the publisher for providing constant support. Lastly, I would like to thank my family for their support in all academic endeavors.

Editor

Genomic insights into head and neck cancer

Tim N. Beck[1,2]* and Erica A. Golemis[1,2]*

Abstract

Head and neck squamous cell carcinoma (HNSCC) is the sixth most common cancer worldwide and is frequently impervious to curative treatment efforts. Similar to other cancers associated with prolonged exposure to carcinogens, HNSCCs often have a high burden of mutations, contributing to substantial inter- and intra-tumor heterogeneity. The heterogeneity of this malignancy is further increased by the rising rate of human papillomavirus (HPV)-associated (HPV+) HNSCC, which defines an etiological subtype significantly different from the more common tobacco and alcohol associated HPV-negative (HPV-) HNSCC. Since 2011, application of large scale genome sequencing projects by The Cancer Genome Atlas (TCGA) network and other groups have established extensive datasets to characterize HPV- and HPV+ HNSCC, providing a foundation for advanced molecular diagnoses, identification of potential biomarkers, and therapeutic insights. Some genomic lesions are now appreciated as widely dispersed. For example, HPV- HNSCC characteristically inactivates the cell cycle suppressors TP53 (p53) and CDKN2A (p16), and often amplifies CCND1 (cyclin D), which phosphorylates RB1 to promote cell cycle progression from G1 to S. By contrast, HPV+ HNSCC expresses viral oncogenes E6 and E7, which inhibit TP53 and RB1, and activates the cell cycle regulator E2F1. Frequent activating mutations in PIK3CA and inactivating mutations in NOTCH1 are seen in both subtypes of HNSCC, emphasizing the importance of these pathways. Studies of large patient cohorts have also begun to identify less common genetic alterations, predominantly found in HPV- tumors, which suggest new mechanisms relevant to disease pathogenesis. Targets of these alterations including AJUBA and FAT1, both involved in the regulation of NOTCH/CTNNB1 signaling. Genes involved in oxidative stress, particularly CUL3, KEAP1 and NFE2L2, strongly associated with smoking, have also been identified, and are less well understood mechanistically. Application of sophisticated data-mining approaches, integrating genomic information with profiles of tumor methylation and gene expression, have helped to further yield insights, and in some cases suggest additional approaches to stratify patients for clinical treatment. We here discuss some recent insights built on TCGA and other genomic foundations.

Keywords: Head and neck cancer, TCGA, HPV, Genomics, Cancer therapy, Cell cycle, Personalized medicine, Tumor heterogeneity

Background

Head and neck squamous cell carcinoma (HNSCC) is the sixth most common cancer, with annual incidence of 600,000 cases worldwide [1]. Anatomically, head and neck cancer regions include the oral cavity, the pharynx (nasopharynx—behind the nose; oropharynx—soft palate, base of the tongue and the tonsils; hypopharynx—the lowest part of the pharynx), the larynx, the paranasal sinuses, the nasal cavity and the salivary glands

[2]. Beyond distinction by anatomic sites, HNSCC is divided into two broad classes: human papillomavirus (HPV)-associated (HPV+) and HPV-negative (HPV-) disease. The majority of HPV-negative HNSCC arises from the larynx and oral cavity [3, 4], although a small fraction of cases originates in the oro- and hypopharynx. HPV+ disease is typically found in the oropharynx, with a minority of cases detected in the larynx and oral cavity [5]. As of 2016, the majority of HNSCC is HPV- disease, and is most commonly associated with tobacco use and heavy alcohol consumption [6]. The exception is oropharyngeal HNSCC, 60-70 % of which is HPV+ in North America and Europe (significant geographic variation

* Correspondence: Tim.Beck@Fccc.edu; Erica.Golemis@fccc.edu
[1]Program in Molecular Therapeutics, Fox Chase Cancer Center, 333 Cottman Ave, Philadelphia, PA 19111, USA
Full list of author information is available at the end of the article

exists in the prevalence of HPV+ disease worldwide [3, 5, 7]). Over 150 types of HPV have been identified, with HPV subtype 16 (HPV–16) identified as the most oncogenic, detected in over 90 % of HPV+ oropharyngeal cancers [8]. HPV+ HNSCC is typically diagnosed in a younger patient population (6th decade of life; [5, 9]) and its prevalence has dramatically increased since the 1980's (then only detected in 16 % of oropharyngeal cancer; [7, 9]). HPV- HNSCC is generally diagnosed in an older patient population (7th decade of life), often presents with locally advanced or metastatic features, and has a relatively poor prognosis compared to HPV+ tumors [5, 10].

Both HPV+ and HPV- HNSCC are treated with a combination of surgery, radiation and adjuvant chemotherapy. Treatment specifics vary depending on anatomic site and disease stage. In general, low stage tumors are treated with surgery, followed by radiation if positive surgery margins are detected. For more advanced cases treatment includes surgery, if possible, followed by radiation with or without adjuvant chemotherapy [1, 9, 11]. In spite of significant improvements, including the introduction of targeted and immunotherapies (most prominently, immune checkpoint inhibitors targeting cytotoxic T-lymphocyte-associated antigen 4 (CTLA-4) and programmed cell death protein 1 (PD-1) [12]), as of 2015 the relative 5-year survival rate is only approximately 25–40 % for HPV- and 70–80 % for HPV + HNSCC [1, 13, 14]. To fully capture the diversity of HNSCC and to gain clinically meaningful insights that can improve treatment, it seems critical to define the full spectrum of molecular alterations and the heterogeneity associated with this pathology.

At no prior point in time has it been possible to describe the molecular landscape of the various, mostly anatomically defined cancers with as much detail and precision as is possible today [15–17], based on concerted efforts to uncover the genomic (most advanced), epigenomic, proteomic and transcriptomic changes that occur as healthy tissue turns malignant, metastatic and resistant to treatment [18]. The Cancer Genome Atlas (TCGA) network and others have periodically published datasets on many cancers [15, 17], including extensive analyses of HPV- and to a lesser degree HPV+ HNSCC (Table 1; [17, 19–24]). Amongst non-lung and non-skin tumor types, head and neck cancer has one of the highest rates of non-synonymous mutations and a high degree of genomic instability [15, 16, 25, 26], which contribute to the enormous heterogeneity of HNSCC [19, 24]. Since large-scale datasets began to appear in 2011 [20, 22], a number of groups have performed integrated bioinformatics, translational, and clinical analyses that leverage the genomic resources, suggesting new research directions. This review summarizes and highlights

potential therapeutic opportunities in HPV- and HPV+ HNSCC based on the analysis of high throughput data published by the TCGA network and others.

Foundational genomic datasets

The pathophysiological differences between HPV+ and HPV- HNSCC necessitate that genomic analyses apply rigorous classification methods for HPV dependence in clinical samples [10, 22, 27]. HPV status is most commonly determined by polymerase chain reaction (PCR) or *in situ* hybridization (*ISH*) to detect HPV genetic material, or by immunohistochemical (IHC) staining for the tumor suppressor p16 (CDKN2A), which is induced as a consequence of HPV-associated transformation [28]. p16 IHC staining is greatly increased as a result of HPV infection, and is a reliable proxy for positive HPV status in primary tumors of the oropharynx [28]. Virally encoded proteins target the cell cycle regulator retinoblastoma 1 gene (RB1), providing one potential feedback mechanisms for enhancing expression of p16 ([29], and discussed further below). Alternatively, it has been shown that upregulation of p16 can also occur as a cellular response to the infection itself, through induction of the histone 3 lysine-27 (H3K27) specific demethylases KDM6A and KDM6B [30–32]. For other anatomic sites, the true positive rate for p16 IHC staining falls below 50 %, reflecting the rarity of HPV-associated tumors outside of the oropharynx [28, 33]. High p16 expression also occurs in about 5 % of HPV- cases, for reasons that are at present unclear [28]. For these reasons, the TCGA network took extensive measures to ensure proper HPV classification of each tumor: in addition to p16 staining and *ISH*, whole HPV genome sequencing as well as HPV RNA-Seq was performed. HPV positive cases were classified as such if > 1000 RNA-Seq reads aligned to viral genes E6 and E7 [19].

The TCGA network analyzed 243 HPV-negative and 36 HPV-positive tumors using multiple platforms (RNA sequencing, DNA sequencing, reverse phase protein array (RPPA), DNA methylation profiling and miRNA sequencing) to define the molecular landscape of this malignancy [19, 34]. Most of the patients in the TCGA cohort were male (~70 %) and heavy smokers (51 mean pack years; [19]), closely resembling the general HPV- HNSCC patient population [1, 11]. Tumors predominantly originated from the oral cavity (*n* = 172; 62 %; 160/172 HPV- and 12/172 HPV+) and the larynx (*n* = 72; 26 %; 71/72 HPV- and 1/72 HPV+), with only a few cases originating from the oropharynx (*n* = 33; 12 %; 11/33 HPV- and 22/33 HPV+) and only two from the hypopharynx (1/2 HPV+ and 1/2 HPV-).

Beyond the work of the TCGA network, additional genomic sequencing studies (Table 1) were performed by Stransky et al. (53 HPV- and 11 HPV+; [22]), Agrawal

Table 1 High-throughput genomic studies of HNSCC. The most frequently altered genes described in seven studies are shown, separated by HPV status when possible

TCGA (2015; [19])[a]	Seiwert et al. (2015; [21])	Lin et al. (2014; [37])[a]	Pickering et al. (2014; [36])[b]	Pickering et al. (2013; [35])	Stransky et al. (2011; [22])[a]	Agrawal et al. (2011; [20])[a]
HPV-	HPV-	N/A (NPC)	N/A (Tongue)	N/A (OSCC)	HPV-	N/A
n = 243	n = 69	n = 128	n = 34 (YT 16, OT 28)	n = 35-40	n = 63	n = 28
TP53 (84 %, M)	TP53 (81 %, M)	TP53 (17 %, M/D)	TP53 (94 %, 57 %, M)	CDKN2A (74 %, D)	TP53 (73 %, M)	TP53 (79 %, M)
CDKN2A (57 %, M/D)	CDKN2A (33, M/D)	CDKN2A/B (13 %, M/D)	CSMD1 (25 %, 75 %, D)	TP53 (66 %, M)	CDKN2A (25 %, M/D[c])	NOTCH1 (14 %, M)
let-7c (40 %, miRNA)	MDM2 (16 %, A)	ARID1A (11 %, M/D)	PIK3CA (0 %, 11 %, M); (30 %, 70 %, A)	FAT1 (46 %, M/D)	SYNE1 (22 %, M)	RELN (14 %, M)
PIK3CA (34 %, M/A)	MLL2 (16 %, M)	SYNE1 (8 %, M)	CDKN2A (6 %, 4 %, M); (55 %, 65 %, D)	TP63 (26 %, A)	CCND1 (22 %, A[c])	SYNE1 (14 %, M)
FADD (32 %, A)	NOTCH 1 (16 %, M)	ATG13 (6 %, M/D)	FADD/CCND1 (40 %, 65 %, A)	CCND1 (23 %, A)	MUC16 (19 %, M)	EPHA7 (11 %, M)
FAT1 (32 %, M/D)	CCND1 (13 %, A)	MLL2 (6 %, M)	FAT1 (6 %, 25 %, M); (50 %, 35 %, D)	MAML1 (23 %, D)	USH2A (18 %, M)	FLG (11 %, M)
CCND1 (31 %, A)	PIK3CA (13 %, M)	PIK3CA (6 %, M/A)	EGFR (20 %, 50 %, A)	EGFR (17 %, A)	FAT1 (14 %, M)	HRAS (11 %, M)
NOTCH1/2/3 (29 %, M/D)	PIK3CB (13 %, M/A)	CCND1 (4 %, A)	NOTCH1 (25 %, 18 %, M)	TNK2 (17 %, A)	LRP1B (14 %, M)	PIK3AP1 (11 %, M)
TP63 (19 %, A)	UBR5 (13 %, M/D)	NOTCH3 (4 %, M)	HLA-A (0 %, 14 %, M)	AKT1 (14 %, A)	ZFHX4 (14 %, M)	RIMBP2 (11 %, M)
EGFR (15 %, M/A)	EGFR (12 %, A)	FGFR2 (4 %, M)	CASP8 (6 %, 11 %, M)	SRC (14 %, A)	NOTCH1 (13 %, M)	SI (11 %, M)
HPV+	HPV+				HPV+	HPV+
n = 36	n = 51				n = 11	n = 4
E6/7 (100 %)	E6/7 (100 %)				E6/E7 (100 %)	E6/E7 (100 %)
PIK3CA (56 %, M/A)	PIK3CA (22 %, M)				PIK3CA (27 %, M)	EPHB3 (25 %, M)
TP63 (28 %, A)	TP63 (16 %, M/A)				RUFY1 (18 %, M)	UNC5D (25 %, M)
TRAF3 (22 %, M/D)	PIK3CB (13 %, M/A)				EZH2 (18 %, M)	NLRP12 (25 %, M)
E2F1 (19 %, A)	FGFR3 (14 %, M)				CDH10 (18 %, M)	PIK3CA (25 %, M)
let-7c (17 %, miRNA)	NF1/2 (12 %, M)				THSD7A (18 %, M)	TM7SF3 (25 %, M)
NOTCH1/3 (17 %, M)	SOX2 (12 %, A)				FAT4 (18 %, M)	ENPP1 (25 %, M)
FGFR3 (11 %, F/M)	ATM (10 %, D)				KMT2D (18 %, M)	NRXN3 (25 %, M)
HLA-A/B (11 %, M/D)	FLG (12 %, M)				ZNF676 (18 %, M)	MICAL2 (25 %, M)
EGFR (6 %, M)	MLL3 (10 %, M)				MUC16 (18 %, M)	

N/A HPV status not available, NPC nasopharyngeal cancer, YT young tongue, OT old tongue, OSCC oral squamous cell carcinoma, M mutation, A amplification, D deletion, F fusion

[a]Data was accessed using cBioportal [38, 39]
[b]values for A and D are approximations
[c]percentages are not based on the 63 cases, because CNAs were not analyzed for all cases

et al. (28 HPV- and 4 HPV+; [20]), Pickering et al. (40 oral squamous cell carcinoma; likely HPV-negative; [35]), Seiwert et al. (69 HPV- and 51 HPV+; [21]), and Pickering et al. (34 squamous cell carcinoma of the oral tongue; likely HPV-negative; [36]). These predominantly relied on a single platform (exome/massively parallel sequencing) for data acquisition. In addition, Lin et al. have sequenced 128 cases of nasopharyngeal carcinomas (NPC; likely HPV-; [37]).

The TCGA dataset [19] is conveniently accessible through cBioportal [38, 39], as are the datasets from Stransky et al., Agrawal et al. [20, 22], and the NPC study [37]. The 279 patient TCGA dataset provides the most extensive tumor profiles, including mutational data from whole exome sequencing, identification of somatic copy number alterations using the GISTIC algorithm [40], mRNA expression data (RNA-Seq V2 RSEM), and protein expression data for a total of 165 combined phosophoproteins and proteins (reverse-phase protein array/microarray; [38, 39, 41]). The other three datasets accessible through cBioPortal predominantly cover somatic mutations. The dataset for Pickering et al. [35] is available through Gene Expression Omnibus (GEO; [42]); the remaining studies provide access to datasets via links provided in the original publications. Table 1 summarizes the top alterations detected in each study for HPV- and, if available, HPV+ cases. Certain alterations were detected across several studies; whereas, a significant number of alterations were not uniformly detected, potentially due to the variation in detection platforms, disease heterogeneity and significant demographic differences.

Common genomic defects: HPV+ and HPV-

Copy number alterations (CNA) are frequent in HNSCC [26] and are highly concordant across most of the genome for HPV- and HPV+ cases [19, 43]. One of the most frequently amplified regions (in approximately 15–30 % of cases [19]) is on chromosome 3q and includes the anti-apoptotic kinase protein kinase C (PIK3CA),

and the transcription factors TP63 and SOX2 [44]. Additional amplifications found in both the HPV+ and HPV- disease subtypes include chromosomes 5p and 8q [19, 43], which encompass telomerase TERT (5p) and the oncogene MYC (8q). Commonly seen deletions prominently cover parts of chromosome 3p and 8p, impacting two tumor suppressor genes: FHIT (3p; expression loss is associated with worse survival in HNSCC [45]) and CSMD1 (8p; [19, 46, 47]). Losses in 3p and 8p and gains in 3q, 5p and 8q are also frequently seen in squamous cell carcinomas (SQCC) of the lung [48], highlighting important genomic similarities between SQCC and HNSCC [19, 43, 48].

The microRNA let-7c, a cell cycle regulator, is frequently inactivated in both HPV- and HPV+ HNSCC in the TCGA cohort (Fig. 1a and b). Depressed expression of let7-c is associated with increased expression of CDK4, CDK6, E2F1 and PLK1, kinases and translational regulators important for progression through the cell cycle [19, 49]. In depth analysis of TCGA microRNA data has been used to test the hypothesis that expression of 28 microRNAs selected based on *in vitro* experiments

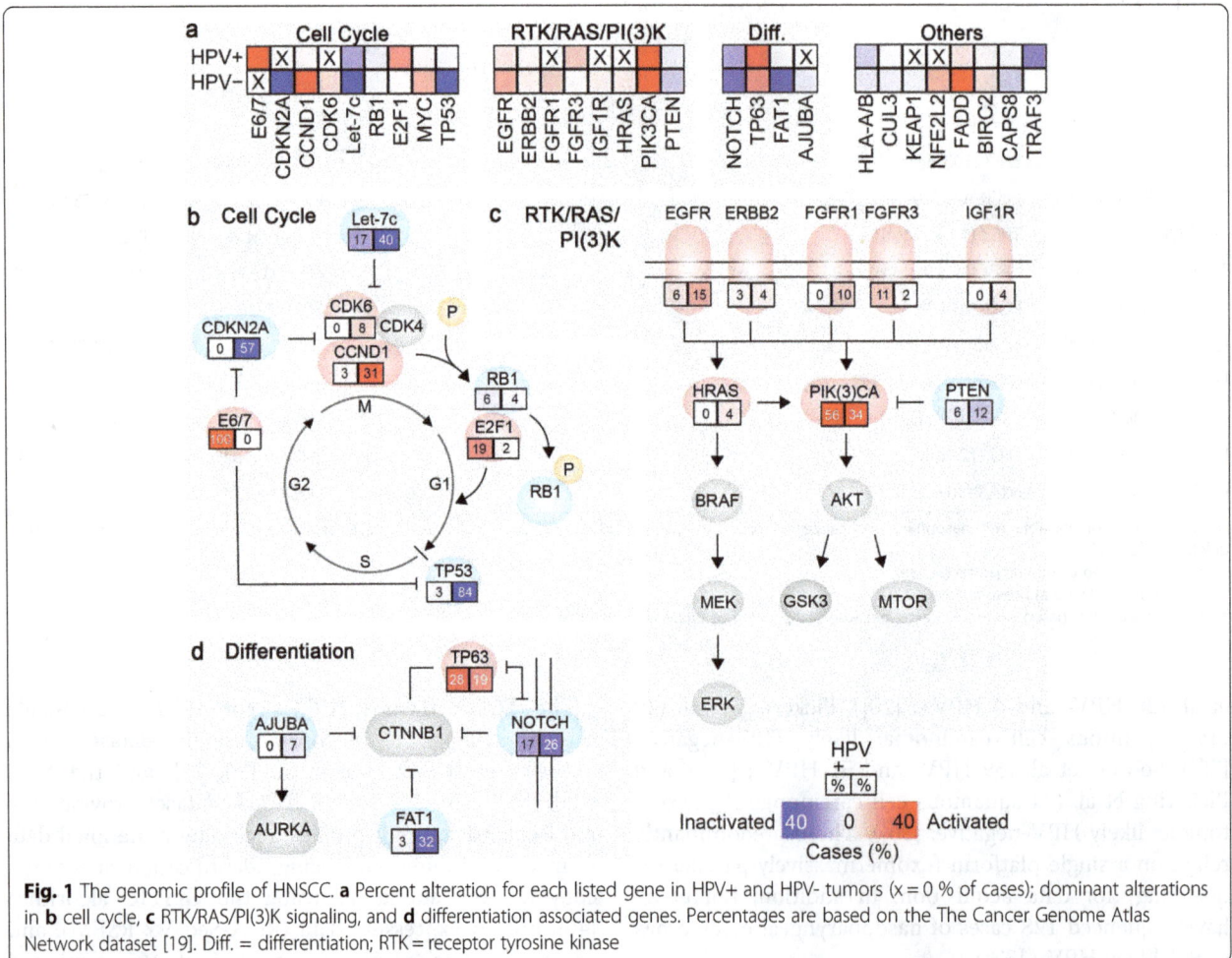

Fig. 1 The genomic profile of HNSCC. **a** Percent alteration for each listed gene in HPV+ and HPV- tumors (x = 0 % of cases); dominant alterations in **b** cell cycle, **c** RTK/RAS/PI(3)K signaling, and **d** differentiation associated genes. Percentages are based on the The Cancer Genome Atlas Network dataset [19]. Diff. = differentiation; RTK = receptor tyrosine kinase

could predict response to radiotherapy [50]. Patients from the TCGA cohort with complete clinical annotations were divided into three groups: radiation with complete response (radiosensitive), radiation with tumor progression (radioresistant), and not irradiated. This analysis suggested that upregulation of miR-016, miR-29, miR-150, miR-1254 and downregulation of let-7e correlated with complete response to radiotherapy. Effects were linked to ATM expression. Higher levels of ATM correlated with increased radio-resistance, based on RPPA data also provided by the TCGA [50]. These interesting findings necessitate validation using additional cohorts, but clearly indicate the potential value of analyzing microRNA expression in HNSCC.

One of the most commonly activated (mutationally or due to amplification of the 3q chromosomal region) genes in both HPV+ and HPV- cases in the TCGA cohorts (56 and 34 %, respectively) and other studies (Table 1; [21–23]) is PIK3CA, encoding the p110α catalytic subunit of phosphinositol-3-kinase (Fig. 1; [19]). In this regard, HNSCC is similar to many other cancers in which PIK3CA is amongst the most commonly mutated genes [18]. PIK3CA encodes a lipid kinase that regulates signal propagation from multiple input sources [51], including many of the receptor tyrosine kinases (RTKs) relevant to HNSCC (Fig. 1c; [19, 52, 53]). Functionally, PIK3CA regulates phosphorylation of AKT1, and mutated PIK3CA has been shown to attenuate apoptotic signals and support tumor invasion [54]. Additionally, mutationally activated PIK3CA has been shown to support cyclin D activity [55]; thus, further emphasizing the tremendous relevance of cell cycle dysregulation in head and neck cancers [43, 56].

Lui et al. performed a focused whole-exome analysis of 151 HNSCC tumors (datasets from Stransky et al. and Agrawal et al., plus 45 additional cases [20, 22]), specifically exploring PI3K pathway mutations for therapeutic opportunities [23], This analysis (which did not assess CNAs) indicated the PI3K pathway was the most frequently mutated oncogenic pathway (30.5 % of tumors, 46/151 [23]). PIK3CA in particular was mutated in 12.6 % of cases (19/151; [23]), which is substantially less than the number of cases with mutated PIK3CA (21 %, 58/279) reported by the TCGA [19]. Nevertheless, assessment of patient derived xenografts expressing wild type PI3KCA or mutant PI3KCA and treated with vehicle or the mTOR/PI3K inhibitor BEZ-235 [57] indicated tumors with mutated PI3KCA were exquisitely sensitive to the small molecule inhibitor, whereas tumors without the mutation did not respond to the treatment [23]. Several studies using pre-clinical models also demonstrated that HNSCC with wild type PI3KCA is sensitive to PI3K/mTOR inhibitors, particularly in combination with a MEK inhibitor or in combination with radiation in the

context of wild type p53 [58, 59]. Development of a large number of PI(3)K inhibitors is ongoing, with several promising compounds currently being tested in clinical trials [60].

Another commonly altered gene in HNSCC is NOTCH1. NOTCH1 is a transmembrane kinase frequently mutationally inactivated (most commonly via missense or truncating mutation) in both HPV+ and HPV- cases (13–26 % and 8–17 %, respectively [19, 21]; Table 1). The role of the NOTCH pathway is complicated and depends on the overall organization of the broader signaling network and on the specific tissue type [61]. Exome sequencing of HNSCC strongly implicated NOTCH1 as a tumor suppressor in this malignancy, as close to 40 % (11/28) of NOTCH1 mutations were truncating mutations predicted to be inactivating [20]. This conclusion was supported by the observation that NOTCH1 knockout mice developed tumors due to increased oncogenic CTNNB1 signaling [62]. Additional work in tongue carcinoma cells observed robust downregulation of CTNNB1 in the background of stable expression of NOTCH1 [63]. Another important feature of NOTCH1 is its participation in reciprocal negative regulation with p63 [64], a member of the p53 family found to be activated with high frequency in HNSCC (19 and 28 % in HPV- and HPV+ cases respectively, mostly due to amplification [19]). In keratinocytes, overexpression of p63 induced cell growth in part by suppression of p21 and thus directly counteracting the growth suppressive input from NOTCH1 [65]. The TCGA data supports this NOTCH1-p63 paradigm in HNSCC, given the high incident of NOTCH1 inactivating mutations and the significant incident of p63 activation. Of note, p63 is transcriptionally activated by two distinct promoters [66]; one of the two resulting p63 variants contains an N-terminal transactivation domain (TAp63), whereas, the other transcript lacks the N-terminal domain and is termed ΔNp63 [66]. The two p63 isoforms are functionally distinct [67], with ΔNp63 acting as a dominant negative regulator of p53 and with TAp63 opposing cell cycle arrest and apoptosis [66, 68]. ΔNp63 is highly expressed in HNSCC [69] and indeed inhibits NOTCH1 activity [65, 70].

HPV-Negative HNSCC

Well prior to the advent of high throughput sequencing, alterations in several genes, including inactivation or deletion of the tumor suppressors CDKN2A (p16; [71]) and TP53 (p53; [72]), and overexpression (via amplification and elevated transcription) of the epidermal growth factor receptor EGFR [73] had been identified as relevant to the pathogenesis of HPV-negative HNSCC. Based on TCGA analysis of genomic-scale data, the two most commonly inactivated genes in HPV- tumors were confirmed as TP53 (84 % of cases [19]; a percentage similar to the one reported by Seiwert et al. (81 % of 69 HPV- tumors; [21]) and Stransky et al. (73 % of 63 HPV-tumors; [22])) and CDKN2A (4–74 % of cases Fig. 1a and b and Table 1; [19, 21, 22]; the broad range is in part due to the lack of CNA data for several of the studies and the difficulties associated with sequencing of GC-rich regions, which are found in CDKN2A [74, 75]).

Due to the high frequency of mutations in TP53 (Table 1), significant effort has been focused on elucidating the prognostic potential of this gene. Some work suggests improved overall survival for patients with wild type TP53 compared to patients with TP53 mutations predicted to be functionally disruptive (i.e., nonsense mutations or missense mutations disruptive to the L2 or L3 DNA-binding domains [76]). Other reports indicated that TP53 status is of low prognostic value when considered independently from other variables [77]. A multi-tiered genomic analysis of 250 HPV-negative tumors in 2014 (TCGA dataset; approximately corresponding to the cohort described above) confirmed that disruptive TP53 mutations correlated with reduced survival; however, in this analysis, cases with TP53 mutations predicted to be non-disruptive also had significantly worse survival outcomes compared to cases with wild type TP53 [78]. Strikingly, this study identified TP53 mutations as frequently co-occurring with deletions of chromosomal region 3p (179 out of 250 cases), with the combination associated with significantly worse survival than was predicted for TP53 mutations or 3p deletions considered independently [78]. Further stratification of the 179 TP53-3p cases showed that elevated expression of miR-548k (a microRNA encoded by a gene proximal to cyclin D1 (CCND1) and the death receptor FADD at 11q13 and described as oncogenic in esophageal squamous cell cancer [79]) predicted further reduction in survival [78].

Efforts to elucidate the prognostic value of different TP53 mutations have also led to the development of a novel computation approach termed the Evolutionary Action score of TP53-coding variants (EAp53; [80–82]). EAp53 stratifies HNSCC patients with tumors harboring TP53 missense mutations based on an estimated degree of risk assigned to each mutation. The foundational principles of this approach are based on previously identified TP53 "gain of function" mutations that enhanced cell transformation and chemotherapy resistance [83]. EAp53 assigns functional sensitivity to sequence variations based on evolutionary substitutions for every sequence position and calculates if substitutions correlate with larger or smaller phylogenetic divergences to determine "risk" [80, 82, 84]. HNSCC patients with p53 mutations classified using EAp53 as high-risk had significantly worse survival outcomes and reduced periods until distant metastases developed [80], as well

as increased resistance to chemotherapy [81]. As larger datasets with clinical annotations become available, it will be critical to refine and validate these models, and to determine if and how TP53 status is suitable to predict efficacy of different therapeutic interventions.

CDKN2A regulates cell cycle progression by blocking the activity of CCND1 (cyclin D1) and its associated kinases, CDK6 and CDK4, which phosphorylate and inactivate the tumor suppressor RB1 (Fig. 1b; [56, 85, 86]). Inactivation of the CDKN2A gene was found in 57 % of HPV- cases in the TCGA cohort [19]; however, other studies produced discordant values for genomic alterations of CDKN2A (ranging from 4 to 74 %; [20–22, 35, 36]; Table 1). Evaluation of CDKN2A status is somewhat complicated by the fact that the gene is GC-rich (> 60 % of bases are cytosine or guanine; [87]). Sequencing GC-rich regions can be problematic because of their higher melting temperature compared to GC-low regions, which is due to base stacking and more stable secondary structure [74, 75]. Methylation-associated inactivation of CDKN2A (further discussed below) is another important factor potentially complicating assessment of the function status of this gene [88–91]. Direct comparison of cases in the TCGA cohort with homozygous deletions or predicted inactivating mutations in CDKN2A versus wild type CDKN2A did not indicate a survival difference. However, as with TP53, subsequent refined analysis of CDKN2A status emphasized that the patient cohort with low mRNA expression of CDKN2A (RNA-seq: z < 3-fold) did have reduced survival ($p = 0.037$; [56]). This observation is in accordance with other work that indicated improved survival for patients with p16-positive non-oropharyngeal squamous cell carcinoma [92]. Further emphasizing the importance of this signaling axis is the fact that CCND1 is the most frequently amplified gene in the TCGA cohort of HPV-HNSCC cases, detected in 31 % of cases (confirming earlier studies [19, 21, 22, 56]). Beck et al. reported that high RNA expression of CCND1 (z > 2-fold) not only correlated with reduced survival in the TCGA dataset [19, 56], but also co-occurred frequently with CDKN2A deletions (co-occurrence ratio: 0.817). Cases harboring both, amplified CCND1 and deleted CDK2N2A had much worse prognosis than cases without these alterations [56].

In the TCGA cohort, EGFR was amplified in 12 % of HPV- cases [19], the same % of cases with EGFR amplification was reported by Seiwert et al. [21]. Seiwert et al. did not report significant incidence of alteration in HER2 (also known as ERBB2), ERBB3 and ERBB4 and the TCGA also only detected alterations of those genes in a small number of cases (4–6 %; [19]). Nevertheless, alterations in ERBB2 or ERBB3 have been directly linked to resistance to EGFR-targeted therapy and are thus of therapeutic relevance [93]. Mining of TCGA data highlighted that RPPA expression of pHER2 correlated with expression of HER2, and both, pHER2 and HER2 expression correlated with protein expression of EGFR [93], providing some patient data in support of *in vivo* results in which dual kinase inhibition of EGFR and HER2 enhances response to cetuximab [94]. In addition, the RTKs FGFR1 and IGF1R were identified with activating mutations in 10 and 4 % of HPV- HNSCC, respectively, while no mutations of these kinases were identified in HPV+ HNSCC tumors (Fig. 1a and c). FGFR1 and IGFR1 participate in a signaling network that includes EGFR and other ERBB family members (Fig. 1c), and both can contribute to resistance to EGFR-targeted therapeutics, the only type of targeted therapy approved for HNSCC [73, 95, 96]. Functioning downstream of these RTKs, the GTPase HRAS was almost exclusively altered in HPV- HNSCC (5 %), propagates pro-proliferation and pro-survival signaling via the BRAF-MEK-ERK axis, and provides alternative input to activate PI3K (Fig. 1c; [97–99]).

For two additional genes, AJUBA and FAT1, almost all detected alterations were found in HPV- tumors (Fig. 1a and d). Both genes are involved in differentiation and are linked to the NOTCH/CTNNB1 signaling pathway as negative regulators [19, 100, 101]. The scaffolding protein AJUBA, inactivated in 7 % of HPV- cases (0 % of HPV+ tumors), has also been implicated in interactions with Aurora-A kinase (AURKA), a critical regulator of mitosis [102]. AURKA is overexpressed in a significant percentage (7 %) of HNSCC cases and correlated with diminished survival in an analysis of provisional TCGA data (significant overlap with the published TCGA dataset; [19, 103]). FAT1 is a member of the cadherin-like protein family and has been described as a suppressor of cancer cell growth based on a role in binding to and antagonizing CTNNB1 [100]. FAT1 had previously been shown to be mutated in roughly 7 % of 60 head and neck tumors [100], but was detected to be inactivated (missense/truncating mutations and homozygous deletions) in a much greater percentage of HPV- cases (32 %; versus inactivated in only 3 % of HPV+ cases; Fig. 1a and d) analyzed by the TCGA network [19]. The discrepancy may be due to a number of reasons, including differences in sample processing, determination of HPV status, demographic factors, different acquisition platforms, and differently constructed analytical pipelines.

The TCGA analysis also identified a set of less well studied alterations associated with oxidative stress, specifically involving CUL3, KEAP1 and NFE2L2 [19]. KEAP1 and NFE2L2 were exclusively altered in HPV- HNSCC (Fig. 1a). KEAP1 was inactivated in 5 % of cases and NFE2L2 was activated in 14 % of cases. Functionally, NFE2L2 is a transcription factor that regulates antioxidant and stress-responsive genes [104]. KEAP1

complexes with the E3 ligase CUL3 (inactivated in 6 % of HPV- cases) to polyubiquitinate NFE2L2 [105]; thus, disruption of canonical KEAP1-CUL3 function promotes NFE2L2 activity [19]. Intriguingly, in lung cancer, a NFE2L2-centric gene signature has been proposed as a valuable prognostic biomarker [106]. This may be relevant because significant molecular similarities between HNSCC and lung squamous cell cancers (SQCC) exist [19, 43, 48, 107], including shared dysregulation of KEAP1 and NFE2L2. Secondary analysis of the TCGA dataset indeed revealed that DNA level alterations of any member of the KEAP1/CUL3/RBX1 complex correlated with significantly reduced survival (median survival of ~35 months versus ~72 months; [108]).

Lastly, the TCGA network detected co-amplification of chromosome regions 11q13 and 11q22. Found within region 11q22, an amplicon previously described in lung, esophageal and cervical cancer [109–111], are the coding sequences for BIRC2 and YAP1. BIRC2 encodes c-IAP1 and is a member of the inhibitor-of-apoptosis family [112]. Functionally, BIRC2 inhibits caspase activity, including the activity of CASP8 [112], and it has been shown that BIRC2 plays an important role in the ubiquitination and degradation of TRAF3 (tumor necrotizing factor receptor-associated factor 3), a negative regulator of NF-kB activity [113]. BIRC2 is more commonly altered in HPV- HNSCC (7 % of cases versus 3 % of cases in HPV+ HNSCC) and, as would have been predicated based on functionality, CASP8 was also frequently detected as inactivated through mutations or homozygous deletion (11 % of HPV- cases; Fig. 1a). YAP1 is a proto-oncogenic transcription factor downstream of BIRC2 and associated with the Hippo pathway [114]. Amongst cancers analyzed by the TCGA, HNSCC had the fifth highest incident of amplified YAP1 (6.3 % of cases). Interestingly, a recent study found that YAP1 amplification strongly correlated with resistance to cetuximab in vitro [115], which may reflect YAP1 associated upregulation of the EGFR ligand amphiregulin; further investigations are needed to fully uncover the precise mechanism of this type of resistance [115, 116]. Amplification of region 11q13 includes the region encoding the Fas-associated death domain gene (FADD; established as frequently overexpressed in HNSCC [117] and found to be amplified in 32 % of HPV- cases analyzed by the TCGA [19]). Importantly, FADD has been implicated in increased lymph node metastasis in HNSCC [117].

HPV-Positive HNSCC

At the molecular level, HPV+ carcinomas significantly differ from HPV- cases, highlighted in great detail by the TCGA network and others [10, 19, 21, 27, 92]. A significant limitation of the TCGA study is the fact that only

36 HPV+ cases were analyzed [19], a limitation partially compensated for by the work of other groups (Table 1; [21, 23, 34, 118]). Further analysis of additional tumors is clearly needed; however, some conclusions can be made in spite of the limited numbers of cases.

HPV+ HNSCC is defined by infection of tumor cells with HPV. HPV DNA can exist either integrated into the human genome or in a nonintegrated form [34, 119]. Upon infection, the HPV genome (8 kb) is first amplified as extrachromosomal circular elements (episomes), some of which may subsequently integrate into one or more location within the host genome [119]. It has been reported that HPV integration sites are randomly distributed throughout the genome [120]. In one study, analysis of 35 of the 36 HPV+ TCGA HNSCC cases identified HPV integration in 25 cases and uncovered distinct gene expression and methylation patterns for HPV integrated versus non-integrated HNSCC, suggesting different pathogenic mechanisms [34]. Another study published similar results for essentially the same group of patients (36 HPV+ HNSCC), and detected HPV DNA integration in 24/36 cases [119]. The general observation regarding HPV integration is not unique to HNSCC, as HPV+ cervical cancers include HPV integrated and nonintegrated cases [121]. Compared to episomal HPV DNA, transcripts derived from integrated viral DNA have been shown to be more stable and more strongly associated with increased proliferative capacity of affected cells [122]. It is likely that HPV integration, particularly if within or proximal to key cancer related genes, is important but not essential for the oncogenicity of HPV: the better understood oncogenic contribution of the virus is the production of different oncoproteins [34].

HPV oncoproteins include E6 and E7 (Fig. 1b; [122]), which perform complementary actions in eliminating negative regulators of the cell cycle. E6 binds p53 and targets this tumor suppressor for proteosomal degradation [123]. Tumor suppressor RB1 interacts with E7, which targets RB1 for degradation through association with the cullin 2-ubiquitin-ligase complex [124–126]. As E6 and E7 function through cell cycle dysregulation by eliminating RB1 and TP53, very few alterations in additional cell cycle regulators occur in HPV+ disease: inactivation of CDKN2A, or TP53, or overexpression of CDK6 or CCND1, occur seldom in HPV+ HNSCC. One exception is the transcription factor E2F1, which is normally inhibited by RB1 (Fig. 1b; [56]); it is the only cell cycle regulator identifier by the TCGA study as being predominantly altered in HPV+ cases (19 % activated via amplification of chromosome 20q11, seen in only in 2 % of HPV- HNSCC; Fig. 1a and b).

Also associated with HPV+ disease is the RTK FGFR3, which is activated in 11 % of cases through either mutation or a gene fusion event, and the aforementioned TNF receptor associated factor TRAF3, inactivated in 22 % of cases (versus 1 % in HPV- disease). The FGFR3 fusion partner is TACC3, a protein critical for nucleation of microtubules at the centrosome [127], aberrantly expressed in some cancers and potentially targetable with small molecules [128]. A FGFR3-TACC3 fusion was first described in glioblastoma [129] and subsequently detected in nasopharyngeal carcinoma and other HNSCCs [130, 131]. This fusion event was detected in two of the 36 HPV+ and zero of the HPV- HNSCC TCGA cases [19]. Constitutive kinase activity of the FGFR3-TACC3 oncogene induces loss of mitotic fidelity and leads to aneuploidy [129, 131]. In cases where present, FGFR3-TACC3 appears to be tumor driving and patients are likely to disproportionally benefit from FGFR3 targeting therapy [131]. TRAF3 has mostly been studied in immunological processes and one of its main functions is regulation of NFkB activity [132]. In subsequent studies in HNSCC, functional analysis of TRAF3 has suggested a tumor suppressive role of the gene when overexpressed, and increased cell proliferation in the context of depleted TRAF3 [133].

Tumor heterogeneity

HPV- and HPV+ HNSCC share one particularly challenging feature: tumor heterogeneity [24]. This aspect of tumor biology has garnered significant attention in recent years because of the immense clinical implications in terms of prognosis, drug resistance and precision medicine [134–136]. Extensive analysis of TCGA data indicates that it is of high relevance in HNSCC [24, 137]. One approach to study HNSCC heterogeneity is based on whole-exome sequencing (WES), which can be used to determine the fraction of total sequenced DNA that contains a given mutant allele: termed mutant-allele fraction (MAF). The width of MAF distribution, normalized to the median MAF value, constitutes the quantitative value of intra-tumor heterogeneity, and has been termed mutant-allele tumor heterogeneity (MATH; [137, 138]). Earlier work indicated that HPV- tumors had significantly higher heterogeneity than HPV+ tumors (though substantial even for HPV+ cases; [137]), which would be predicated based on the frequency of and genomic instability associated with TP53 mutations, increased age and continuous tobacco use [24].

Provocatively, in a ten-variable multivariate analysis of TCGA HNSCC data incorporating MATH scores, no prognostic significance of HPV status, N classification or TP53 mutational status was determined [138]. While the lack of significance in the multivariate analysis does not suggest irrelevance of the three parameters, it strongly suggests that further work is needed to unravel these variables and to determine how much each parameter truly impacts disease progression and survival in the context of appreciated heterogeneity. For example, disruptive TP53 mutations [78] are strongly associated with higher intra-tumor heterogeneity as calculated by MATH (i.e., high MATH scores), and both TP53 mutational status and high MATH scores, based on univariate analysis, indicated reduced survival [78, 137].

Additional innovative and detailed analysis by McGranahan et al. utilized TCGA datasets for nine tumor types, including HNSCC, to highlight important aspects of cancer evolution and clonality [24]. In order to determine if specific alterations were clonal (present in most/all tumor cells sequenced and therefore considered "early" mutations) or subclonal (present in a small fraction of cells and considered "late" mutations) McGranahan et al. used exome sequencing data and single-nucleotide polymorphism arrays to calculate the confidence interval of the cancer cell fraction (CCF; proportion of cancer cells harboring a given mutation; [139–141]) for a given mutation. A 95 % confidence interval of ≥ 1 was used to define clonal ("early") mutations, and mutations with a confidence interval of less than 1 were defined as subclonal ("late") mutations [24, 140–142]. In HNSCC, the majority of driver mutations were clonal, and CDKN2A and TP53 were identified as almost exclusively clonal. Based on the proportion of mutations, three mutational signatures (previously defined [25]) were identified for HNSCC: 1) a signature with C > T transitions at CpG sites associated with spontaneous deamination of methylated cytosines that strongly correlated with patient age at diagnosis and was most prevalently linked to "early" mutations; 2) a signature indicative of up-regulation of APOBEC cytosine deaminases [143], seen in both "early" and "late" mutations, although with significant prominence in "late" mutations; and 3) a signature associated with smoking induced mutations, seen predominantly with "early" mutations [24]. McGranahan et al. did not differentiate between HPV+ and HPV- cases, which future studies should do, particularly given that previous analysis of TCGA data detected evidence that HPV infection was strongly associated with APOBEC-mediated mutagenesis in HNSCC [144]. Furthermore, the same study suggested that APOEC-mediated mutagenesis significantly contributes to helical domain E545K and E542K gain of function mutations in PIK3CA, one of the most frequently altered genes in HNSCC (32 out of 58 PIK3CA mutations in the TCGA cohort are E545K/E542K mutations; [19, 21, 144, 145]).

As an emerging concept for this disease, consideration of germline variants may be relevant to fully appreciate tumor heterogeneity. Recent analysis of TCGA data suggested that 15 % (44 out of 291 cases; incompletely congruent with the published TCGA dataset [19]) of HNSCC cases have rare germline truncations, including truncations in several genes important in the Fanconi Anemia Pathway, specifically FANCA and FANCM, which are involved in DNA repair [146, 147]. FANCM mutations significantly correlated with increased somatic mutational frequency in the complete HNSCC cohort (mean age was 60.9 +/− 12.4 years; based on personal correspondence with authors), whereas, FANCA had a similar correlation with the frequency of somatic mutations, but specific in cases defined as younger age (mean age was 46.3 +/− 7.0 years) of onset (no indication regarding HPV status; [146]). Recent studies using murine models have implicated MYH9 as a gene that induces oral squamous cell carcinoma in the context of germline mutations or knockout [148, 149]. MYH9 encodes for non-muscle myosin II-A (NM II-A), best known for its roles as a cytoskeletal protein and during embryonic development [150]. Intriguingly, MYH9 may also acts as a tumor suppressor, by regulating stabilization and nuclear retention of p53 [149]. MYH9 and MYH10 were mutated in 4 and 5 % of cases, respectively within the TCGA cohort of 279 patients [148]. No correlation with HPV status was detected. Success of future clinical efforts, particularly for targeted therapeutics, will likely heavily depend on consideration of heterogeneity and cancer evolution, guided by studies of spatio-temporal differences in genomic alterations, including presence or absence of germline mutations [134, 151].

Therapeutic insights

The majority of patients with HNSCC are treated with surgery and/or radiation and in some cases adjuvant chemotherapy [1, 3, 11, 27]. Treatment approaches for HPV- and HPV+ cases remain very similar [1]. However, because of the better prognosis and the younger age of onset associated with HPV+ disease, therapeutic de-intensification, currently only available as part of clinical trials, for the treatment of patients with HPV+ HNSCC is being actively explored [27, 152]. Thus far, the only targeted therapeutic approved to treat HNSCC is the monoclonal antibody cetuximab, designed to target the extracellular region of EGFR (Fig. 2; [153]). The clinical impact of cetuximab has been significant in some patients [154], but relatively modest overall [2, 73, 155]. Several small molecules, for example lapatinib (targeting EGFR and HER2; [156]), afatinib (targeting EGFR and HER2; [157]) and others (reviewed in [153]), have shown some promise in the treatment of HNSCC. Inter- and intra-disease heterogeneity are likely determining factors that have thus far held back greater success of available therapeutics, and represents one of the key challenges to overcome [19, 24, 151]. Consideration of a single gene, based on a single biopsy, does not seem sufficient to maximize therapeutic interventions [73]. For example, consideration of EGFR expression and/or amplification does not correspond with response to EGFR inhibitors

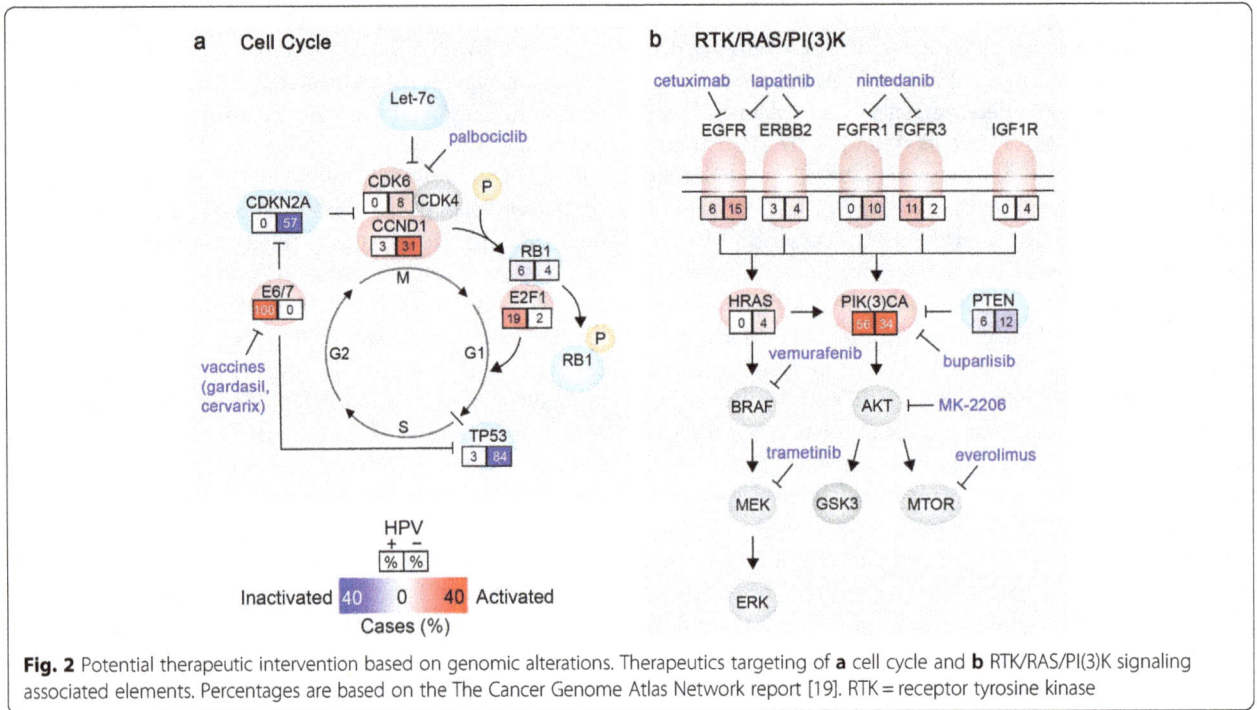

Fig. 2 Potential therapeutic intervention based on genomic alterations. Therapeutics targeting of **a** cell cycle and **b** RTK/RAS/PI(3)K signaling associated elements. Percentages are based on the The Cancer Genome Atlas Network report [19]. RTK = receptor tyrosine kinase

[107]. Data provided by the TCGA and others suggest that targeting EGFR may not be efficacious in the context of extensively altered parallel or downstream signaling components, including cell cycle regulators, due to overlapping functional contributions [73, 158].

Figure 2 summarizes potentially promising targets other than EGFR, based on available genomics data. The drugs shown in Fig. 2 are examples of drugs currently in clinical development for the treatment of HNSCC; recent reviews provide more complete lists of available drugs for each target [3, 159–161]. The near universality of cell cycle dysregulation in HNSCC strongly recommends investigation of CDK inhibitors [19, 56]. HPV-HNSCC with functional CDKN2A and high levels of phosphorylated RB1 may present the ideal molecular background for effective treatment with CDK4/6 inhibitors (Fig. 2; [56]). Furthermore, therapeutic targeting of aberrant cell cycle activity may partially circumvent the challenge presented by heterogeneity, given that clonal status analysis of the TCGA HNSCC cohort indicated that genes associated with cyclin-dependent kinases have 0 % of mutations arise in subclonal populations [24], which suggests that cell cycle alterations arise early during tumor development and are present in most if not all tumor cells. A large number of CDK inhibitors are currently in development [162] and the possibility of RB1 phosphorylation status as a response predictive biomarker is encouraging [56]. PI3K [NCT01816984], FGFR [NCT02558387], BRAF [NCT01286753], MEK [NCT01553851], AKT [NCT01349933] and mTOR [NCT010

51791] are further targets of potential therapeutic relevance (Fig. 2b; [102, 103, 163, 164]). Additional promising pre-clinical work has explored Second Mitochondria-derived Activator of Caspases (SMAC)-mimetics, antagonists of inhibitors of apoptosis, which seem particularly effective against HNSCC models with FADD/BIRC2 alterations [165, 166]; particularly meaningful considering the aforementioned high incident of FADD/BIRC2 alterations in HNSCC (Table 1).

The perhaps most exciting recent development in the treatment of cancer is immunotherapy [167]. Immunotherapy, specifically checkpoint blockade, has been tremendously successful in some cases of non-small cell lung cancer [168, 169], malignant melanoma [170] and other cancers [171, 172]. Checkpoint inhibitors seem to be particularly effective against tumors with high rates of mutation, which suggests that a subpopulation of patients with HNSCC would benefit form this type of therapy. Furthermore, HNSCC appears to be an immunosuppressive disease commonly associated with lymphopenia [173, 174] and in a few cases (7 % of HPV- and 11 % of HPV+ HNSCC in the TCGA cohort) presenting with specific mutations in HLA alleles and the antigen processing machinery to reduce tumor immunodetection [19]. A substantial number of clinical trials are currently exploring the applicability of immunotherapy for the treatment of HNSCC, with primary focus on immune checkpoint blockade via CTLA-4 and PD1 [12]. In brief, CTLA-4 and PD1 are expressed by T-cells and function as negative regulators of T-cell activity, a process required for normal immunologic homeostasis. Tumor cells frequently engage CTLA-4 or PD1 to modulate T-cell activity and escape immunodetection [172, 175]. Immune checkpoint blockade inhibits interaction of tumor cells with CTLA-4 or PD1; thus, blocking inactivation of T-cells [175]. Regarding HNSCC, several phase III studies are currently exploring the utility of checkpoint inhibitors; specifically, the humanized monoclonal PD-1 specific antibody pembrolizumab [NCT02564263, NCT02358031, NCT02252042], recently approved for the treatment of melanoma and lung cancer (two cancer types with high mutational burden; [25, 26, 176–178]) and tremelimumab (fully human antibody against CTLA-4) with or without durvalumab (Fc optimized monoclonal antibody against the PD1 ligand 1; NCT02551159). Initial results are expected to be published in the near future [12]. It will be important to determine if distinct molecular lesions found in HNSCC, as summarized above, are prognostic for response to these new treatments. In the case of immunotherapy, considerations beyond the tumor may also be particularly important; for example, early laboratory studies have shown that the composition of the intestinal microbiota significantly impacts the efficacy of CTLA-4/PD-1 inhibitors [179, 180].

Methylation in HNSCC

Future endeavors are likely to include more extensive elucidation of the role of DNA methylation in HNSCC, in part to substantiate publications based on the TCGA dataset. DNA methylation is important in the regulation of gene expression, and aberrant methylation has been described for essentially all cancer types and as a critical aspect of cancer genomics [181, 182]. Previously published work suggests that HPV+ HNSCC has significantly differentiated CpG island methylation compared to HPV- cases, reflecting the notion that HPV+ and HPV- HNSCC are distinct diseases on the genomic, transcriptomic and methylomic level [183–185]. Comparative analyses of available HPV+ TCGA cases revealed specific hypermethylated regions downstream of CDKN2A, which correlated with increased transcription of CDKN2A variant p14 (ARF; [184]). CDKN2A is also frequently methylated (23–67 % of cases; [91]) to silence expression of this tumor suppressor [88, 90, 186]; although, degree of methylation and expression changes can vary significantly among individual tumors [187]. The mechanistic and clinical ramifications of this observation are not yet understood. Another study of HPV+ HNSCC reported that a promoter methylation signature of 5 genes, three with high methylation (GATA4, GRIA4, IRX4) and two with low methylation (ALDH1A2 and OSR2), correlated strongly with improved survival [188].

The signature was validated across multiple cohorts. Methylation patters in HPV+ HNSCC are significantly distinct for cases with integrated HPV DNA and episomal DNA [34, 119], a potentially important factor not always considered.

Interestingly, prominent differential methylation of three members of the zinc finger gene family, ZNF14, ZNF160 and ZNF420, has been identified as suitable to detect HNSCC with 100 % specificity in primary tissue and saliva samples; subsequently, the three ZNF methylation signature was validated using the 273 TCGA cohort [185]. For most of the methylomics driven studies of HNSCC [183, 185, 188, 189], few cases were analyzed (particularly for HPV+ cases) and additional work is needed to better understanding and interpret the various methylation patterns. How methylomics data is going to be integrated into clinical practice for HNSCC remains to be seen, although prognostic and diagnostic potential of such information is apparent in some cancer types [181, 185, 190]. No DNA methylation markers for HNSCC have been accepted for clinical use to date [185].

Conclusions

Detailed profiling of HNSCC by the TCGA network and other research groups has greatly enhanced our understanding of this malignancy. First and foremost, the composite results have highlighted the tremendous inter- and intra-tumor heterogeneity, complicated by the increasing incidence of HPV-associated tumors. Efforts have started to focus on classifying tumors based on molecular profiles [191–193]; however, inroads in terms of improved survival have not substantially materialized yet. The next phase is likely to require multi-platform analysis of many more HPV- and HPV+ tumors, ideally sufficient to cover each anatomic site to enable actionable conclusions. In parallel, laboratory research and clinical trials have to continue to provide data that can guide therapeutic strategies based on molecularly defined parameters and higher-order interactions. Progress continues to be made and the status quo for patients with HNSCC is likely to continue to improve over the next decade.

The greatest potential therapeutic advantage to come from the detailed parsing of HNSCC heterogeneity is advanced and eventually precise treatment with immunotherapy. For example, consistent identification of tumors with highly immunogenic alterations would significantly help guide therapeutic decision-making [194]. Immunotherapy has been remarkably successful against many types of cancer, with particularly striking successes against other carcinogen-associated cancers, such as lung cancer [169, 195] and melanoma [170, 196]. High mutation burden, common for many sub-types of HNSCC [19, 24, 25], and carcinogen-associated genomic profiles seems to correlate with higher efficacy of immunotherapy [194, 197]. Leveraging and advancing current knowledge to optimize selection of HNSCC cases for treatment with immunotherapy should be a top priority and could greatly enhance the many ongoing clinical trials [12]. The perhaps most promising approach to eradicate HPV+ HNSCC is extended use of the available vaccine, which currently appears to be successful in reducing rates of cervical cancer [198, 199] and would presumably be as successful in reducing the rate of HPV+ HNSCC.

Abbreviations
AJUBA: protein coding gene located at 14q11.2; adaptor/scaffolding protein; AKT: also known as AKT1, v-akt murine thymoma viral oncogenes homolg 1; codes for serine-threonine protein kinase and is located at 14q32.32; ALDH1A2: aldehyde dehydrogenase 1 family member A2; enzyme that catalyzes the synthesis of retinoic acid from retinaldehyde; APOBEC: apolipoprotein B mRNA editing enzyme, catalytic polypeptide-like; family of C-to-U editing cydidine deaminase enzymes located on chromosome 22; AURKA: aurora kinase A; protein is involved in cell cycle-regulation and microtubule formation; located at 20q13; BEZ-235: ATP-competitive inhibitor; imidazoquinoline derivative targeting PI3K/mTor; also known as dactolisib; BIRC2: baculoviral IAP repeat containing 2; member of a family of proteins involved in inhibiting cell death; located at 11q22; BRAF: B-Raf proto-oncogene; member of the raf/mil family of serine/theonine kinases; located at 7q34; C > T transition: a point mutation that changes the pyrimidine thymine to the pyrimidine cytosine; CASP8: caspase 8, apoptosis-related cysteine peptidase; involved in programmed cell death; located at 2q33-q34; CCF: cancer cell fraction; used to infer the size of a subpopulation affected by somatic mutations from genomic data; CCND1: cyclin D1; member of the cyclin family associated with the regulation of CDKs; located at 11q13; CDK4: cyclin-dependent kinase 4; catalytic subunit of the protein kinase complex required for G1 cell cycle progression; located at 12q14; CDK6: cyclin-dependent kinase 6; catalytic subunit of the protein kinase complex required for G1 cell cycle progression; located at 7q21–q22; CDKN2A: cyclin-dependent kinase inhibitor 2A; codes for p16; inhibitor of CDK4; at least three alternatively spliced protein coding variants have been reported; located at 9p21; chromosome p: *petit*; shorter arm of the chromosome; chromosome q: longer arm of the chromosome; CNA: copy number alteration; gains or losses of large segments of the genome; CpG: cytosine and guanine separated by exactly one phosphate; amiable to methylation; CSMD1: CUB and Sushi multiple domains 1; located at 8p23.2; CTLA4: cytotoxic T-lymphocyte-associated protein 4; immunoglobulin; transmits inhibitory signal to T-cells; located at 2q33; CTNNB1: catenin beta 1; part of adherens junctions and signaling; located at 3p21; CUL3: cullin 3; component of an E3 ubiquitin ligase complex; located at 2q36.2; DNA: deoxyribonucleic acid; E2F1: E2F transcription factor 1; involved in cell cycle control; located at 20q11.2; E6: transforming protein; targeted p53; associated with human papillomavirus infection; E7: transforming protein; targets RB1; associated with human papillomavirus infection; EAp53: Evolutionary Action score of TP53-coding variants; computational approach to estimate the risk of various TP53 mutations in order to predict survival and treatment response; EGFR: epidermal growth factor receptor; member of the ERBB family of receptor tyrosine kinases; located at 7p12; EML4-ALK: fusion gene composed of echinoderm microtubule-associated protein-like 4 and anaplastic lymphoma kinase; chromosome 2p inversion; ERBB2: erb-b2 receptor tyrosine kinase 2; also known as HER2 or NEU; no lignd-binding domain; located at 17q12; ERBB3: erb-b2 receptor tyrosine kinase 3; also known as HER3; no active kinase domain; located at 12q13; ERBB4: erb-b2 receptor tyrosine kinase 4; also known as HER4; located at 2q33.3-q34; ERK: officially known as MAPK1; mitogen-activated protein kinase 1; member of the MAP kinase family; located at 22q11.21; FADD: Fas associated via death domain; adaptor protein that interacts with surface receptors to mediate apoptosis; located at 11q13.3; FAT1: FAT atypical cadherin 1; member of the cadherin superfamily; located at 4q35; FGFR1: fibroblast growth factor receptor 1; receptor tyrosine kinase; located at 8p11.23-p11.22; FGFR3: fibroblast growth factor receptor 3;

receptor tyrosine kinase; located at 4p16.3; FHIT: fragile histidine triad; codes for triphospate hydrolase required for purine metabolism; located at 3q14.2; G1: gap 1 phase; first phase of the cell cycle and part of interphase; GATA4: GATA binding protein 4; member of the GATA family of zinc-finger transcription factors; located at 8p23.1-p22; GEO: Gene Expression Omnibus; public genomic data repository; GISTIC: Genomic Identification of Significant Targets in Cancer; algorithm designed to identify likely driver somatic copy-number alterations by evaluating the amplitude and frequency of events; GRIA4: glutamate receptor, ionotropic, AMPA 4; AMPA (alpha-amino-3-hydroxy-5-methyl-4-isoxazole propionate sensitive glutamate receptor; subject to RNA editing; located at 11q22; GTPase: family of enzymes that hydrolyze guanosine triphosphate (GTP); important for signal transduction in cancer cells; HLA: human leukocyte antigen; encode proteins essential to the immune system; chromosome 6; HNSCC: head and neck squamous cell carcinoma; HPV: human papillomavirus; DNA virus; HPV subtype 16 is most commonly associated with HNSCC; HPV-16: high-risk human papillomavirus subtype and the subtype most commonly associated with cervical, anal and oropharyngeal cancer; HRAS: Harvey rat sarcoma viral oncogenes homolog; member of the Ras oncogenes family with intrinsic GTPase activity; located at 11p15.5; IGF1R: insulin like growth factor 1 receptor; tyrosine kinase receptor; located at 11q26.3; IHC: immunohistochemistry; antibody-based tissue staining; IRX4: Iroquois homeobox 4; located at 5p15.3; ISH: *in situ* hybridization; uses labeled complementary DNA or RNA to localize specific DNA or RNA in tissue; KEAP1: kelch like ECH associated protein 1; interacts with NFE2L2 in a redox-sensitive manner; located at 19p13.2; let-7c: MIRLET7C also known as microRNA let-7c; short non-coding RNA involved in post-translational regulation of genes; located at 21q21.1; MAF: mutant-allele fraction; fractional of total sequenced DNA with a given mutant allele based on whole-exome sequencing; MATH: mutant-allele tumor heterogeneity; width of the mutant-allele fraction distribution normalized to the median MAF value; MEK: mitogen-activated protein kinase kinase; group of kinases also known as MAP2K; MAPKK or MKK; miRNA: micro RNA; small non-coding RNA molecule; mRNA: messenger ribonucleic acid; mTOR: mechanistic target of rapamycin; serine/threonine phosphatidylinositol kinase-related protein; located at 1p36.2; MYC: v-myc avian myelocytomatosis viral oncogenes homolog; nuclear phosphoprotein and transcription factor; located at 8q24.21; MYH9: Nonmuscle Myosin Heavy Chain II-A (also known as NMHC-II-A); cytoskeleton protein; N classification: part of the TNM classification of malignant tumours staging notation system; describes cancer positive regional lymph nodes; ranges from N0 (tumor cells absent from regional lymph nodes) to N3 (tumor cells detected in distant lymph nodes); NFE2L2: transcription factor; regulates expression of genes with antioxidant response elements; located at 2q31; NFkB: NFKB1; nuclear factor of kappa light polypeptide gene enhancer in B-cells 1; transcription regulator; located at 4q24; NOTCH: highly conserved signaling pathway; may also refer to NOTCH1; a type 1 single pass transmembrane receptor; located at 9q34.3; NPC: nasopharyngeal cancer; originates in the upper part of the throat behind the nose and near the base of the skull; OSCC: oral squamous cell carcinoma; OSR2: odd-skipped related transcription factor 2; located at 8q22.2; p14(ARF): alternative reading frame protein product of the CDKN2A locus; inhibits the E3 ubiquitin protein ligase MDM2 (p53 degradation); PCR: polymerase chain reaction; PD-1: PDCD1; programmed cell death 1; member of the immunoglobulin superfamily expressed on pro-B and T cells; located at 2q37.3; PI(3)K: phosphatidylinositol-4,5-bisphosphate 3-kinase; family of intracellular enzymes; PI3KCA: phosphatidylinositol-4,5-bisphosphate 3-kinase catalytic subunit alpha; codes for p110α; the catalytic subunit; located at 3q26.3; PLK1: polo-like kinase 1; serine/threonine kinase; highly expressed during mitosis; located at 16p12.2; RB1: retinoblastoma 1; negative regulator of the cell cycle; located at 13q14.2; RNA-Seq: RNA sequencing; next-generation sequencing to detect and quantify RNA; RPPA: reverse phase protein array; high-throughput antibody-based protein detection technique; RTK: receptor tyrosine kinases; large family of transmembrane tyrosine kinases; S: synthesis phase; phase of the cell cycle during which DNA is replicated; follows G1 and precedes G2; SOX2: SRY-box 2; transcription factor; located at 3q26.3-q27; SQCC: squamous cell carcinomas; TACC3: transforming, acidic coiled-coil containing protein 3; motor spindle protein; located at 4p16.3; TCGA: the Cancer Genome Atlas; TERT: telomerase reverse transcriptase; ribonucleoprotein polymerase; maintains telomere ends; located at 5p15.33; TP53: tumor protein p53; transcription factor and tumor suppressor; located at 17p13.1; TP63: tumor protein p63; p53 family transcription factor; located at 3q28; TP73: tumor protein p73; member of the p53 family of transcription factors; located at 1p36.3; TRAF3: TNF receptor associated factor 3; member of the TNF receptor associated factor protein family; located at 14q32.32; WES: whole exome sequencing; technique for sequencing protein-coding genes; YAP1: Yes associated protein 1; nuclear effector of the Hippo pathway; located at 11q13; ZNF14: zinc finger protein 14; located at 19p13.11; ZNF160: zinc finger protein 160; located at 19q13.42; ZNF420: zinc finger protein 420; located at 19q13.12; ΔNp63α: isoform of the p53 homologue TP63 that lacks (ΔN) the transactivation domain.

Acknowledgements

The authors were supported by U54 CA149147, R21 CA181287, R21 CA191425 and P50 CA083638 from the NIH (to EAG), the Ruth L. Kirschstein NRSA F30 fellowship (F30 CA180607) from the NIH (to TNB) and NCI Core Grant P30 CA006927 (to Fox Chase Cancer Center).

Authors' contributions

Conception and design: TNB. Collection and assembly of data: TNB. Data analysis and interpretation: Both authors. Manuscript writing: Both authors. Both authors read and approved the final manuscript.

Competing interests

The authors declare that they have no competing interests.

Author details

[1]Program in Molecular Therapeutics, Fox Chase Cancer Center, 333 Cottman Ave, Philadelphia, PA 19111, USA. [2]Program in Molecular and Cell Biology and Genetics, Drexel University College of Medicine, Philadelphia, PA 19129, USA.

References

1. Pfister DG, Spencer S, Brizel DM, Burtness B, Busse PM, Caudell JJ, Cmelak AJ, Colevas AD, Dunphy F, Eisele DW et al. Head and Neck Cancers, Version 1.2015 Featured Updates to the NCCN Guidelines. J Natl Compr Canc Netw. 2015;13(7):847–56.
2. Burtness B, Golemis EA. Overview: the pathobiology of head and neck cancer. In: Burtness B, Golemis EA, editors. Molecular determinants of head and neck cancer. 1st ed. New York: Springer New York; 2014. p. 1–5.
3. Dillon MT, Harrington KJ. Human papillomavirus-negative pharyngeal cancer. J Clin Oncol. 2015;33(29):3251–61.
4. Chaturvedi AK, Anderson WF, Lortet-Tieulent J, Curado MP, Ferlay J, Franceschi S, Rosenberg PS, Bray F, Gillison ML. Worldwide trends in incidence rates for oral cavity and oropharyngeal cancers. J Clin Oncol. 2013;31(36):4550–9.
5. Gillison ML, Chaturvedi AK, Anderson WF, Fakhry C. Epidemiology of human papillomavirus-positive head and neck squamous cell carcinoma. J Clin Oncol. 2015;33(29):3235–42.
6. Hashibe M, Brennan P, Benhamou S, Castellsague X, Chen C, Curado MP, Dal Maso L, Daudt AW, Fabianova E, Fernandez L et al. Alcohol drinking in never users of tobacco, cigarette smoking in never drinkers, and the risk of head and neck cancer: pooled analysis in the International Head and Neck Cancer Epidemiology Consortium. J Natl Cancer Inst. 2007;99(10):777–89.
7. Mehanna H, Beech T, Nicholson T, El-Hariry I, McConkey C, Paleri V, Roberts S. Prevalence of human papillomavirus in oropharyngeal and nonoropharyngeal head and neck cancer–systematic review and meta-analysis of trends by time and region. Head Neck. 2013;35(5):747–55.
8. Chung CH, Bagheri A, D'Souza G. Epidemiology of oral human papillomavirus infection. Oral Oncol. 2014;50(5):364–9.
9. Maxwell JH, Grandis JR, Ferris RL. HPV-Associated Head and Neck Cancer: unique features of epidemiology and clinical management. Annu Rev Med. 2016;67:91–101.
10. Ang KK, Harris J, Wheeler R, Weber R, Rosenthal DI, Nguyen-Tan PF, Westra WH, Chung CH, Jordan RC, Lu C et al. Human papillomavirus and survival of patients with oropharyngeal cancer. New Engl J Med. 2010;363(1):24–35.
11. Ang KK, Chen A, Curran Jr WJ, Garden AS, Harari PM, Murphy BA, et al. Head and neck carcinoma in the United States: first comprehensive report of the Longitudinal Oncology Registry of Head and Neck Carcinoma (LORHAN). Cancer. 2012;118(23):5783–92.
12. Ferris RL. Immunology and immunotherapy of head and neck cancer. J Clin Oncol. 2015;33(29):3293–304.
13. Huang SH, Xu W, Waldron J, Siu L, Shen X, Tong L, Ringash J, Bayley A, Kim J, Hope A et al. Refining American Joint Committee on Cancer/Union for International Cancer Control TNM stage and prognostic groups for human papillomavirus-related oropharyngeal carcinomas. J Clin Oncol. 2015;33(8):836–45.
14. O'Rorke MA, Ellison MV, Murray LJ, Moran M, James J, Anderson LA. Human papillomavirus related head and neck cancer survival: a systematic review and meta-analysis. Oral Oncol. 2012;48(12):1191–201.
15. Garraway LA, Lander ES. Lessons from the cancer genome. Cell. 2013;153(1):17–37.
16. Vogelstein B, Papadopoulos N, Velculescu VE, Zhou S, Diaz Jr LA, Kinzler KW. Cancer genome landscapes. Science. 2013;339(6127):1546–58.
17. Cancer Genome Atlas Research N, Weinstein JN, Collisson EA, Mills GB, Shaw KR, Ozenberger BA, Ellrott K, Shmulevich I, Sander C, Stuart JM. The Cancer Genome Atlas Pan-Cancer analysis project. Nat Genet. 2013; 45(10):1113–20.
18. Hoadley KA, Yau C, Wolf DM, Cherniack AD, Tamborero D, Ng S, Leiserson MDM, Niu BF, McLellan MD, Uzunangelov V et al. Multiplatform analysis of 12 cancer types reveals molecular classification within and across tissues of origin. Cell. 2014;158(4):929–44.
19. Cancer Genome Atlas N. Comprehensive genomic characterization of head and neck squamous cell carcinomas. Nature. 2015;517(7536):576–82.
20. Agrawal N, Frederick MJ, Pickering CR, Bettegowda C, Chang K, Li RJ, Fakhry C, Xie TX, Zhang J, Wang J et al. Exome sequencing of head and neck squamous cell carcinoma reveals inactivating mutations in NOTCH1. Science. 2011;333(6046):1154–7.
21. Seiwert TY, Zuo ZX, Keck MK, Khattri A, Pedamallu CS, Stricker T, Brown C, Pugh TJ, Stojanov P, Cho J et al. Integrative and Comparative Genomic Analysis of HPV-Positive and HPV-Negative Head and Neck Squamous Cell Carcinomas. Clin Cancer Res. 2015;21(3):632–41.
22. Stransky N, Egloff AM, Tward AD, Kostic AD, Cibulskis K, Sivachenko A, Kryukov GV, Lawrence MS, Sougnez C, McKenna A et al. The mutational landscape of head and neck squamous cell carcinoma. Science. 2011; 333(6046):1157–60.
23. Lui VW, Hedberg ML, Li H, Vangara BS, Pendleton K, Zeng Y, Lu Y, Zhang Q, Du Y, Gilbert BR et al. Frequent mutation of the PI3K pathway in head and neck cancer defines predictive biomarkers. Cancer Discov. 2013;3(7):761–9.
24. McGranahan N, Favero F, de Bruin EC, Birkbak NJ, Szallasi Z, Swanton C. Clonal status of actionable driver events and the timing of mutational processes in cancer evolution. Sci Transl Med. 2015;7(283):283ra54.
25. Alexandrov LB, Nik-Zainal S, Wedge DC, Aparicio SA, Behjati S, Biankin AV, Bignell GR, Bolli N, Borg A, Borresen-Dale AL et al. Signatures of mutational processes in human cancer. Nature. 2013;500(7463):415–21.
26. Ciriello G, Miller ML, Aksoy BA, Senbabaoglu Y, Schultz N, Sander C. Emerging landscape of oncogenic signatures across human cancers. Nat Genet. 2013;45(10):1127–33.
27. Bhatia A, Burtness B. Human papillomavirus-associated oropharyngeal cancer: defining risk groups and clinical trials. J Clin Oncol. 2015;33(29): 3243–50.
28. Vokes EE, Agrawal N, Seiwert TY. HPV-Associated Head and Neck Cancer. J Natl Cancer Inst. 2015;107(12):djv344.
29. Leemans CR, Braakhuis BJ, Brakenhoff RH. The molecular biology of head and neck cancer. Nat Rev Cancer. 2011;11(1):9–22.
30. McLaughlin-Drubin ME, Crum CP, Munger K. Human papillomavirus E7 oncoprotein induces KDM6A and KDM6B histone demethylase expression and causes epigenetic reprogramming. Proc Natl Acad Sci U S A. 2011; 108(5):2130–5.
31. Munger K, Jones DL. Human papillomavirus carcinogenesis: an identity crisis in the retinoblastoma tumor suppressor pathway. J Virol. 2015; 89(9):4708–11.
32. Agger K, Cloos PA, Rudkjaer L, Williams K, Andersen G, Christensen J, Helin K. The H3K27me3 demethylase JMJD3 contributes to the activation of the INK4A-ARF locus in response to oncogene- and stress-induced senescence. Genes Dev. 2009;23(10):1171–6.
33. Gillison ML, D'Souza G, Westra W, Sugar E, Xiao W, Begum S, Viscidi R. Distinct risk factor profiles for human papillomavirus type 16-positive and human papillomavirus type 16-negative head and neck cancers. J Natl Cancer Inst. 2008;100(6):407–20.
34. Parfenov M, Pedamallu CS, Gehlenborg N, Freeman SS, Danilova L, Bristow CA, Lee S, Hadjipanayis AG, Ivanova EV, Wilkerson MD et al. Characterization

of HPV and host genome interactions in primary head and neck cancers. Proc Natl Acad Sci U S A. 2014;111(43):15544–9.

35. Pickering CR, Zhang J, Yoo SY, Bengtsson L, Moorthy S, Neskey DM, Zhao M, Ortega Alves MV, Chang K, Drummond J et al. Integrative genomic characterization of oral squamous cell carcinoma identifies frequent somatic drivers. Cancer Discov. 2013;3(7):770–81.

36. Pickering CR, Zhang JX, Neskey DM, Zhao M, Jasser SA, Wang JP, Ward A, Tsai CJ, Alves MVO, Zhou JH et al. Squamous cell carcinoma of the oral tongue in young Non-smokers is genomically similar to tumors in older smokers. Clin Cancer Res. 2014;20(14):3842–8.

37. Lin DC, Meng X, Hazawa M, Nagata Y, Varela AM, Xu L, Sato Y, Liu LZ, Ding LW, Sharma A et al. The genomic landscape of nasopharyngeal carcinoma. Nat Genet. 2014;46(8):866–71.

38. Gao JJ, Aksoy BA, Dogrusoz U, Dresdner G, Gross B, Sumer SO, Sun YC, Jacobsen A, Sinha R, Larsson E et al. Integrative analysis of complex cancer genomics and clinical profiles using the cBioPortal. Sci Signal. 2013;6(269):pl1.

39. Cerami E, Gao J, Dogrusoz U, Gross BE, Sumer SO, Aksoy BA, et al. The cBio cancer genomics portal: an open platform for exploring multidimensional cancer genomics data. Cancer Discov. 2012;2(5):401–4.

40. Mermel CH, Schumacher SE, Hill B, Meyerson ML, Beroukhim R, Getz G. GISTIC2.0 facilitates sensitive and confident localization of the targets of focal somatic copy-number alteration in human cancers. Genome Biol. 2011;12(4):R41.

41. Masuda M, Yamada T. Signaling pathway profiling by reverse-phase protein array for personalized cancer medicine. Biochim Biophys Acta. 2015;1854(6):651–7.

42. Barrett T, Wilhite SE, Ledoux P, Evangelista C, Kim IF, Tomashevsky M, et al. NCBI GEO: archive for functional genomics data sets-update. Nucleic Acids Res. 2013;41(D1):D991–5.

43. Hayes DN, Van Waes C, Seiwert TY. Genetic landscape of human papillomavirus-associated head and neck cancer and comparison to tobacco-related tumors. J Clin Oncol. 2015;33(29):3227–34.

44. Walter V, Yin X, Wilkerson MD, Cabanski CR, Zhao N, Du Y, et al. Molecular subtypes in head and neck cancer exhibit distinct patterns of chromosomal gain and loss of canonical cancer genes. PLoS One. 2013;8(2):e56823.

45. Tai SK, Lee JI, Ang KK, El-Naggar AK, Hassan KA, Liu D, et al. Loss of FHIT expression in head and neck squamous cell carcinoma and its potential clinical implication. Clin Cancer Res. 2004;10(16):5554–7.

46. Ma C, Quesnelle KM, Sparano A, Rao S, Park MS, Cohen MA, et al. Characterization CSMD1 in a large set of primary lung, head and neck, breast and skin cancer tissues. Cancer Biol Ther. 2009;8(10):907–16.

47. Scholnick SB, Richter TM. The role of CSMD1 in head and neck carcinogenesis. Genes Chromosomes Cancer. 2003;38(3):281–3.

48. Cancer Genome Atlas Research N. Comprehensive genomic characterization of squamous cell lung cancers. Nature. 2012;489(7417):519–25.

49. Liu Z, Long XB, Chao C, Yan C, Wu QY, Hua SN, Zhang YJ, Wu AB, Fang WY. Knocking down CDK4 mediates the elevation of let-7c suppressing cell growth in nasopharyngeal carcinoma. Bmc Cancer. 2014;14:274.

50. Liu N, Boohaker RJ, Jiang C, Boohaker JR, Xu B. A radiosensitivity MiRNA signature validated by the TCGA database for head and neck squamous cell carcinomas. Oncotarget. 2015;6(33):34649–57.

51. Thorpe LM, Yuzugullu H, Zhao JJ. PI3K in cancer: divergent roles of isoforms, modes of activation and therapeutic targeting. Nat Rev Cancer. 2015;15(1):7–24.

52. Vivanco I, Sawyers CL. The phosphatidylinositol 3-Kinase AKT pathway in human cancer. Nat Rev Cancer. 2002;2(7):489–501.

53. Elkabets M, Pazarentzos E, Juric D, Sheng Q, Pelossof RA, Brook S, et al. AXL mediates resistance to PI3K alpha inhibition by activating the EGFR/PKC/mTOR axis in head and esophageal squamous cell carcinomas. Cancer Cell. 2015;27(4):533–46.

54. Samuels Y, Diaz Jr LA, Schmidt-Kittler O, Cummins JM, Delong L, Cheong I, et al. Mutant PIK3CA promotes cell growth and invasion of human cancer cells. Cancer Cell. 2005;7(6):561–73.

55. Halilovic E, She QB, Ye Q, Pagliarini R, Sellers WR, Solit DB, et al. PIK3CA mutation uncouples tumor growth and cyclin D1 regulation from MEK/ERK and mutant KRAS signaling. Cancer Res. 2010;70(17):6804–14.

56. Beck TN, Kaczmar J, Handorf E, Nikonova A, Dubyk C, Peri S, et al. Phospho-T356RB1 predicts survival in HPV-negative squamous cell carcinoma of the head and neck. Oncotarget. 2015;6(22):18863–74.

57. Brachmann SM, Hofmann I, Schnell C, Fritsch C, Wee S, Lane H, et al. Specific apoptosis induction by the dual PI3K/mTor inhibitor NVP-BEZ235 in HER2 amplified and PIK3CA mutant breast cancer cells. Proc Natl Acad Sci U S A. 2009;106(52):22299–304.

58. Mohan S, Vander Broek R, Shah S, Eytan DF, Pierce ML, Carlson SG, et al. MEK Inhibitor PD-0325901 Overcomes Resistance to PI3K/mTOR Inhibitor PF-5212384 and potentiates antitumor effects in Human Head and Neck Squamous Cell Carcinoma. Clin Cancer Res. 2015;21(17):3946–56.

59. Herzog A, Bian YS, Vander Broek R, Hall B, Coupar J, Cheng H, et al. PI3K/mTOR Inhibitor PF-04691502 Antitumor Activity Is Enhanced with Induction of Wild-Type TP53 in Human Xenograft and Murine Knockout Models of Head and Neck Cancer. Clin Cancer Res. 2013;19(14):3808–19.

60. Rodon J, Dienstmann R, Serra V, Tabernero J. Development of PI3K inhibitors: lessons learned from early clinical trials. Nat Rev Clin Oncol. 2013;10(3):143–53.

61. Dotto GP. Crosstalk of Notch with p53 and p63 in cancer growth control. Nat Rev Cancer. 2009;9(8):587–95.

62. Nicolas M, Wolfer A, Raj K, Kummer JA, Mill P, van Noort M, et al. Notch1 functions as a tumor suppressor in mouse skin. Nat Genet. 2003;33(3):416–21.

63. Duan L, Yao J, Wu X, Fan M. Growth suppression induced by Notch1 activation involves Wnt-beta-catenin down-regulation in human tongue carcinoma cells. Biol Cell. 2006;98(8):479–90.

64. Dotto GP. Notch tumor suppressor function. Oncogene. 2008;27(38):5115–23.

65. Okuyama R, Ogawa E, Nagoshi H, Yabuki M, Kurihara A, Terui T, et al. p53 homologue, p51/p63, maintains the immaturity of keratinocyte stem cells by inhibiting Notch1 activity. Oncogene. 2007;26(31):4478–88.

66. Yang AN, Kaghad M, Wang YM, Gillett E, Fleming MD, Dotsch V, et al. p63, a p53 homolog at 3q27-29, encodes multiple products with transactivating, death-inducing, and dominant-negative activities. Mol Cell. 1998;2(3):305–16.

67. Wu G, Nomoto S, Hoque MO, Dracheva T, Osada M, Lee CC, et al. DeltaNp63alpha and TAp63alpha regulate transcription of genes with distinct biological functions in cancer and development. Cancer Res. 2003;63(10):2351–7.

68. Westfall MD, Pietenpol JA. p63: Molecular complexity in development and cancer. Carcinogenesis. 2004;25(6):857–64.

69. Melino G. p63 is a suppressor of tumorigenesis and metastasis interacting with mutant p53. Cell Death Differ. 2011;18(9):1487–99.

70. Zangen R, Ratovitski E, Sidransky D. Delta Np63 alpha levels correlate with clinical tumor response to cisplatin. Cell Cycle. 2005;4(10):1313–5.

71. Riese U, Dahse R, Fiedler W, Theuer C, Koscielny S, Ernst G, et al. Tumor suppressor gene p16 (CDKN2A) mutation status and promoter inactivation in head and neck cancer. Int J Mol Med. 1999;4(1):61–5.

72. Greenblatt MS, Bennett WP, Hollstein M, Harris CC. Mutations in the p53 tumor suppressor gene: clues to cancer etiology and molecular pathogenesis. Cancer Res. 1994;54(18):4855–78.

73. Burtness B, Bauman JE, Galloway T. Novel targets in HPV-negative head and neck cancer: overcoming resistance to EGFR inhibition. Lancet Oncol. 2013;14(8):e302–9.

74. Jensen MA, Fukushima M, Davis RW. DMSO and betaine greatly improve amplification of GC-rich constructs in de novo synthesis. PLoS One. 2010;5(6):e11024.

75. Kozarewa I, Ning Z, Quail MA, Sanders MJ, Berriman M, Turner DJ. Amplification-free Illumina sequencing-library preparation facilitates improved mapping and assembly of (G + C)-biased genomes. Nat Methods. 2009;6(4):291–5.

76. Poeta ML, Manola J, Goldwasser MA, Forastiere A, Benoit N, Califano JA, et al. TP53 mutations and survival in squamous-cell carcinoma of the head and neck. N Engl J Med. 2007;357(25):2552–61.

77. Masica DL, Li S, Douville C, Manola J, Ferris RL, Burtness B, et al. Predicting survival in head and neck squamous cell carcinoma from TP53 mutation. Hum Genet. 2015;134(5):497–507.

78. Gross AM, Orosco RK, Shen JP, Egloff AM, Carter H, Hofree M, et al. Multi-tiered genomic analysis of head and neck cancer ties TP53 mutation to 3p loss. Nat Genet. 2014;46(9):939–43.

79. Song Y, Li L, Ou Y, Gao Z, Li E, Li X, et al. Identification of genomic alterations in oesophageal squamous cell cancer. Nature. 2014;509(7498):91–5.

80. Neskey DM, Osman AA, Ow TJ, Katsonis P, McDonald T, Hicks SC, et al. Evolutionary action score of TP53 identifies high-risk mutations associated with decreased survival and increased distant metastases in head and neck cancer. Cancer Res. 2015;75(7):1527–36.

81. Osman AA, Neskey DM, Katsonis P, Patel AA, Ward AM, Hsu TK, et al. Evolutionary action score of TP53 coding variants is predictive of platinum response in head and neck cancer patients. Cancer Res. 2015; 75(7):1205–15.

82. Katsonis P, Lichtarge O. A formal perturbation equation between genotype and phenotype determines the evolutionary action of protein-coding variations on fitness. Genome Res. 2014;24(12):2050–8.

83. Brosh R, Rotter V. When mutants gain new powers: news from the mutant p53 field. Nat Rev Cancer. 2009;9(10):701–13.

84. Lichtarge O, Wilkins A. Evolution: a guide to perturb protein function and networks. Curr Opin Struc Biol. 2010;20(3):351–9.

85. Weinberg RA. The retinoblastoma protein and cell cycle control. Cell. 1995; 81(3):323–30.

86. Burke JR, Hura GL, Rubin SM. Structures of inactive retinoblastoma protein reveal multiple mechanisms for cell cycle control. Gene Dev. 2012;26(11): 1156–66.

87. Wong SQ, Li J, Salemi R, Sheppard KE, Do H, Tothill RW, et al. Targeted-capture massively-parallel sequencing enables robust detection of clinically informative mutations from formalin-fixed tumours. Sci Rep. 2013;3:3494.

88. Demokan S, Chuang A, Suoglu Y, Ulusan M, Yalniz Z, Califano JA, et al. Promoter methylation and loss of p16INK4a gene expression in head and neck cancer. Head Neck-J Sci Spec. 2012;34(10):1470–5.

89. El-Naggar AK, Lai S, Clayman G, Lee JK, Luna MA, Goepfert H, et al. Methylation, a major mechanism of p16/CDKN2 gene inactivation in head and neck squamous carcinoma. Am J Pathol. 1997;151(6):1767–74.

90. Reed AL, Califano J, Cairns P, Westra WH, Jones RM, Koch W, et al. High frequency of p16 (CDKN2/MTS-1/INK4A) inactivation in head and neck squamous cell carcinoma. Cancer Res. 1996;56(16):3630–3.

91. Ha PK, Califano JA. Promoter methylation and inactivation of tumour-suppressor genes in oral squamous-cell carcinoma. Lancet Oncol. 2006;7(1): 77–82.

92. Chung CH, Zhang Q, Kong CS, Harris J, Fertig EJ, Harari PM, et al. p16 protein expression and human papillomavirus status as prognostic biomarkers of nonoropharyngeal head and neck squamous cell carcinoma. J Clin Oncol. 2014;32(35):3930–U3212.

93. Pollock NI, Grandis JR. HER2 as a therapeutic target in head and neck squamous cell carcinoma. Clin Cancer Res. 2015;21(3):526–33.

94. Quesnelle KM, Grandis JR. Dual kinase inhibition of EGFR and HER2 overcomes resistance to cetuximab in a novel in vivo model of acquired cetuximab resistance. Clin Cancer Res. 2011;17(18):5935–44.

95. Ratushny V, Astsaturov I, Burtness BA, Golemis EA, Silverman JS. Targeting EGFR resistance networks in head and neck cancer. Cell Signal. 2009;21(8):1255–68.

96. Marshall ME, Hinz TK, Kono SA, Singleton KR, Bichon B, Ware KE, et al. Fibroblast growth factor receptors are components of autocrine signaling networks in head and neck squamous cell carcinoma cells. Clin Cancer Res. 2011;17(15):5016–25.

97. Wellbrock C, Karasarides M, Marais R. The RAF proteins take centre stage. Nat Rev Mol Cell Biol. 2004;5(11):875–85.

98. Weber CK, Slupsky JR, Herrmann C, Schuler M, Rapp UR, Block C. Mitogenic signaling of Ras is regulated by differential interaction with Raf isozymes. Oncogene. 2000;19(2):169–76.

99. Logue JS, Morrison DK. Complexity in the signaling network: insights from the use of targeted inhibitors in cancer therapy. Gene Dev. 2012; 26(7):641–50.

100. Morris LGT, Kaufman AM, Gong YX, Ramaswami D, Walsh LA, Turcan S, et al. Recurrent somatic mutation of FAT1 in multiple human cancers leads to aberrant Wnt activation. Nat Genet. 2013;45(3):253–61.

101. Haraguchi K, Ohsugi M, Abe Y, Semba K, Akiyama T, Yamamoto T. Ajuba negatively regulates the Wnt signaling pathway by promoting GSK-3beta-mediated phosphorylation of beta-catenin. Oncogene. 2008;27(3):274–84.

102. Nikonova AS, Astsaturov I, Serebriiskii IG, Dunbrack RL, Golemis EA. Aurora A kinase (AURKA) in normal and pathological cell division. Cell Mol Life Sci. 2013;70(4):661–87.

103. Mehra R, Serebriiskii IG, Burtness B, Astsaturov I, Golemis EA. Aurora kinases in head and neck cancer. Lancet Oncol. 2013;14(10):e425–35.

104. Jaramillo MC, Zhang DD. The emerging role of the Nrf2-Keap1 signaling pathway in cancer. Genes Dev. 2013;27(20):2179–91.

105. Cullinan SB, Gordan JD, Jin JO, Harper JW, Diehl JA. The Keap1-BTB protein is an adaptor that bridges Nrf2 to a Cul3-based E3 ligase: Oxidative stress sensing by a Cul3-Keap1 ligase. Mol Cell Biol. 2004;24(19):8477–86.

106. Qian Z, Zhou T, Gurguis CI, Xu X, Wen Q, Lv J, et al. Nuclear factor, erythroid 2-like 2-associated molecular signature predicts lung cancer survival. Sci Rep. 2015;5:16889.

107. Hammerman PS, Hayes DN, Grandis JR. Therapeutic insights from genomic studies of head and neck squamous cell carcinomas. Cancer Discov. 2015; 5(3):239–44.

108. Martinez VD, Vucic EA, Thu KL, Pikor LA, Lam S, Lam WL. Disruption of KEAP1/CUL3/RBX1 E3-ubiquitin ligase complex components by multiple genetic mechanisms: association with poor prognosis in head and neck cancer. Head Neck-J Sci Spec. 2015;37(5):727–34.

109. Choschzick M, Tabibzada AM, Gieseking F, Woelber L, Jaenicke F, Sauter G, et al. BIRC2 amplification in squamous cell carcinomas of the uterine cervix. Virchows Arch. 2012;461(2):123–8.

110. Imoto I, Tsuda H, Hirasawa A, Miura M, Sakamoto M, Hirohashi S, et al. Expression of cIAP1, a target for 11q22 amplification, correlates with resistance of cervical cancers to radiotherapy. Cancer Res. 2002;62(17):4860–6.

111. Imoto I, Yang ZQ, Pimkhaokham A, Tsuda H, Shimada Y, Imamura M, et al. Identification of cIAP1 as a candidate target gene within an amplicon at 11q22 in esophageal squamous cell carcinomas. Cancer Res. 2001;61(18): 6629–34.

112. Phillips AH, Schoeffler AJ, Matsui T, Weiss TM, Blankenship JW, Zobel K, et al. Internal motions prime cIAP1 for rapid activation. Nat Struct Mol Biol. 2014; 21(12):1068–74.

113. Vallabhapurapu S, Matsuzawa A, Zhang WZ, Tseng PH, Keats JJ, Wang HP, et al. Nonredundant and complementary functions of TRAF2 and TRAF3 in a ubiquitination cascade that activates NIK-dependent alternative NF-kappa B signaling. Nat Immunol. 2008;9(12):1364–70.

114. Stanger BZ. Quit your YAPing: a new target for cancer therapy. Gene Dev. 2012;26(12):1263–7.

115. Jerhammar F, Johansson AC, Ceder R, Welander J, Jansson A, Grafstrom RC, et al. YAP1 is a potential biomarker for cetuximab resistance in head and neck cancer. Oral Oncol. 2014;50(9):832–9.

116. Zhang JM, Ji JY, Yu M, Overholtzer M, Smolen GA, Wang R, et al. YAP-dependent induction of amphiregulin identifies a non-cell-autonomous component of the Hippo pathway. Nat Cell Biol. 2009;11(12):1444–U1134.

117. Pattje WJ, Melchers LJ, Slagter-Menkema L, Mastik MF, Schrijvers ML, Gibcus JH, et al. FADD expression is associated with regional and distant metastasis in squamous cell carcinoma of the head and neck. Histopathology. 2013; 63(2):263–70.

118. Lechner M, Frampton GM, Fenton T, Feber A, Palmer G, Jay A, et al. Targeted next-generation sequencing of head and neck squamous cell carcinoma identifies novel genetic alterations in HPV+ and HPV- tumors. Genome Med. 2013;5(5):49.

119. Khoury JD, Tannir NM, Williams MD, Chen YX, Yao H, Zhang JP, et al. Landscape of DNA virus associations across human malignant cancers: analysis of 3775 cases using RNA-Seq. J Virol. 2013;87(16):8916–26.

120. Wentzensen N, Vinokurova S, Doeberitz MV. Systematic review of genomic integration sites of human papillomavirus genomes in epithelial dysplasia and invasive cancer of the female lower genital tract. Cancer Res. 2004; 64(11):3878–84.

121. Hu Z, Zhu D, Wang W, Li W, Jia W, Zeng X, et al. Genome-wide profiling of HPV integration in cervical cancer identifies clustered genomic hot spots and a potential microhomology-mediated integration mechanism. Nat Genet. 2015;47(2):158–63.

122. Moody CA, Laimins LA. Human papillomavirus oncoproteins: pathways to transformation. Nat Rev Cancer. 2010;10(8):550–60.

123. Thomas M, Pim D, Banks L. The role of the E6-p53 interaction in the molecular pathogenesis of HPV. Oncogene. 1999;18(53):7690–700.

124. Huh K, Zhou XB, Hayakawa H, Cho JY, Libermann TA, Jin JP, et al. Human papillomavirus type 16 E7 oncoprotein associates with the cullin 2 ubiquitin ligase complex, which contributes to degradation of the retinoblastoma tumor suppressor. J Virol. 2007;81(18):9737–47.

125. Dyson N, Howley PM, Munger K, Harlow E. The human papilloma virus-16 E7-oncoprotein is able to bind to the retinoblastoma gene-product. Science. 1989;243(4893):934–7.

126. Chung CH, Gillison ML. Human papillomavirus in head and neck cancer: its role in pathogenesis and clinical implications. Clin Cancer Res. 2009;15(22): 6758–62.

127. Singh P, Thomas GE, Gireesh KK, Manna TK. TACC3 protein regulates microtubule nucleation by affecting gamma-tubulin ring complexes. J Biol Chem. 2014;289(46):31719–35.

128. Yao R, Kondoh Y, Natsume Y, Yamanaka H, Inoue M, Toki H, et al. A small compound targeting TACC3 revealed its different spatiotemporal contributions for spindle assembly in cancer cells. Oncogene. 2014;33(33): 4242–52.

129. Singh D, Chan JM, Zoppoli P, Niola F, Sullivan R, Castano A, et al. Transforming Fusions of FGFR and TACC Genes in Human Glioblastoma. Science. 2012;337(6099):1231–5.

130. Wu YM, Su F, Kalyana-Sundaram S, Khazanov N, Ateeq B, Cao X, et al. Identification of targetable FGFR gene fusions in diverse cancers. Cancer Discov. 2013;3(6):636–47.

131. Yuan L, Liu ZH, Lin ZR, Xu LH, Zhong Q, Zeng MS. Recurrent FGFR3-TACC3 fusion gene in nasopharyngeal carcinoma. Cancer Biol Ther. 2014;15(12):1613–21.

132. Hacker H, Tseng PH, Karin M. Expanding TRAF function: TRAF3 as a tri-faced immune regulator. Nat Rev Immunol. 2011;11(7):457–68.

133. Zhang J, Chen H, Yang X, Guven E, Nussinov R, Chen Z, VanWaes C. Defective TRAF3 modulates alternative NF-kB signaling and cytokine expression to promote cancer cell survival in HPV positive head and neck cancer (TUM10P.1049). J Immunol. 2015;194:211.30.

134. McGranahan N, Swanton C. Biological and therapeutic impact of intratumor heterogeneity in cancer evolution. Cancer Cell. 2015;27(1):15–26.

135. Alizadeh AA, Aranda V, Bardelli A, Blanpain C, Bock C, Borowski C, et al. Toward understanding and exploiting tumor heterogeneity. Nat Med. 2015; 21(8):846–53.

136. Gerlinger M, Rowan AJ, Horswell S, Larkin J, Endesfelder D, Gronroos E, et al. Intratumor heterogeneity and branched evolution revealed by multiregion sequencing. N Engl J Med. 2012;366(10):883–92.

137. Mroz EA, Rocco JW. MATH, a novel measure of intratumor genetic heterogeneity, is high in poor-outcome classes of head and neck squamous cell carcinoma. Oral Oncol. 2013;49(3):211–5.

138. Mroz EA, Tward AM, Hammon RJ, Ren Y, Rocco JW. Intra-tumor genetic heterogeneity and mortality in head and neck cancer: analysis of data from the Cancer Genome Atlas. Plos Med. 2015;12(2):e1001786.

139. Landau DA, Carter SL, Getz G, Wu CJ. Clonal evolution in hematological malignancies and therapeutic implications. Leukemia. 2014;28(1):34–43.

140. Landau DA, Carter SL, Stojanov P, McKenna A, Stevenson K, Lawrence MS, et al. Evolution and impact of subclonal mutations in chronic lymphocytic leukemia. Cell. 2013;152(4):714–26.

141. Lohr JG, Stojanov P, Carter SL, Cruz-Gordillo P, Lawrence MS, Auclair D, et al. Widespread genetic heterogeneity in multiple myeloma: implications for targeted therapy. Cancer Cell. 2014;25(1):91–101.

142. Carter SL, Cibulskis K, Helman E, McKenna A, Shen H, Zack T, et al. Absolute quantification of somatic DNA alterations in human cancer. Nat Biotechnol. 2012;30(5):413–21.

143. Swanton C, McGranahan N, Starrett GJ, Harris RS. APOBEC enzymes: mutagenic fuel for cancer evolution and heterogeneity. Cancer Discov. 2015;5(7):704–12.

144. Henderson S, Chakravarthy A, Su X, Boshoff C, Fenton TR. APOBEC-mediated cytosine deamination links PIK3CA helical domain mutations to human papillomavirus-driven tumor development. Cell Rep. 2014;7(6):1833–41.

145. Zhao L, Vogt PK. Helical domain and kinase domain mutations in p110alpha of phosphatidylinositol 3-kinase induce gain of function by different mechanisms. Proc Natl Acad Sci U S A. 2008;105(7):2652–7.

146. Lu C, Xie M, Wendl MC, Wang J, McLellan MD, Leiserson MD, et al. Patterns and functional implications of rare germline variants across 12 cancer types. Nat Commun. 2015;6:10086.

147. Moldovan GL, D'Andrea AD. How the Fanconi Anemia pathway guards the genome. Annu Rev Genet. 2009;43:223–49.

148. Conti MA, Saleh AD, Brinster LR, Cheng H, Chen Z, Cornelius S, et al. Conditional deletion of nonmuscle myosin II-A in mouse tongue epithelium results in squamous cell carcinoma. Sci Rep. 2015;5:14068.

149. Schramek D, Sendoel A, Segal JP, Beronja S, Heller E, Oristian D, et al. Direct in Vivo RNAi Screen Unveils Myosin IIa as a Tumor Suppressor of Squamous Cell Carcinomas. Science. 2014;343(6168):309–13.

150. Ma X, Adelstein RS. The role of vertebrate nonmuscle Myosin II in development and human disease. Bioarchitecture. 2014;4(3):88–102.

151. Bozic I, Reiter JG, Allen B, Antal T, Chatterjee K, Shah P, et al. Evolutionary dynamics of cancer in response to targeted combination therapy. Elife. 2013;2:e00747.

152. Mirghani H, Amen F, Blanchard P, Moreau F, Guigay J, Hartl DM, et al. Treatment de-escalation in HPV-positive oropharyngeal carcinoma: ongoing trials, critical issues and perspectives. Int J Cancer. 2015;136(7):1494–503.

153. Liu H, Cracchiolo JR, Beck TN, Serebriiskii IG, Golemis EA. EGFR inhibitors as therapeutic agents in head and neck cancer. In: Burtness B, Golemis EA, editors. Molecular determinants of head and neck cancer. 1st ed. New York: Springer New York; 2014. p. 55–90.

154. Vermorken JB, Mesia R, Rivera F, Remenar E, Kawecki A, Rottey S, et al. Platinum-based chemotherapy plus cetuximab in head and neck cancer. N Engl J Med. 2008;359(11):1116–27.

155. Burtness B, Goldwasser MA, Flood W, Mattar B, Forastiere AA, Eastern Cooperative Oncology G. Phase III randomized trial of cisplatin plus placebo compared with cisplatin plus cetuximab in metastatic/recurrent head and neck cancer: an eastern cooperative oncology group study. J Clin Oncol. 2005;23(34):8646–54.

156. Harrington K, Berrier A, Robinson M, Remenar E, Housset M, de Mendoza FH, et al. Randomised Phase II study of oral lapatinib combined with chemoradiotherapy in patients with advanced squamous cell carcinoma of the head and neck: rationale for future randomised trials in human papilloma virus-negative disease. Eur J Cancer. 2013;49(7):1609–18.

157. Machiels JP, Haddad RI, Fayette J, Licitra LF, Tahara M, Vermorken JB, et al. Afatinib versus methotrexate as second-line treatment in patients with recurrent or metastatic squamous-cell carcinoma of the head and neck progressing on or after platinum-based therapy (LUX-Head & Neck 1): an open-label, randomised phase 3 trial. Lancet Oncol. 2015;16(5): 583–94.

158. Chong CR, Janne PA. The quest to overcome resistance to EGFR-targeted therapies in cancer. Nat Med. 2013;19(11):1389–400.

159. Dorsey K, Agulnik M. Promising new molecular targeted therapies in head and neck cancer. Drugs. 2013;73(4):315–25.

160. Suh Y, Amelio I, Guerrero Urbano T, Tavassoli M. Clinical update on cancer: molecular oncology of head and neck cancer. Cell Death Dis. 2014;5:e1018.

161. Sacco AG, Cohen EE. Current treatment options for recurrent or metastatic head and neck squamous cell carcinoma. J Clin Oncol. 2015;33(29):3305–13.

162. Asghar U, Witkiewicz AK, Turner NC, Knudsen ES. The history and future of targeting cyclin-dependent kinases in cancer therapy. Nat Rev Drug Discov. 2015;14(2):130–46.

163. Shaw AT, Hsu PP, Awad MM, Engelman JA. Tyrosine kinase gene rearrangements in epithelial malignancies. Nat Rev Cancer. 2013;13(11):772–87.

164. Huang M, Shen AJ, Ding J, Geng MY. Molecularly targeted cancer therapy: some lessons from the past decade. Trends Pharmacol Sci. 2014;35(1):41–50.

165. Matzinger O, Viertl D, Tsoutsou P, Kadi L, Rigotti S, Zanna C, et al. The radiosensitizing activity of the SMAC-mimetic, Debio 1143, is TNF alpha-mediated in head and neck squamous cell carcinoma. Radiother Oncol. 2015;116(3):495–503.

166. Eytan DF, Snow GE, Carlson SG, Schiltz S, Chen Z, Van Waes C. Combination effects of SMAC mimetic birinapant with TNFalpha, TRAIL, and docetaxel in preclinical models of HNSCC. Laryngoscope. 2015;125(3):E118–24.

167. Mahoney KM, Rennert PD, Freeman GJ. Combination cancer immunotherapy and new immunomodulatory targets. Nat Rev Drug Discov. 2015;14(8):561–84.

168. Gettinger SN, Horn L, Gandhi L, Spigel DR, Antonia SJ, Rizvi NA, et al. Overall Survival and Long-Term Safety of Nivolumab (Anti-Programmed Death 1 Antibody, BMS-936558, ONO-4538) in Patients With Previously Treated Advanced Non-Small-Cell Lung Cancer. J Clin Oncol. 2015;33(18):2004–U2032.

169. Borghaei H, Paz-Ares L, Horn L, Spigel DR, Steins M, Ready NE, et al. Nivolumab versus Docetaxel in advanced nonsquamous non-small-cell lung cancer. N Engl J Med. 2015;373(17):1627–39.

170. Hodi FS, O'Day SJ, McDermott DF, Weber RW, Sosman JA, Haanen JB, et al. Improved survival with ipilimumab in patients with metastatic melanoma. N Engl J Med. 2010;363(8):711–23.

171. Le DT, Uram JN, Wang H, Bartlett BR, Kemberling H, Eyring AD, et al. PD-1 blockade in tumors with mismatch-repair deficiency. N Engl J Med. 2015; 372(26):2509–20.

172. Postow MA, Callahan MK, Wolchok JD. Immune checkpoint blockade in cancer therapy. J Clin Oncol. 2015;33(17):1974–82.

173. Kuss I, Hathaway B, Ferris RL, Gooding W, Whiteside TL. Decreased absolute counts of T lymphocyte subsets and their relation to disease in squamous cell carcinoma of the head and neck. Clin Cancer Res. 2004;10(11):3755–62.

174. Jie HB, Schuler PJ, Lee SC, Srivastava RM, Argiris A, Ferrone S, et al. CTLA-4(+) regulatory T cells increased in cetuximab-treated head and neck cancer

patients suppress NK cell cytotoxicity and correlate with poor prognosis. Cancer Res. 2015;75(11):2200–10.

175. Pardoll DM. The blockade of immune checkpoints in cancer immunotherapy. Nat Rev Cancer. 2012;12(4):252–64.

176. Robert C, Schachter J, Long GV, Arance A, Grob JJ, Mortier L, et al. Pembrolizumab versus ipilimumab in advanced melanoma. N Engl J Med. 2015;372(26):2521–32.

177. Garon EB, Rizvi NA, Hui RN, Leighl N, Balmanoukian AS, Eder JP, et al. Pembrolizumab for the treatment of non-small-cell lung cancer. New Engl J Med. 2015;372(21):2018–28.

178. Ribas A, Puzanov I, Dummer R, Schadendorf D, Hamid O, Robert C, et al. Pembrolizumab versus investigator-choice chemotherapy for ipilimumab-refractory melanoma (KEYNOTE-002): a randomised, controlled, phase 2 trial. Lancet Oncol. 2015;16(8):908–18.

179. Sivan A, Corrales L, Hubert N, Williams JB, Aquino-Michaels K, Earley ZM, et al. Commensal Bifidobacterium promotes antitumor immunity and facilitates anti-PD-L1 efficacy. Science. 2015;350(6264):1084–9.

180. Vetizou M, Pitt JM, Daillere R, Lepage P, Waldschmitt N, Flament C, et al. Anticancer immunotherapy by CTLA-4 blockade relies on the gut microbiota. Science. 2015;350(6264):1079–84.

181. Weisenberger DJ. Characterizing DNA methylation alterations from the Cancer Genome Atlas. J Clin Invest. 2014;124(1):17–23.

182. Jones PA, Baylin SB. The epigenomics of cancer. Cell. 2007;128(4):683–92.

183. Lleras RA, Smith RV, Adrien LR, Schlecht NF, Burk RD, Harris TM, et al. Unique DNA methylation loci distinguish anatomic site and HPV status in head and neck squamous cell carcinoma. Clin Cancer Res. 2013; 19(19):5444–55.

184. Schlecht NF, Ben-Dayan M, Anayannis N, Lleras RA, Thomas C, Wang Y, et al. Epigenetic changes in the CDKN2A locus are associated with differential expression of P16INK4A and P14ARF in HPV-positive oropharyngeal squamous cell carcinoma. Cancer Med. 2015;4(3):342–53.

185. Gaykalova DA, Vatapalli R, Wei Y, Tsai HL, Wang H, Zhang C, et al. Outlier analysis defines zinc finger gene family DNA methylation in tumors and saliva of head and neck cancer patients. PLoS One. 2015; 10(11):e0142148.

186. Timmermann S, Hinds PW, Munger K. Re-expression of endogenous p16(ink4a) in oral squamous cell carcinoma lines by 5-aza-2 '-deoxycytidine treatment induces a senescence-like state. Oncogene. 1998;17(26):3445–53.

187. Shi H, Chen X, Lu C, Gu CM, Jiang HW, Meng RW, Niu X, Huang YX, Lu MX. Association between P16(INK4a) promoter methylation and HNSCC: a meta-analysis of 21 published studies. Plos One. 2015;10(4):e0122302.

188. Kostareli E, Holzinger D, Bogatyrova O, Hielscher T, Wichmann G, Keck M, et al. HPV-related methylation signature predicts survival in oropharyngeal squamous cell carcinomas. J Clin Invest. 2013;123(6):2488–501.

189. Shi H, Chen X, Lu C, Gu C, Jiang H, Meng R, et al. Association between P16INK4a promoter methylation and HNSCC: a meta-analysis of 21 published studies. PLoS One. 2015;10(4):e0122302.

190. Chen X, Liu L, Mims J, Punska EC, Williams KE, Zhao W, et al. Analysis of DNA methylation and gene expression in radiation-resistant head and neck tumors. Epigenetics. 2015;10(6):545–61.

191. Le Tourneau C, Kamal M, Tsimberidou AM, Bedard P, Pierron G, Callens C, Rouleau E, Vincent-Salomon A, Servant N, Alt M, et al. Treatment algorithms based on tumor molecular profiling: the essence of precision medicine trials. J Natl Cancer Inst. 2016;108(4):djv362.

192. Le Tourneau C, Paoletti X, Servant N, Bieche I, Gentien D, Rio Frio T, et al. Randomised proof-of-concept phase II trial comparing targeted therapy based on tumour molecular profiling vs conventional therapy in patients with refractory cancer: results of the feasibility part of the SHIVA trial. Br J Cancer. 2014;111(1):17–24.

193. Rodon J, Soria JC, Berger R, Batist G, Tsimberidou A, Bresson C, et al. Challenges in initiating and conducting personalized cancer therapy trials: perspectives from WINTHER, a Worldwide Innovative Network (WIN) Consortium trial. Ann Oncol. 2015;26(8):1791–8.

194. Brown SD, Warren RL, Gibb EA, Martin SD, Spinelli JJ, Nelson BH, et al. Neo-antigens predicted by tumor genome meta-analysis correlate with increased patient survival. Genome Res. 2014;24(5):743–50.

195. Brahmer J, Reckamp KL, Baas P, Crino L, Eberhardt WE, Poddubskaya E, et al. Nivolumab versus Docetaxel in advanced squamous-cell non-small-cell lung cancer. N Engl J Med. 2015;373(2):123–35.

196. Wolchok JD, Kluger H, Callahan MK, Postow MA, Rizvi NA, Lesokhin AM, et al. Nivolumab plus ipilimumab in advanced melanoma. N Engl J Med. 2013;369(2):122–33.

197. Rizvi NA, Hellmann MD, Snyder A, Kvistborg P, Makarov V, Havel JJ, et al. Cancer immunology. Mutational landscape determines sensitivity to PD-1 blockade in non-small cell lung cancer. Science. 2015;348(6230): 124–8.

198. Hariri S, Markowitz LE, Dunne EF, Unger ER. Population impact of HPV vaccines: summary of early evidence. J Adolesc Health. 2013;53(6): 679–82.

199. Baldur-Felskov B, Dehlendorff C, Munk C, Kjaer SK. Early impact of human papillomavirus vaccination on cervical neoplasia–nationwide follow-up of young Danish women. J Natl Cancer Inst. 2014;106(3):djt460.

2

Biomarker driven treatment of head and neck squamous cell cancer

Nnamdi Eze[1]* , Ying-Chun Lo[2] and Barbara Burtness[3]

Abstract: Treatment modalities of head and neck squamous cell cancer include surgery, radiation, chemotherapy, targeted agents and immune checkpoint inhibition. Treatment is often toxic and can affect long-term function and quality of life. In this context, identification of biomarker data that can help tailor therapy on an individualized basis and reduce treatment-related toxicity would be highly beneficial. A variety of predictive biomarkers have been discovered and are already utilized in clinical practice, while many more are being explored. We will review p16 overexpression as a surrogate biomarker in HPV-associated head and neck cancer and plasma EBV DNA as a biomarker in nasopharyngeal carcinoma, the two established biomarkers currently utilized in clinical practice. We will also examine novel predictive biomarkers that are in clinical development and may shape the future landscape of targeted head and neck cancer therapy. These emerging biomarkers include the tyrosine kinases and their signaling pathway, immune checkpoint biomarkers, tumor suppressor abnormalities, and molecular predictors of hypoxia-targeted therapy. We will also look at futuristic biomarkers including detection of circulating DNA from clinical specimens and rapid tumor profiling. We will highlight the ongoing effort that will see a shift from prognostic to predictive biomarker development in head and neck cancer with the goal of delivering individualized cancer therapy.

Trial registration: N/A.

Keywords: Head and neck squamous cell cancer (HNSCC), Biomarkers, Human papilloma virus (HPV), Epidermal growth factor receptor (EGFR), Epstein Barr virus (EBV), Cetuximab, Nasopharyngeal carcinoma (NPC), Phosphatase and tensin homolog (PTEN), Phosphoinositide 3- kinase (PI3K)

Background

Head and neck squamous cell cancer (HNSCC) is a heterogeneous group of cancers accounting for about 3% of all cancers in the United States. Each year, an estimated 61,000 people develop HNSCC, of whom about 13,000 die [1]. Treatment modalities include surgery, radiation, chemotherapy, targeted agents and immune checkpoint inhibition. For the many patients who are cured, late sequelae of treatment can affect function, quality of life and possibly even non-cancer mortality [2–4]. In this context, indicators of biologic behavior and treatment sensitivity could prove enormously helpful in tailoring therapy on an individualized basis. This is the rationale behind the search for predictive and prognostic biomarkers in HNSCC. The National Cancer Institute (NCI) defines a biomarker as "a biological molecule found in blood, other body fluids, or tissues that is a sign of a normal or abnormal process or of a condition or disease; and may be used to see how well the body responds to a treatment for a disease or condition" [5]. Although biomarkers of Human Papilloma Virus (HPV) association have emerged as validated, standard biomarkers in this disease, numerous studies point to the potential utility of biomarkers in predicting outcome and selecting therapy. This review focuses on prognostic and predictive biomarkers that drive therapeutic choices in HNSCC. We will look at established biomarkers that are standard of care in clinical practice, as well as novel biomarkers that are in clinical development.

Established biomarkers

With the identification of HPV as an etiologic agent in a subset of HNSCC, p16 overexpression by immunohistochemistry (IHC) as a surrogate marker of HPV association

* Correspondence: nnamdi.eze@yale.edu
[1]Section of Medical Oncology, Department of Internal Medicine, Yale University School of Medicine and Yale Cancer Center, 333 Cedar Street, Room WWW-221, P.O. Box 208028, New Haven, CT 06520, USA
Full list of author information is available at the end of the article

has become the most robust HNSCC biomarker employed in clinical practice. Plasma Epstein Barr Virus (EBV) Deoxyribonucleic Acid (DNA) also plays a role as a predictive and prognostic biomarker specifically in nasopharyngeal carcinoma (NPC) patients.

HPV status in oropharyngeal SCC (OPSCC)

HPV-initiated HNSCC is a biologically distinct category of HNSCC with significantly better prognosis and treatment outcome compared to HPV-negative HNSCC [6–8]. p16 overexpression by IHC is an outstanding surrogate marker of HPV association in OPSCC [9] and is well established as a prognostic biomarker of favorable outcome in HNSCC. p16, a tumor suppressor protein that is encoded by *CDKN2A gene*, regulates cell cycle by inhibiting the phosphorylation of the retinoblastoma (Rb) tumor suppressor protein by cyclin dependent kinases (CDK) 4 and 6. This leads to inactivation of factor E2F1, an important component of cell-cycle progression. In the setting of HPV-associated tumors, the HPV E7 viral oncoprotein promotes rapid degradation of Rb, and as Rb usually regulates p16, the disruption of Rb permits increased p16 expression [6, 10]. Expression of p16 is therefore up-regulated in HPV-positive cancer and frequently lost in HPV-negative tumors.

Several studies have shown that patients with HPV-associated OPSCC have a better prognosis than patients with HPV-negative tumors, with significantly decreased risk of death (40–60% reduction) and relapse (60–70% reduction) in HPV-associated tumors compared to HPV-negative tumors, when treated with multimodality therapies [7, 8, 11–13]. HPV-positive cancers also have better outcome following induction chemotherapy (IC), radiation and chemoradiation for OPSCC patients. A prospective analysis of the association of tumor HPV status and therapeutic response and survival among 96 patients with stage III/IV HNSCC of oropharynx or larynx treated with IC followed by concurrent chemoradiotherapy on the ECOG 2399 phase II trial showed that patients with HPV-ISH-positive or p16-positive tumors had significantly higher response rates (RR) after IC and after paclitaxel-based chemoradiotherapy compared with patients with HPV-negative tumors. After a median follow-up of 39.1 months, patients with HPV-associated tumors also had significantly improved overall survival (OS) and lower risks of progression than those with HPV-negative tumors [8]. In the recent E1308 phase II trial, 90 patients with HPV16 and/or p16-positive stage III-IV OPSCC received three cycles of IC with cisplatin, paclitaxel, and cetuximab, after which patients with primary-site complete clinical response (cCR) received intensity-modulated radiation therapy (IMRT) 54 Gy with weekly cetuximab, while those with less than cCR received 69.3 Gy and cetuximab. The primary end-point was two-year progression-free survival (PFS). Fifty-six patients (70%) achieved a primary-site cCR to IC and 51 patients continued to cetuximab with IMRT 54 Gy. After median follow-up of 35.4 months, two-year PFS and OS rates were 80% and 94%, respectively, for patients with primary-site cCR treated with 54 Gy of radiation (n = 51); and 96% and 96%, respectively, for patients with < T4, < N2c, and <10 pack-year smoking history who were treated with ≤54 Gy of radiation (n = 27). At 12 months, significantly fewer patients treated with a radiation dose ≤54 Gy had difficulty swallowing solids (40% v 89%; P = 0.011) or had impaired nutrition (10% v 44%; P = 0.025). The study therefore suggests that for IC responders, reduced-dose IMRT with concurrent cetuximab should be considered in favorable-risk patients with HPV-associated OPSCC since de-intensification with radiation dose reduction resulted in significantly improved swallowing and nutritional status [14]. Another biomarker analysis studied the association of HPV with clinical outcomes in recurrent or metastatic (R/M) HNSCC patients treated on two clinical trials: E1395, a phase III trial of cisplatin and paclitaxel versus cisplatin and 5-fluorouracil, and E3301, a phase II trial of irinotecan and docetaxel [15]. HPV DNA was detected by ISH and p16 status was evaluated by IHC. Sixty-four patients were analyzed for HPV ISH and 65 for p16. Eleven tumors (17%) were HPV-positive, 12 (18%) were p16-positive, whereas 52 (80%) were both HPV and p16-negative. There was significantly improved objective response rate (ORR) for HPV-positive versus HPV-negative (55% vs 19%; P = 0.022), and for p16-positive versus p16-negative (50% vs. 19%; P = 0.057) tumors. There was also improved median survival for HPV-positive versus HPV-negative patients (12.9 vs. 6.7 months; P = 0.014), and for p16-positive versus p16-negative patients (11.9 vs. 6.7 months; P = 0.027). After adjusting for other covariates, hazard ratio (HR) for OS was 2.69 (P = 0.048) and 2.17 (P = 0.10), favoring HPV-positive and p16-positive patients, respectively [15]. HPV is therefore a favorable prognostic factor in R/M HNSCC.

The predictive role of HPV status with specific therapy has been less well understood. Epidermal growth factor receptor (EGFR) inhibitors in particular have been studied in this regard. Subset analysis of the SPECTRUM phase III trial of chemotherapy with or without the anti-EGFR antibody panitumumab in R/M HNSCC suggested that p16-negative patients had benefit to addition of the human anti-EGFR antibody, panitumumab, unlike p16-positive patients [11]. However, the significance of the data has been called into question because of the limited cohort of p16-positive patients across subsites and the high rates of p16 positivity outside the oropharynx, as well as by the fact that pantitumumab has not prolonged survival in HNSCC in any trial in any line of therapy.

Biomarker analysis of HPV-association conducted on the similarly designed EXTREME phase III trial of chemotherapy with or without cetuximab showed that the benefits of chemotherapy and cetuximab over chemotherapy alone appeared to be independent of HPV/p16 status. This analysis was however limited by the small number of patients with HPV-positive (5%) and p16-positive (10%) tumors [13]. A secondary analysis of the MCL-9815 (Bonner) phase III trial examined the association of HPV DNA status and p16 expression with outcomes in patients with OPSCC treated with cetuximab plus RT versus RT alone in the definitive setting [13]. Although sample sizes precluded conclusive tests of interaction in this study, the results suggest that regardless of p16 status, patient's outcomes were improved by the addition of cetuximab to RT compared with RT alone. Interestingly, the benefit of cetuximab in the p16-positive population was more pronounced compared to the p16-negative population, with improved locoregional control (LRC) and OS with the addition of cetuximab to RT compared with RT alone in p16-positive (HPV-associated) OPSCC. The HR for LRC and OS for HPV-associated were 0.31 (95% CI; 0.11–0.88) and 0.38 (95% CI; 0.15–0.94) respectively compared to HR of 0.78 (95% CI; 0.49–1.25) and 0.93 (95% CI; 0.59–1.48) in HPV-negative patients [13].

HPV status and p-16 in non-OPSCC

The clinical significance of p16 positivity in non-OPSCC is less clear than for OPSCC, however patients with p16-positive non-OPSCC have better outcomes than patients with p16-negative non-OPSCC, similar to findings in patients with OPSCC. In a retrospective analysis of non-OPSCC tumors from 332 patients enrolled on three RTOG studies, overall p16 expression was positive in 19.3% of the non-OPSCC tumors with the rates of p16 positivity of 14.1%, 24.2% and 19% for RTOG 0129, 0234 and 0522 studies, respectively [16]. In this study, patients with p16-positive non-OPSCC tumors had a better prognosis compared with those who were p16-negative, after adjusting for known prognostic factors including age, sex, T stage and N stage. For PFS, the adjusted HR was 0.63 (95% CI 0.42–0.95, $P = 0.03$), while for OS the adjusted HR was 0.56 (95% CI 0.35–0.89, $P = 0.01$). Comparing OPSCC and non-OPSCC patients from the same studies, p16-positive OPSCC have better survival than patients with p16-positive non-OPSCC (HR for OS of 0.48; 95% CI 0.30–0.78), but patients with p16-negative OPSCC and non-OPSCC have similar survival, even after adjustment of prognostic variables (HR for OS of 0.97; 95% CI 0.74–1.24). A recent study suggested that HNSCC associated with HPV genotypes other than HPV-16 have inferior survival, and that determination of HPV genotypes in HNSCC could provide a more robust risk stratification than p16 IHC findings or HPV-16

detection alone, especially in the era of treatment deintensification for HPV-associated HNSCC [17]. In this study, 551 HNSCC tumors from the cancer genome atlas (TCGA) were analyzed, along with corresponding patient data, looking at 179 distinct HPV genotypes. Seventy-three tumors expressed HPV transcripts, among which 61 (84%) were HPV-16 genotype and twelve (16%) were HPV-other genotypes. The study showed that three-year OS was significantly worse for the non-HPV-16 cohort (49%) compared to the HPV-16 cohort (88%), $P = 0.003$ [17]. However, the significance of the data has been called into question because 41% of HPV-other genotypes were detected outside the oropharynx, the prognostic impact of observed differences in viral gene expression found in the study remains unclear, and the clinically validated biomarker p16 was available only for one-third of HPV-other genotype cases [18]. Further prospective studies of HPV-other genotypes in OPSCC will be required before we can conclude that HPV genotype alone can serve as patient selection factor precluding treatment de-intensification.

Plasma EBV in nasopharyngeal carcinoma

NPC is the predominant tumor type arising in the epithelial lining of the nasopharynx, and differs from other HNSCC in epidemiology, histology, natural history, and response to therapy [19]. The World Health Organization (WHO) classifies NPC into the three histopathologic types, including the keratinizing SCC subtype (WHO type I), the differentiated, non-keratinizing sub-type (WHO type II) and the undifferentiated, non-keratinizing subtype (WHO type III) [20]. The sporadic form of NPC is most commonly the keratinizing subtype (WHO type I) while the endemic form of NPC is commonly the undifferentiated, non-keratinizing subtype (WHO type III). This endemic form is strongly associated with EBV and has a more favorable prognosis than other types [19]. The incidence of NPC demonstrates a marked geographical variation. It is rare in the United States and Western Europe, but endemic in Southern China, while intermediate-risk regions include Southeast Asia, North Africa, the Middle East, and the Arctic [19]. There is a multifactorial etiology, which to an extent explains the geographic variation of incidence. In endemic populations, risk appears to be due to an interaction of several factors including EBV infection, environmental factors such as smoking, and genetic predisposition. Smoking may be involved in the pathogenesis of NPC by causing EBV reactivation [21, 22]. A study in China showed that smoking is associated with increased risk of NPC Chinese patients with 20–40 and 40 or more pack-years vs. never smokers (OR = 1.52, 95% CI = 1.22–1.88 and OR = 1.76, 95% CI = 1.34 to 2.32, respectively; $P < 0.001$) [23]. In vitro analysis showed that exposure of cells to cigarette smoke extract promoted EBV replication, induced the expression of the immediate-early transcriptional activators *Zta* and *Rta*, and increased transcriptional expression of its lytic gene products, *BFRF3* and *gp350* [23]. In the US and Europe, NPC is more commonly associated with alcohol and tobacco usage, which are classic risk factors for other HNSCC [24].

The role of EBV as a primary etiologic agent in the pathogenesis of NPC is well established [25]. EBV DNA and EBV gene expression has been identified in precursor lesions and tumor cells. NPC cells express a specific subgroup of EBV-latent proteins, including EBNA-1 and two integral membrane proteins, LMP-1 and LMP-2, along with the BamHI-A fragment of the EBV genome. Patients with NPC also demonstrate specific immunologic responses to various gene products of EBV, particularly immunoglobulin A (IgA) antibodies directed against the EBV viral capsid antigen [25, 26]. This association of NPC with EBV infection has been harnessed to develop noninvasive diagnostic tests, some of which have been explored as clinical biomarkers. Plasma EBV DNA is currently the most reliable and accurate predictive and prognostic biomarker for NPC and has utility in diagnosis, prognosis, surveillance and assessment of response to therapy. Pre-treatment EBV DNA was a found in 96% of NPC patients in Hong Kong, and high levels of EBV DNA was associated with advanced disease, disease relapse and worse outcome [27, 28]. Elevated post-treatment EBV DNA is a strong negative prognostic factor in prospective trials of RT alone, concurrent chemoradiotherapy or IC followed by RT [29, 30]. A prospective study evaluated the use of serial plasma EBV DNA on the long-term survival of non-metastatic NPC patients treated with IMRT +/− adjunct chemotherapy by time-dependent

receiver operating characteristics (TD-ROC) [31]. Baseline plasma EBV was assessed, then repeated at 8 weeks and 6 months after IMRT, after which survival outcome was analyzed. Results revealed that post-IMRT undetectable plasma EBV DNA accurately predicted almost all survival endpoints and early post-IMRT plasma EBV DNA should be regarded as a new sentinel time point to consider further intensified treatment or not after completion of chemo IMRT. NCT02135042 (NRG-HN001) is an ongoing randomized phase II/III study evaluating individualized treatment for NPC based on biomarker EBV DNA expression [32]. The study is based on two cohorts of patients with a diagnosis of stage II-IVB non-metastatic NPC and detectable pre-treatment plasma EBV DNA. In the persistently detectable plasma EBV DNA cohort (phase II), the primary objective is to determine whether substituting adjuvant CDDP and 5-FU with gemcitabine and paclitaxel will result in superior PFS. In the second cohort, the undetectable plasma EBV DNA cohort (phase III), the primary objective is to determine whether omitting adjuvant CDDP and 5-FU (observation alone in the adjuvant setting) will result in non-inferior OS compared to those patients that receive conventional treatment with adjuvant CDDP and 5-FU chemotherapy.

Emerging/novel biomarkers

The landscape of HNSCC treatment is changing with the emergence of tumor biomarkers, some of which are potential pharmacologic targets. Downstream abnormalities associated with constitutive activation and signaling of the EGFR pathway may be an important therapeutic target in HNSCC especially in HPV-negative tumors (Fig. 1).

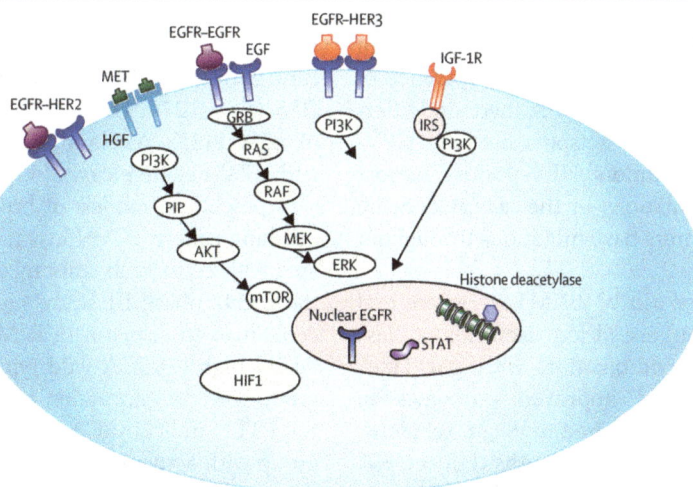

Fig. 1 EGFR and receptor tyrosine kinase signaling in head and neck cancer. Resistance to EGFR inhibition may arise via signaling from redundant tyrosine kinases, such as HER family members, as well as downstream signaling activation. These may be important biomarkers predicting therapeutic response in head and neck cancer

Targeting receptor tyrosine kinases and their signaling pathways

Dysregulation of EGFR signaling has been shown to stimulate tumor cell proliferation, inhibit apoptosis, and promote angiogenesis and metastatic spread; and aberrations of the EGFR pathway are a common feature of HNSCC and are associated with worse prognosis [33]. Based on current genome-wide sequencing data, only a few oncogenes in HNSCC are immediately targetable with drugs in clinical development. These include *EGFR, PIK3CA, FGFR, MET* and *CCND1*.

PI3K/MTOR pathway

Genetic aberrations of the phosphoinositide 3- kinase (PI3K) pathway are common in HNSCC [34]. Phosphatidylinositol-4, 5-biphosphate 3-kinase, catalytic subunit alpha (*PIK3CA*) encodes p110α, a catalytic subunit of PI3K and activated PI3K triggers downstream effects on transcription, protein synthesis, metabolism, proliferation and apoptosis [35]. It was shown in correlative studies from the E2303 trial of cetuximab-based induction and chemo-radiotherapy in locally advanced HNSCC that PI3K/AKT pathway activation is associated with inferior PFS and OS and may predict resistance to EGFR-targeted therapy [36]. Previous data suggested *PIK3CA* mutations in approximately 8% of HNSCC samples [37], but more recent data from TCGA study identified *PIK3CA* mutations in 21% of HNSCC samples, with 73% of the *PIK3CA* mutations localized to hotspots that promote activation [38]. HPV-negative samples were noted to have 18% *PIK3CA* mutations whereas HPV-positive samples harbored 38% *PIK3CA* mutations. Additionally, *PIK3CA* mutations and/or amplifications were observed in 37% of the HNSCC (34% of HPV-negative and 56% of HPV-positive) samples. Approximately 25% of the mutated *PIK3CA* cases displayed concurrent amplification; while additional 20% of tumors displayed focal amplification without evidence of mutation [38]. The data also suggest that there are differences in the *PIK3CA* mutation hotspots between HPV-positive and HPV-negative tumors. HPV-positive tumors were observed to have mutations in the helical domain, whereas HPV-negative tumors have mutations throughout the entire gene [38].

The PI3K inhibitor buparlisib (BKM120) is an oral pan-PI3K inhibitor that targets all four isoforms of class I PI3K. When used in combination with paclitaxel, buparlisib has demonstrated improved outcomes in patients with R/M HNSCC compared to paclitaxel alone, with a median PFS of 4.6 versus 3.5 months (HR = 0.65), a median OS of 10.4 versus 6.5 months (HR = 0.72), as well as improved ORR 39% versus 14% [39]. Data regarding PIK3CA mutational status and PTEN content were not presented, and although it is not presently known whether patient selection will be required for this therapy, it is likely that buparlisib/paclitaxel combination will emerge as a treatment option for R/M HNSCC.

PTEN

A common downstream abnormality associated with activation and signaling in HNSCC is loss of phosphatase and tensin homolog (PTEN) expression. PTEN is a key negative regulator of the PI3K/AKT/mTOR pathway and PTEN loss results in unrestrained signaling of this pathway [35]. There is loss of PTEN expression in about 30% of HNSCC, either via *PTEN* mutation or post-translational modification, [40–42] and this may be associated with worse outcome in HNSCC [41]. In a study on HPV-positive OPSCC, PTEN loss (assessed by FISH) was identified in 7/21 (33%) cases, suggesting PTEN loss may be independent of HPV status [43]. Another study analyzed DNA samples obtained from 252 formalin-fixed paraffin-embedded (FFPE) HNSCC tumor samples using next-generation sequencing-based (NGS) clinical assay [44]. HPV status was determined by presence of the HPV DNA sequence and corroborated with high-risk HPV ISH and p16 IHC staining in a subset of tumors. This study demonstrated *PTEN* genomic alterations (PTEN mutation or loss) in 15% of HPV-positive and 5% of HPV-negative tumors [44]. In another recent study, the expression of PTEN, p53, PIK3CA, Akt and mTOR (all evaluated by IHC) were investigated according to HPV status (evaluated by ISH) in 65 tonsillar SCC tumors. [45] This study demonstrated that total PTEN (nuclear and cytoplasmic) expression was more frequently observed in HPV-positive compared to HPV-negative tonsillar SCC cases (*P* = 0.037), with predominant PTEN distribution in the nucleus. Overall, PTEN expression was lost in 47% of tumors and preserved in 53% of tumors. PTEN was negative in 27% of HPV-positive compared to 57% of HPV-negative tumors. The study also showed a significant correlation between nuclear PTEN expression and DFS (*P* = 0.27). There was no difference in expression of p53, PIK3, Akt and mTOR between HPV-positive and HPV-negative cases [45].

In preclinical models of breast, prostate and non-small cell lung cancer, PTEN loss has been shown to be associated with cetuximab resistance [46]. Biomarker analysis of the E5397 phase III study suggested that the addition of cetuximab to cisplatin in R/M HNSCC improved PFS in PTEN high/PIK3CA wild type patients (representing the group with non-activation of PI3K pathway; *P* = 0.07) but not PTEN null/PIK3CA mutant patients (representing the group with activation of PI3K pathway; *P* = 0.6) [47]. This suggests that there may be cetuximab resistance when the PI3K pathway is activated downstream of EGFR. LUX-Head and Neck 1 studied another active EGFR inhibitor, afatinib, in patients with previously treated R/M HNSCC, demonstrating improved PFS but not significantly improved OS in this population [48]. Biomarker analysis suggests that afatinib utility could be improved with the use of biomarker patient enrichment. PTEN, p16 and HER3 status are evaluated by IHC while EGFR amplification is evaluated by FISH. Overall, the study appeared to show a more pronounced effect on outcome with afatinib vs. MTX in p16- negative, EGFR-amplified, HER3-low and PTEN-high tumors. However, the p16 data were underpowered as the sample size of p16-positive patients was small in this study. In PTEN high tumors, afatinib showed a significantly improved PFS when compared to MTX, with a median PFS of 2.9 vs. 1.4 months (HR of 0.36; 95% CI 0.16–0.81, $P = 0.014$). In HER3 low tumors, afatinib also demonstrated a significantly improved PFS compared to MTX, with a median PFS of 2.9 vs. 2.0 months (HR of 0.47; 95% CI 0.25–0.86, $P = 0.014$) [48, 49].

EGFR over-expression

EGFR over-expression is a negative prognostic factor after radiotherapy but has not been validated as predictive biomarker [50]. The E5397 phase III trial of cisplatin plus placebo versus cisplatin plus cetuximab for first-line treatment of R/M HNSCC suggested it might have a predictive role [47]. In this study, almost all the patients had EGFR over-expression. The RR only improved from 6% to 12% ($P = 0.99$) with addition of cetuximab in patients with very high EGFR expression (IHC 3+ in 80–100% of cells). In contrast, there was a more dramatic improvement in RR, from 12% to 41% ($P = 0.03$), with addition of cetuximab in patients with low to moderate EGFR expression (IHC 3+ in 0–79% of cells). Although, the interaction between EGFR and treatment group was not found to be statistically significant in a logistic regression analysis of response, there appeared to be reduced benefit of cetuximab in patients with very high EGFR expression compared to patients with low to moderate EGFR expression. Based on this study, highest EGFR expression intensity and density appear to define a group, representing about a third of the cohort, with lesser sensitivity to EGFR inhibition.

FGFR

The fibroblast growth factor receptor (FGFR) signaling pathway plays a role in cellular differentiation, proliferation, apoptosis, migration, angiogenesis and wound repair. FGF binding to members of this family of transmembrane tyrosine kinase receptors with four members (FGFR1–4) leads to FGFR dimerization and activation of downstream signaling pathways including MAPK, PI3K/AKT/MTOR, and STAT pathways [51]. Activating mutations, amplification and translocation resulting in fusion genes involving these receptors have been reported in

many cancers, including HNSCC. FGFR1 amplification or mutation is seen in 10% of HPV-negative HNSCC, while FGFR3 mutations or fusions occur in 11% of HPV-positive HNSCC [38]. FGFR inhibition has been extensively studied in HNSCC and targeting FGFRs is a promising therapeutic strategy in HNSCC. The FGFR inhibitor PD173074 was shown to reduce cell proliferation and increase cell apoptosis in HNSCC in vitro and in vivo [52]. Selective FGFR inhibitors are being evaluated in several cancers harboring FGFR amplification and mutation. BGJ398 is a pan FGFR kinase inhibitor that has been tested in a phase I dose escalation study in patients with advanced solid malignancies harboring either FGFR1 or FGFR2 amplification or FGFR3 mutations (NCT01004224) [53]. An ongoing JNJ-42756493 phase I study includes efforts to optimize dose and schedule and to analyze biomarkers. Expansion cohorts are currently enrolling patients with FGFR-aberrant tumors, including HNSCC (NCT01703481) [54].

Cyclin D1

Cyclin D1 is encoded by CCND1 and is a cell-cycle protein that regulates the key G1-to-S phase transition through formation of complexes with CDKs, such as CDK 4 and 6. The cyclin D1-CDK4/6 complex phosphorylates Rb on tyrosine residue 356 (phospho-^{T356}), inactivating Rb and releasing the inhibition of cell cycle progression by Rb [55]. Alterations in cyclin D-CDK4/6-Rb pathway such as CCND1 amplification can lead to uncontrolled tumor cell proliferation via sustained activation of CDK 4/6 and inactivation of Rb [55, 56]. In a recent TCGA study, 28% of HNSCC had CCND1 amplification, with 77/243 (32%) in HPV-negative and 2/36 (6%) in HPV-positive samples [57]. Over-expression of cyclin D1 and amplification of CCND1 in HNSCC are associated with poor prognosis and resistance to cisplatin and EGFR inhibition [58, 59]. Targeting of cyclin D1 is not currently feasible, though inhibition of its binding partners CDK4 and/or CDK6, might have a future role in patients with CCND1 amplification. EGFR activity has been shown to regulate cell-cycle progression via ERK1/2-dependent induction of cyclin D1 [55]. A recent study investigated EGFR and HER2 expression in the context of Rb, phospho-^{T356} Rb, cyclin D1, and CDK6 in in 99 HPV-negative HNSCC patient samples and correlated this with clinical data [60]. The study demonstrated that Rb inactivation, reflected by phosphorylation of Rb, inversely correlated with expression of EGFR in HNSCC samples. Stratification of high EGFR expressors by expression levels of cyclin D1, CDK6, or the cyclin D1/CDK6-regulatory protein p16 (CDKN2A) identified groups with significant survival differences, consistent with prior studies that demonstrated improved survival in HNSCC with low levels of cyclin D1 and in those with low phosho-^{T356} Rb [61, 62]. In this study, simultaneous inhibition of Rb phosphorylation with the CDK4/6 inhibitor, palbociclib, and of EGFR activity with dual tyrosine kinase inhibitors (TKI), lapatinib or afatinib, was also performed [60]. These drug combinations showed synergistic inhibitory effects on the proliferation of HNSCC cells, suggesting that combinations of CDK and EGFR inhibitors may be particularly useful in EGFR and phosphorylated Rb-expressing or cyclin D1/CDK6-overexpressing HPV-negative HNSCC. Combined consideration of phosho-^{T356} Rb status and EGFR expression may therefore be useful as predictive biomarkers in this context and should be explored further as predictive biomarkers to select patients for therapy with EGFR/HER2 and/or CDK inhibitors.

C-MET

Hepatocyte growth factor receptor (HGFR) or c-MET is encoded by the *MET* gene and it is a RTC associated with enhanced migration, invasion and angiogenesis when overexpressed in cancer. Although considerable evidence implicates the MET-HGF axis as a therapeutic target in HNSCC [63], appropriate assays to detect aberrations in MET and its ligand HGF are lacking and further investigation is warranted.

Immune checkpoint related biomarkers

PD-L1, PD-L2 and IFN-gamma are potential immune biomarkers shown to correlate with response to immunotherapy in R/M HNSCC [64]. Pembrolizumab has shown promising efficacy in R/M HNSCC in the phase I KEYNOTE-012 study. In this study, analysis of PD-L1 showed an increase in ORR between PD-L1 positive versus PD-L1 negative tumors ($P = 0.23$) when both tumor and stromal cells were used to score PD-L1 [65]. Assessing RNA expression of IFN-gamma related genes using a six-gene signature (*CXCL9*, *CXCL10*, *IDO1*, *IFNG*, *HLA-DRA* and *STAT1*) identified in a melanoma cohort in the KEYNOTE-001 study [66], showed that all six IFN-gamma related genes had significantly higher mean expression values in pembrolizumab-responders compared to non-responders [65]. Exploratory analyses suggest that PD-L2 and IFN-gamma signature may be associated with clinical response in pembrolizumab and may offer additional strategies to improve prediction of response. In the recent Phase III CheckMate-141 study, nivolumab, an anti-PD-1 monoclonal antibody, was shown to improve OS in patients with platinum-refractory R/M HNSCC compared to single agent therapy of the investigator's choice, consisting of MTX, docetaxel or cetuximab [64]. Patients with PD-L1 expression >1% had significantly longer median OS (8.7 months vs. 4.6 months, HR: 0.55, 95% CI: 0.36–0.83) with nivolumab than with investigator's choice.

Tumor suppressor abnormalities
TP53

TP53 is the most commonly mutated gene in HNSCC and is present in about 50–80% of HNSCC [67, 68]. Disruptive *TP53* mutation in tumor DNA has been shown to correlate with worse prognosis after surgical treatment of HNSCC [68]. The p53 protein is a transcription factor and tumor suppressor protein encoded by *TP53*. Loss of p53 function occurs in more than 90% of HNSCC through loss of heterozygosity, interaction with HPV viral oncoprotein E6 or increased expression of MDM2 (seen in about 5% of HNSCC and promotes rapid degradation of p53 protein) [37, 69]. An inverse relationship between the presence of a *TP53* mutation and the presence of HPV DNA in OPSCC may be due to the contribution of high-risk HPV infection, in which p53 is rapidly degraded after interacting with E6 [68, 70, 71]. Inhibition of WEE1, a G2-M cell-cycle regulator, can render synthetic lethality in *TP53*-mutant tumors because cells without functional p53 lack an effective G1 checkpoint and rely heavily on the G2 checkpoint regulators, such as WEE1, resulting in increased sensitivity of *TP53*-mutant cells to WEE1 inhibitors. Thus, *TP53* mutations need to be further investigated as a predictive biomarkers and therapeutic target in HNSCC [72].

Notch

The Notch pathway consists of four receptors, Notch 1–4. Activation of the Notch pathway leads to different effects in different cell types. *NOTCH-1* is believed to play a role in regulating normal cell differentiation and has dual functions with both oncogenic and tumor suppressor activity. In epithelial tissue, including HNSCC, *NOTCH-1* appears to act as a tumor suppressor gene [37, 73]. Two independent whole exome sequencing studies report *NOTCH1* mutations in about 14% and 15% of HNSCC respectively [37, 74], and these studies hypothesize that *NOTCH1* functions as a tumor suppressor in HNSCC based on its mutational characteristics. Evidence also suggest that the majority of the mutations identified in exome sequencing are likely inactivating or loss of function mutations that affect the EGF-like ligand binding domain or the *NOTCH* intracellular domain [37, 73]. In one of the studies that examined 32 patients with mostly pre-treated HNSCC tumors, *NOTCH1* was the second most frequently mutated gene found, next to *TP53*, with alterations present in 15% of patients [74]. In this study, 28 *NOTCH1* mutations were identified and nearly 40% of these *NOTCH1* mutations were predicted to truncate the gene product, again suggesting that *NOTCH1* may function as a tumor suppressor gene rather than an oncogene in this tumor type. Other reports also suggest that a subset of HNSCC may have activating *NOTCH1* mutations [75], with overexpression of downstream Notch effectors noted in 32% of HNSCC evaluated for DNA-copy number, methylation and gene expression of the 47 Notch signaling pathway genes. This indicates that the Notch1 pathway could be a potential therapeutic target in a subset of HNSCC. Therapeutic targeting of *NOTCH-1* in HNSCC remains an evolving field.

Tumor hypoxia as predictive biomarker in HNSCC

A hypoxic microenvironment is a common feature in HNSCC, and contributes to the development of tumor aggression and metastasis, playing a key role in radio-resistance, chemo-resistance, and poor prognosis. Acute hypoxic stress leads to the development of an aggressive cancer phenotype with high metastatic rate, resistance to therapeutic agents, and higher tumor recurrence rates [76]. This is mostly mediated by hypoxia inducible factor-1- alpha (HIF-1α), which is over-expressed in HNSCC, and plays a central role in hypoxia-induced therapeutic resistance in HNSCC through its role in initiating angiogenesis and regulating cellular metabolism to overcome hypoxia [77]. Therefore, HIF-1α and its downstream proteins are potential predictive biomarkers and therapeutic targets in HNSCC. Strategies to overcome hypoxia-induced therapeutic resistance include the use of hypoxic cell cytotoxins like tirapazamine (TPZ), enhancing oxygen delivery using hyperbaric oxygen, and use of hypoxic cell radiosensitizers. TPZ is reduced to a reactive radical when exposed to hypoxic conditions, leading to single- and double-strand DNA breaks. In contrast, this reactive radical is oxidized to the inert parent compound in normal oxygen tension. A prospective trial [78] evaluated the combination of TPZ with cisplatin and radiation in advanced HNSCC using ^{18}F fluoromisonidazole PET imaging as a biomarker to measure hypoxia levels. The study demonstrated that hypoxia levels decreased with treatment and showed that combination of TPZ with cisplatin and radiotherapy led to durable clinical responses with three-year EFS of 69%, a three-year local PFS of 88%, and a three-year OS of 69%. In another phase II trial, it was demonstrated that patients treated with TPZ, cisplatin and radiation had higher three-year EFS and three-year locoregional PFS than patients treated with cisplatin, fluorouracil and radiation, with less radiation-induced toxicities [79]. A prospective study assessed the efficacy of misonidazole, a hypoxic cell radiosensitizer, in 626 patients with pharynx and larynx carcinoma and showed that patients with pharyngeal carcinoma treated with misonidazole exhibited a significantly better control disease rate than patients treated with placebo [80]. However, the clinical use of misonidazole is limited because it caused significant peripheral neuropathy in 26% of the patients. Another phase III clinical study assessed the efficacy and tolerance of nimorazole in combination with primary radiotherapy in 422 patients with pharynx and supraglottic larynx carcinoma, and showed that patients treated with nimorazole displayed a better locoregional control and OS than patients that received placebo [81]. These findings suggest that hypoxia biomarkers have the potential to predict response to hypoxic-cell radiosensitizers or cytotoxins. Although attempts to target tissue hypoxia, including TPZ, have not been successful in large phase III trials, patient selection via biomarkers of hypoxia was not employed in these trials and would merit further exploration.

Tumor hypoxia and interleukin-8 (IL-8)

Attempts have been made to identify molecular predictors for hypoxia-targeted therapy. IL-8 has been shown to be an independent prognostic factor in HNSCC patients irrespective of treatment. A randomized study investigated the prognostic and predictive significance of IL-8 and hepatocyte growth factor (HGF or scatter factor), a hypoxia- induced secretory protein that binds c-MET and regulates IL-8 expression, on the efficacy of TPZ [82]. Four hundred and ninety-eight patients with Stage III–IV HNSCC were randomized to receive radiotherapy with cisplatin (control arm) or cisplatin plus TPZ (treatment arm). Eligibility criteria included plasma sample availability for HGF, IL-8 assay by ELISA and no major radiation deviations. Analyses included adjustment for major prognostic factors. p16 staining was performed on available tumors. Findings suggest that IL-8 is an independent prognostic factor irrespective of treatment and that there is an interaction between treatment arm and HGF level. Elevated IL-8 level was associated with worse OS irrespective of treatment. Elevated HGF was associated with significantly worse OS in the control but not in the TPZ/CIS arm ($P = 0.053$). Similar trends were observed in analyses restricted to p16-negative patients. Four subgroups defined by high and low HGF/IL-8 levels were examined for TPZ effect and TPZ/CIS appeared to be beneficial for patients with high HGF and IL-8, but adverse for low HGF and high IL-8. This highlights the complexity of hypoxia targeting in unselected patients.

Futuristic biomarkers

With advancements in digital genomic technologies, such as digital PCR and BEAMing, reliable detection of circulating DNA from clinical specimens has become feasible, and is a potential future predictive biomarker in HNSCC therapy.

Liquid biopsies

Evaluation of DNA aberrations in blood samples can be quite beneficial as it can be a challenge to obtain tumor DNA in clinical settings. Highly sensitive and specific assays are required to detect mutant DNA fragments in the blood. With advancements in digital genomic technologies, such as digital PCR, tagged-amplicon deep sequencing, pyrophosphorolysis-activated polymerization, and BEAMing, reliable detection of circulating DNA from clinical specimens has become feasible [83]. DNA from blood can be obtained by two methods, either as circulating tumor DNA (ctDNA) or from circulating tumor cells (CTC).

A recent study used digital PCR–based technologies to evaluate the ability of ctDNA to detect tumors in 640 patients with various localized and metastatic cancer types, including HNSCC [84]. ctDNA was detectable in more than 75% of patients with advanced HNSCC, and was often present in patients without detectable circulating tumor cells, suggesting that these two biomarkers are distinct entities. Using liquid biopsies, it has been shown that RAS mutations may account for acquired resistance to EGFR-targeting in a substantial proportion of HNSCC patients, even though these tumors are rarely mutated at baseline. A recent study analyzed the activating RAS mutations in tumor tissue of cetuximab-naive HNSCC patients by NGS and compared this with liquid biopsies taken during and after cetuximab/platinum/5-fluorouracil treatment [85]. Baseline data showed that tumors of cetuximab-naive patients were mostly unmutated, except for HRAS mutations in 4.3% of patients. Liquid biopsies revealed acquired KRAS, NRAS or HRAS mutations in more than one-third of patients after cetuximab exposure. Almost half of patients with on-treatment disease progression showed acquired RAS mutations, while no RAS mutations were found in the non-progressive subset of patients, indicating that acquisition of RAS mutant clones correlated significantly with clinical resistance to EGFR-inhibition. These novel assays can be applied in the early detection of cancer, surveillance after treatment, early identification of resistance to targeted agents, and to explore mechanisms of resistance without invasive tissue sampling.

Genomic profiling

Rapid tumor profiling with sequencing of panels of several hundred cancer relevant genes is now commercially available for use in clinical practice. The relevance of this approach to management of HNSCC has not been demonstrated, given the predominance of mutations in tumor suppressor genes. A recent study compared the genomic profile of the HNSCC tumors obtained through routine clinical practice with sequencing data from frozen tumors in TCGA and University of Chicago public datasets studied in research setting [44], and the findings suggest that the selected gene analysis using FFPE tumors obtained through clinical practice yield comparable assessment of genomic alterations to frozen tumors, demonstrating the feasibility of comprehensive genomic

profiling in a clinical setting. However, the clinical significance of these genomic alterations requires further investigation through application of these genomic profiles as integral biomarkers in clinical trials.

MicroRNAs

MicroRNAs (miRNA) are a family of small, non-coding, endogenously synthesized, single-strand RNAs which are responsible for post-transcriptional regulation of mRNA expression, and have been shown to play an important role in cellular differentiation, proliferation, apoptosis, and carcinogenesis [86]. MiRNAs can be accurately measured in plasma and are potential non-invasive biomarkers for early detection of HNSCC. They are also one of the promising candidates for development of development of novel and therapeutic approaches in HNSCC. However, studies evaluating the diagnostic accuracy of miRNAs in HNSCC detection have been conflicting and inconclusive and miRNAs have not been proven to play a definite role in prognosis or predicting response to therapy in HNSCC [87].

HNSCC biomarkers and racial disparities

There appear to be racial disparities, not only in the incidence and outcome of HNSCC, but also in the role of biomarkers in HNSCC. Many biomarker studies in HNSCC involve mostly Caucasian populations and it remains unclear if these biomarkers are applicable to non-Caucasian populations. No biomarker till date has been specifically validated in African American or other minority populations in the United States. Many prior studies suggest higher rates of HPV- associated OPSCC among Caucasians than AA [88, 89] but that may in part be due to the fact that majority of studies on HPV-associated OPSCC have been reported in Caucasian patients, with paucity of data in African American (AA) cohorts. A recent study examined the prevalence and outcomes of HPV-associated OPSCC in an AA cohort and demonstrated that HPV OPSCC is strongly present in this AA cohort. Interestingly, the study also identified an unexpectedly frequent molecular subtype in this AA cohort, HPV-positive/p16-negative tumors, with demonstrated worse outcomes than HPV-positive/p16-positive OPSCC [90]. Therefore, given these disparities, larger studies evaluating specific biomarkers in HNSCC are warranted in non-Caucasian populations.

Conclusion

In this era of individualized medicine and biomarker-driven cancer therapy, it is important to explore robust biomarker data and incorporate them in patient selection for HNSCC therapy. We have well established prognostic biomarkers in clinical practice; however, we need to direct efforts towards development and implementation of predictive biomarkers that will aid patient selection for specific HNSCC therapies. The current standard therapies for HNSCC are either too toxic or have low response rates, and are thus not beneficial to all patients. The emphasis should be to improve patient survival and reduce treatment-related toxicity through the identification predictive biomarkers, in addition to development of specific therapies targeting these biomarkers. In patients with poor prognosis, we need to develop strategies to prevent and control recurrence and distant metastasis. A variety of predictive biomarkers have been discovered and are already utilized in clinical practice, while many more are being explored as therapeutic targets. Moving forward, it will be necessary for clinicians to educate themselves in order to understand basic technologies used in biomarker studies. Each biomarker needs to be critically assessed and standardized prior to application to patient care. Currently, there is no validated biomarker for minority populations in current clinical practice. Biomarkers that specifically target non- white populations should also be an area of future research as these groups of patients may be under-represented in large research studies. Unfortunately, although the technology and science are available, the clinical research, health-care policy and insurance policy are lagging behind, limiting the implementation of these emerging biomarkers. Nevertheless, we are optimistic that the goal of delivering individualized cancer therapy for patients with HNSCC is within our reach.

Abbreviations
cCR: Complete clinical response; CDK: Cyclin dependent kinase; CTC: Circulating tumor cells; ctDNA: Circulating tumor DNA; DNA: Deoxyribonucleic acid; EBV: Epstein Barr virus; EGFR: Epidermal growth factor receptor; FFPE: Formalin-fixed paraffin-embedded; FGFR: Fibroblast growth factor receptor; HGFR: Hepatocyte growth factor receptor (HGFR); HIF-1α: Hypoxia inducible factor-1- alpha; HNSCC: Head and neck squamous cell cancer; HPV: Human papilloma virus; HR: Hazard ratio; IC: Induction chemotherapy; Ig: Immunoglobulin; IHC: Immunohistochemistry; IMRT: Intensity modulated radiation therapy; LRC: Locoregional control; NCI: National Cancer Institute; NGS: Next-generation sequencing-based; NPC: Nasopharyngeal cancer; OPSCC: Oropharyngeal squamous cell cancer; OS: Overall survival; PFS: Progression free survival; PI3K: Phosphoinositide 3- kinase; PIK3CA: Phosphatidylinositol-4, 5-biphosphate 3-kinase, catalytic subunit alpha; PTEN: Phosphatase and tensin homolog; R/M: Recurrent/metastatic; Rb: Retinoblastoma; RR: Response rate; TD-ROC: Time-dependent receiver operator characteristics; TKI: Tyrosine kinase inhibitors; TPZ: Tiparazamine; WHO: World Health Organization

Acknowledgements
Not applicable.

Funding
Not applicable.

Authors' contributions
NE drafted the manuscript, YL contributed to the manuscript; BB conceived the article and supervised the writing of the manuscript. All authors read and approved the final manuscript.

Competing interests
The authors declare that they have no competing interests.

Author details
[1]Section of Medical Oncology, Department of Internal Medicine, Yale University School of Medicine and Yale Cancer Center, 333 Cedar Street, Room WWW-221, P.O. Box 208028, New Haven, CT 06520, USA. [2]Department of Pathology, Yale University School of Medicine, New Haven, CT, USA. [3]Section of Medical Oncology, Department of Internal Medicine, Yale University School of Medicine and Yale Cancer Center, New Haven, CT, USA.

References
1. Siegel RL, et al. Cancer statistics, 2016. CA Cancer J Clin. 2016;66(1):7–30.
2. Trotti A. Toxicity in head and neck cancer: a review of trends and issues. Int. J. Rad Oncol Biol Phys. 2000;47(1):1–12.
3. Garden A, Harris J, Trotti A, et al. Long-term results of concomitant boost radiation plus concurrent cisplatin for advanced head and neck carcinomas: a phase II trial of the radiation therapy oncology group (RTOG 99-14). Int J Rad Oncol Biol Phys. 2008;71(5):1351–5.
4. Forastiere A, et al. Long-term results of RTOG 91-11: a comparison of three nonsurgical treatment strategies to preserve the larynx in patients with locally advanced larynx cancer. J Clin Oncol. 2013;31:845–52.
5. National Cancer Institute. NCI dictionary of cancer terms. 2005. https://www.cancer.gov/publications/dictionaries/cancer-terms.
6. Ang KK, et al. Human papillomavirus and survival of patients with oropharyngeal cancer. N Engl J Med. 2010;363:24–35.
7. Ragin CC, Taioli E. Survival of squamous cell carcinoma of the head and neck in relation to human papillomavirus infection: review and meta-analysis. Int J Cancer. 2007;121:1813–20.
8. Fakhry C, et al. Improved survival of patients with HPV- positive HNSCC in a prospective trial. J Natl Cancer Inst. 2008;100:261–9.
9. Gillison ML, et al. Tobacco smoking and increased risk of death and progression for patients with p16-positive and p16-negative oropharyngeal cancer. J Clin Oncol. 2012;30(17):2102–11.
10. Vokes EE, et al. HPV-associated head and neck cancer. J Natl Cancer Inst. 2015;107:djv344.
11. Vermorken JB, et al. Cisplatin and fluorouracil with or without panitumumab in patients with recurrent or metastatic squamous cell carcinoma of the head and neck (SPECTRUM): an open –label phase 3 randomized trial. Lancet Oncol. 2013;14:697–710.
12. Vermoken JB, et al. Impact of tumor HPV status on outcome in patients with recurrent and/or metastatic squamous cell carcinoma of the head and neck receiving chemotherapy with or without cetuximab: retrospective analysis of the phase III EXTREME trial. Ann Oncol. 2014;25:801–7.
13. Rosenthal D, et al. Association of human papillomavirus and p16 status with outcomes in the IMCL-9815 phase III registration trial for patients with locoregionally advanced oropharyngeal squamous cell carcinoma of the head and neck treated with radiotherapy with or without cetuximab. J Clin Oncol. 2016;34(12):1300–8.
14. Marur S, et al. E1308: phase II trial of induction chemotherapy followed by reduced-dose radiation and weekly Cetuximab in patients with HPV-associated resectable squamous cell carcinoma of the oropharynx- ECOG-ACRIN cancer research group. J Clin Oncol. 2016;35(5):490–7. doi: 10.1200/JCO.2016.68.3300.
15. Argiris A, et al. Prognostic significance of human papillomavirus in recurrent or metastatic head and neck cancer: an analysis of eastern cooperative oncology group trials. Ann Oncol. 2014;25(7):1410–6. doi:10.1093/annonc/mdu167. Epub 2014 May 5

16. Chung CH, et al. p16 expression and human papillomavirus status as prognostic biomarkers of non-oropharyngeal head and neck squamous cell carcinoma. J Clin Oncol. 2014;32:3930.

17. Bratman SV, et al. Human papillomavirus genotypes association with survival in head and neck Squamous cell carcinoma. JAMA Oncol. 2016;2(6):823–6. doi:10.1001/jamaoncol.2015.6587.

18. Psyrri A, et al. Human papillomavirus genotypes conferring poor prognosis in head and neck squamous cell carcinoma. JAMA Oncol. 2017;3(1):125. doi:10.1001/jamaoncol.2016.3409.

19. Chang ET, Adami HO. The enigmatic epidemiology of nasopharyngeal carcinoma. Cancer Epidemiol Biomark Prev. 2006;15:1765.

20. Barnes L, et al. Pathology and genetics of head and neck tumors. In: World Health Organization classification of tumors. Lyon: IARC Press; 2005.

21. Chua M, et al. Nasopharyngeal carcinoma. Lancet. 2016;387:1012.

22. Hsu WL, et al. Independent effect of EBV and cigarette smoking on nasopharyngeal carcinoma: a 20-year follow-up study on 9,622 males without family history in Taiwan. Cancer Epidemiol Biomark Prev. 2009;18:1218.

23. Xu FH, et al. An epidemiological and molecular study of the relationship between smoking, risk of nasopharyngeal carcinoma and Epstein-Barr virus activation. J Natl Cancer Inst. 2012;104:1396.

24. Vaughan TL, et al. Nasopharyngeal cancer in low-risk population: defining risk factors by histological type. Cancer Epidemiol Biomark Prev. 1996;5:587.

25. Raghupathy R et al. Epstein-Barr virus as a paradigm in nasopharyngeal cancer: from lab to clinic. Am Soc Clin Oncol Educ Book. 2014;149-53. doi:10.14694/EdBook_AM.2014.34.149.

26. Raab-Traub N. Novel mechanisms of EBV-induced oncogenesis. Curr Opin Virol. 2012;2:453–8.

27. Lo YM, et al. Quantitative analysis of cell-free Epstein-Barr virus DNA in plasma of patients with nasopharyngeal carcinoma. Cancer Res. 1999;59:1188.

28. Lo YM, et al. Molecular prognostication of nasopharyngeal carcinoma by quantitative analysis of circulating Epstein-Barr virus DNA. Cancer Res. 2000;60:6878–81.

29. Lin JC, et al. Quantification of plasma Epstein-Barr virus DNA in patients with advanced nasopharyngeal carcinoma. N Engl J Med. 2004;350:2461–70.

30. Chan, A.T et al. Phase II study of neoadjuvant carboplatin and paclitaxel followed by radiotherapy and concurrent cisplatin in patients with locoregionally advanced nasopharyngeal carcinoma: therapeutic monitoring with plasma Epstein-Barr virus DNA. J Clin Oncol. 2004;22(15):3053–60.

31. Lee et al, ASCO Annual meeting. Serial early post-IMRT undetectable plasma EBV DNA to predict outcomes in non-metastatic nasopharyngeal cancer. J Clin Oncol. 33, 2015 (suppl; abstr 6007).

32. Lee N, NRG-HN001: Randomized Phase II and Phase III Studies of Individualized Treatment for Nasopharyngeal Carcinoma Based on Biomarker Epstein Barr Virus (EBV) Deoxyribonucleic Acid (DNA). https://www.rtog.org/ClinicalTrials/ProtocolTable/StudyDetails.aspx?study=1305.

33. Jorissen RN, et al. Epidermal growth factor receptor: mechanisms of activation and signaling. Exp Cell Res. 2003;284:31–53.

34. Seiwert TY et al. Genomic profiling of a clinically annotated cohort of locoregionally advanced head and neck cancers treated with definitive chemoradiotherapy. J Clin Oncol. 2012; 30 (suppl: abstr 5517).

35. Engelman JA. Targeting PI3K signaling in cancer: opportunities, challenges and limitations. Nat Rev Cancer. 2009;9:550–62.

36. Psyrri A, et al. Prognostic biomarkers in phase II trial of cetuxiamb containing induction and chemoradiation in respectable HNSCC: eastern cooperative oncology group E2303. Clin Ca Res. 2014;20(11):3023–32.

37. Stansky N, et al. The mutational landscape of head and neck squamous cell carcinoma. Science. 2011;333:1157–60.

38. Network CGA. Comprehensive genomic characterization of head and neck squamous cell carcinomas. Nature. 2015;517(7536):576–82.

39. Soulieres D et al. ASCO Annual Meeting. BERIL-1: A phase II, placebo-controlled study of buparlisib (BKM120) plus paclitaxel in patients with platinum-pretreated recurrent/metastatic HNSCC. J Clin Oncol. 34, 2016: (suppl; abstr 6008).

40. Squarize CH, et al. PTEN deficiency contributes to the development and progression of head and neck cancer. Neoplasia. 2013;15(5):461–71.

41. Lee JI, et al. Loss of PTEN expression as a prognostic marker for tongue cancer. Arch Otolaryngol Head Neck Surg. 2001;127(12):1441–5. doi:10.1001/archotol.127.12.1441.

42. Shao X, et al. Mutational analysis of the PTEN gene in head and neck squamous cell carcinoma. Int J Cancer. 1998;77(5):684–8.

43. Chiosea SI, et al. PIK3CA, HRAS and PTEN in human papillomavirus positive oropharyngeal squamous cell carcinoma. BMC Cancer. 2013;13:602. doi:10.1186/1471-2407-13-602.

44. Chung CH, et al. Genomic alterations in head and neck squamous cell carcinoma determined by cancer gene-targeted sequencing. Ann Oncol. 2015;26(6):1216–23. doi:10.1093/annonc/mdv109.

45. Chun SH, et al. Divergence of P53, PTEN, AKT and mTOR expression in tonsillar cancer. Head Neck. 2014;37(5):636–43. doi:10.1002/hed.23643.

46. Holsinger PC, et al. Biomarker- directed therapy of squamous carcinomas of the head and neck: targeting PI3K/PTEN/mTOR pathway. J Clin Oncol. 2013;31(9):e137–40.

47. Burtness B, et al. A phase III randomized trial of cisplatin plus placebo compared with cisplatin plus cetuximab in metastatic/recurrent head and neck cancer: an eastern cooperative oncology group study. J Clin Oncol. 2005;23(34):8646–54.

48. Cohen E, et al. Tumor biomarker association with clinical outcomes in recurrent and/or metastatic head and neck squamous cell carcinoma patients treated with afatinib versus methotrexate: LUX-Head & Neck 1. Int J Rad Oncol. 2016;94(4):868–9.

49. Machiels JH, et al. Afatinib versus methotrexate as second-line treatment in patients with recurrent or metastatic squamous-cell carcinoma of the head and neck progressing on or after platinum-based therapy (LUX-Head & Neck 1): an open-label, randomized phase 3 trial. Lancet Oncol. 2015;16(5):583–94.

50. Ang KK, et al. Impact of epidermal growth factor receptor expression and pattern of relapse in patients with advanced head and neck carcinoma. Cancer Res. 2002;62:7350–6.

51. Turner N, Grose R. Fibroblast growth factor signaling: from development to cancer. Nat Rev Cancer. 2010;10:116–29.

52. Sweeny L, et al. Inhibition of fibroblasts reduced head and neck cancer growth by targeting fibroblast growth factor receptor. Laryngoscope. 2012;122(7):1539–44. doi:10.1002/lary.23266.

53. NCT01004224: A dose escalation study in adult patients with advanced solid malignancies. US National Library of Medicine. ClinicalTrials.gov [online]. https://clinicaltrials.gov/ct2/show/NCT01703481?term=NCT01703481&rank=1.

54. Tabernero J, et al. Phase 1 Dose-escalation study of JNJ-42756493, an oral pan-fibroblast growth factor receptor inhibitor, in patients with advanced solid tumors. J Clin Oncol. 2015;33(30)3401-8. doi:10.1200/JCO.2014.60.7341.

55. Ewen M, Lamb J. The activities of cyclin D1 that drives tumorigenesis. Trends Mol Med. 2004;10:158–62.

56. Choi YJ, Anders L. Signaling through cyclin D-dependent kinases. Oncogene. 2014;33:1890–903.

57. Memorial Sloan Kettering Cancer Center. cBioPortal for Cancer Genomics [online]. 2014; http://www.cbioportal.org/.

58. Hayes DN, et al. The cancer genome atlas: integrated analysis of genome alterations in squamous cell carcinoma of the head and neck. J Clin Oncol. 2013;31:609. doi:10.1200/jco.2013.31.15_suppl.6009.

59. Kalish LH, et al. Degulated cyclin d1 expression is associated with decreased efficacy of the selective EGFR TKI gefetinib in HNSCC cell lines. Clin Cancer Res. 2004;10:7764–74.

60. Beck TN, et al. EGFR and RB1 as dual biomarkers in HPV-negative head and neck cancer. Mol Cancer Ther. 2016;15(10):2486-97. doi:10.1158/1535-7163.MCT-16-0243.

61. Beck TN, et al. Phospho-T356RB1 predicts survival in HPV-negative squamous cell carcinoma of the head and neck. Oncotarget. 2015;6:18863–74.

62. Akervall J, et al. Cyclin D1 overexpression versus response to induction chemotherapy in squamous cell carcinoma of the head and neck- preliminary report. Acta Oncol. 2011;40:505–11.

63. Seiwert T, et al. The MET receptor tyrosine kinase is a potential novel therapeutic agent for head and neck squamous cell carcinoma. Cancer Res. 2009;69:3021–31.

64. Chow L, et al. 2016 ASCO Annual meeting. Biomarkers and response to pembrolizumab in recurrent/metastatic head and neck squamous cell carcinoma. J Clin Oncol. 34, 2016 (suppl; abstr 6010).

65. Seiwert TY, et al. Safety and clinical activity of pembrolizumab for treatment of recurrent or metastatic squamous cell carcinoma of the head and neck (KEYNOTE-012): an open-label, multicentre, phase 1b trial. The Lancet Oncol. 2016;17(7):956–65.

66. Ribas A, et al. Association of response to programmed death receptor 1 (PD-1) blockade with pembrolizumab (MK-3475) with an interferon-inflammatory

immune gene signature. J Clin Oncol. 2015;33(15):3001. doi:10.1200/jco.2015.
33.15_suppl.3001.

67. Vousden KH, Lane DP. P53 in health and disease. Nat Rev Mol Cell Biol.
2007;8:275–83.

68. Poeta ML, et al. TP53 mutations and survival in squamous cell carcinoma of
the head and neck. N Engl J Med. 2007;357:2552–61.

69. Haupt Y, et al. Mdm2 promotes the rapid degradation of p53. Nature. 1997;
387:296–9.

70. Gillison ML, et al. Evidence for a causal association between human
papillomavirus and a subset of head and neck cancers. J Natl Cancer Inst.
2000;92(9):709–20.

71. Scheffner M, et al. The HPV-16 E6 and E6-AP complex functions as an
ubiquitin-protein ligase in the ubiquitination of p53. Cell. 1993;73(3):495–505.

72. Moser R, et al. Functional kinomics identifies candidate therapeutic targets
in HNSCC. Clin Cancer Res. 2014;20:4274–88.

73. Sathyan KM, et al. H-Ras mutation modulates the expression of major cell
cycle regulatory proteins and disease prognosis in oral carcinoma. Mod
Pathol. 2007;20:1141.

74. Agrawal N, et al. Exome sequencing of head and neck squamous cell
carcinoma reveals inactivating mutations in NOTCH1. Science. 2011;
333(6046):1154–7. doi:10.1126/science.1206923.

75. Sun W, et al. Activation of the NOTCH pathway in head and neck cancer.
Cancer Res. 2014;74:1091–104.

76. Nordsmark M, et al. Prognostic value of tumor oxygenation in 397 head and
neck tumors after primary radiation therapy. Radiother Oncol. 2005;77:18–24.

77. Semenza GL. HIF-1 and human disease: one highly involved factor. Genes
Dev. 2000;14:1983–91.

78. Rischin D, et al. Phase I trial of concurrent tirapazamine, cisplatin, and
radiotherapy in patients with advanced head and neck cancer. J Clin Oncol.
2001;19(2):535–42.

79. Rischin D, et al. Tirapazamine, cisplatin, and radiation versus fluorouracil,
cisplatin, and radiation in patients with locally advanced head and neck
cancer: a randomized phase II trial of the trans-Tasman radiation oncology
group (TROG 98.02). J Clin Oncol. 2005;23(1):79–87.

80. Overgaard J, et al. Misonidazole combined with split-course radiotherapy in
the treatment of invasive carcinoma of larynx and pharynx: report from the
DAHANCA 2 study. Int J Radiation Oncol Bio Phys. 1989;16(4):1065–8.

81. Overgaard J, et al. A randomized double blind phase III study of nimorazole
as a hypoxic radiosensitizer of primary radiotherapy in supraglottic larynx
and pharynx carcinoma. Results of the Danish head and neck cancer study
(DAHANCA) protocol 5-85. Radiother Oncol. 1998;46(2):135–46.

82. Le Q-T, et al. Prognostic and predictive significance of plasma HGF and
IL8 in a phase III trial of chemoradiation with or without tirapazamine
in locoregionally advanced head and neck cancer. Clin Cancer Res.
2012;18(6):1798–807.

83. Meyerson M, et al. Advances in understanding cancer genomes through
second-generation sequencing. Nat Rev Genet. 2010;11:685–96.

84. Bettogowda C, et al. Detection of circulating tumor DNA in early-and
late-stage human malignancies. Sci Transl Med. 2014;6:224ra24.

85. Braig F, et al. Liquid biopsy monitoring uncovers acquired RAS-mediated
resistance to cetuximab in a substantial proportion of patients with head
and neck squamous cell carcinoma. Oncotarget. 2016;7(28):42988–95. doi:
10.18632/oncotarget.8943.

86. Kent OA, Mendell JT. A small piece in the cancer puzzle: microRNAs as
tumor suppressors and oncogenes. Oncogene. 2006;25:6188–96.

87. Zhang M, et al. Identification of microRNAs as diagnostic biomarkers in
screening of head and neck cancer: a meta-analysis. Genet Mol Res. 2015;
14(4):16562–76. doi:10.4238/2015.December.11.3.

88. Weinberger PM, et al. Human papillomavirus-active head and neck cancer
and ethnic health disparities. Laryngoscope. 2010;120:1531–7. doi:10.1002/
lary.20984.

89. Jiron J, et al. Racial disparities in human papillomavirus (HPV) associated
head and neck cancer. Am J Otolaryngol. 2014;35:147–53. doi:10.1016/j.
amjoto.2013.09.004.

90. Liu JC, et al. High prevalence of discordant HPV and p16 Oropharynx
squamous cell carcinomas in an African American cohort. Head Neck. 2016;
38(Suppl 1):E867–72. doi:10.1002/hed.24117.

3

The cylindromatosis (*CYLD*) gene and head and neck tumorigenesis

Krista Roberta Verhoeft[1], Hoi Lam Ngan[2] and Vivian Wai Yan Lui[3*]

Abstract

Germline *CYLD* mutation is associated with the development of a rare inheritable syndrome, called the *CYLD* cutaneous syndrome. Patients with this syndrome are distinctly presented with multiple tumors in the head and neck region, which can grow in size and number over time. Some of these benign head and neck tumors can turn into malignancies in some individuals. *CYLD* has been identified to be the only tumor suppressor gene reported to be associated with this syndrome thus far. Here, we summarize all reported *CYLD* germline mutations associated with this syndrome, as well as the reported paired somatic *CYLD* mutations of the developed tumors. Interestingly, whole-exome sequencing (WES) studies of multiple cancer types also revealed *CYLD* mutations in many human malignancies, including head and neck cancers and several epithelial cancers. Currently, the role of *CYLD* mutations in head and neck carcinogenesis and other cancers is poorly defined. We hope that this timely review of recent findings on *CYLD* genetics and animal models for oncogenesis can provide important insights into the mechanism of head and neck tumorigenesis.

Keywords: Head and Neck Cancer, Cylindromatosis (*CYLD*), The *CYLD* cutaneous syndrome, Turban Tumor Syndrome, Brooke-Spiegler Syndrome (BSS), Multiple Familial Trichoepithelioma (MFT1), Familial Cylindromatosis (FC), tumorigenesis, Deubiquitinating (DUB), Nuclear Factor-kB (NF-kB), TNF-receptor associated factor (TRAF) proteins, and B-cell lymphoma 3 (Bcl-3)

Abbreviations: DMBA, 7,12-dimethybenza(a)anthracene; TPA, 12-O-tetradecanoylphorbol-13-acetate; BCAC, Basal cell adenocarcinoma; BCAC-HG, Basal cell adenocarcinoma-like pattern high grade; BCAC-LG, Basal cell adenocarcinoma-like pattern low-grade; BCC, Basal cell carcinoma; Bcl-3, B-cell lymphoma 3; BSS, Brooke-Spiegler Syndrome; CAP350, Centrosome-Associated Protein 350; cIAP1/2, Cellular inhibitor of apoptosis 1 and 2; JNK, c-Jun NH(2)-terminal kinase; CCD, Clear cell differentiation; CYLD, Cylindromatosis; CAP-GLY, Cytoskeletal-associated proteinglycine-conserved; DUB, Deubiquitinating; DSS, Dextran sulphate sodium; DEN, Diethylnitrosamine; Dvl, Dishevelled; FC, Familial Cylindromatosis; FISH, Fluorescence in-situ hybridization; HNSCC, Head & neck squamous cell carcinoma; Hes1, Hes Family BHLH Transcription Factor 1; HDAC6, Histone-deacetylase 6; HPV, Human Papilloma virus; T, Individual tumor; IACs, Invasive adenocarcinomas; IKKα/IKKβ, IkB Kinase α and β; LOH, Loss of heterozygosity; LRP6, Low-density lipoprotein receptor-related protein 6; LEF/TCF, Lymphoid enhancer factor/T-cell factor; K, Lysine; MEFs, Mouse embryonic fibroblasts; Md, Mild; MKK7, Mitogen-Activated Protein Kinase 7; MFT1, Multiple Familial Trichoepithelioma 1; NGS, Next generation sequencing; NIK, NF-kappa-B inducing kinase; NEMO, NF-kB essential modulator; NF-kB, Nuclear Factor-kB; PTCH1, Patched 1; PDGFR-α, Platelet-derived growth factor receptor; RIP1, Receptor-interacting protein 1; RB1, Retinoblastoma 1; RIG1, Retinoic acid-inducible gene-1; S, Severe; SMO, Smoothened; snail1, Snail family transcriptional repressor 1; Shh, Sonic Hedgehog; Shh/Ptch1, Shh/Patched 1; SCCs, Squamous cell carcinomas; SUFU, Suppressor of Fused; TAB1, TGF-beta activated kinase 1;

(Continued on next page)

---

* Correspondence: vlui002@cuhk.edu.hk
[3]School of Biomedical Sciences, Faculty of Medicine, the Chinese University of Hong Kong, Hongkong, SAR, Hong Kong
Full list of author information is available at the end of the article

(Continued from previous page)

TAK1, TGF-β-activated kinase 1; TRAF, TNF receptor associate factor; TRADD, TNFRSF1AAssociated Via Death Domain; TRIP, TRAF interacting protein; TRPA1, Transient receptor potential cation channel A1; TRK, Tropomyosin kinase; TNFR, Tumor necrosis factor receptor; TNF-α, Tumor necrosis factor-α; TP53, Tumor protein 53; UCH, Ubiquitin C-terminal Hydrolase; Ubs, Ubiquitins; VEGF-A, Vascular endothelial growth factor-A; VS, Very severe; WES, Whole-exome sequencing

Introduction

Understanding of genetic diseases that are closely linked to tumor development can provide important insights into the biology of human tumorigenesis and treatment. To date, only a handful of human genetic diseases are uniquely associated with predisposition of head and neck tumor formation. In this focused review, we will provide an up-to-date summary of the cylindromatosis (*CYLD*) gene defects in a genetic disease called the *CYLD* cutaneous syndrome. This genetic syndrome is, in particular, characterized by multiple tumor formation in the head and neck region often with early age onset. Some of these tumors will remain benign, while some can turn malignant. Interestingly, *CYLD* genetic aberrations have recently been reported by recent whole-exome sequencing (WES) studies in head and neck cancers, and some other cancers, thus revealing its potential involvement in human carcinogenesis. Therefore, it is timely to review the genomic aberrations of *CYLD* in this particular genetic disease, which will deepen our understanding of human tumorigenesis, in particular, of the head and neck.

The *CYLD* gene

The *CYLD* gene (chr 16q12.1) codes for a 107 kDa cytoplasmic deubiquitinating (DUB) enzyme, which removes ubiquitin molecules from various signaling proteins, and regulates the activities of many cellular and signaling processes. This gene was first discovered and cloned in 2000 by Bignell et al. with prior evidence suggesting the existence of a potential tumor suppressor gene on chr 16q12-q13 linked to a peculiar cutaneous disease characterized by multiple tumors in the head and neck region [1]. Subsequent functional studies revealed multiple roles of CYLD in the regulation of inflammation, immunity, cell cycle progression, spermatogenesis, osteoclastogenesis, ciliogenesis, migration and potentially tumorigenesis [1-4]. To date, several major signaling pathways have been found to be linked with or regulated by CYLD, which include the Nuclear Factor-kB (NF-kB), Wnt/β-catenin and c-Jun NH(2)-terminal kinase (JNK) pathways, and potentially others [5-7]. Genetic alterations of *CYLD* could result in aberrant activation or inhibition of these signaling pathways, which may contribute to disease pathology.

The CYLD cutaneous syndrome

In 1842, a rare cutaneous disease was first described in a female patient, named Frances Massenger, who developed multiple tumors in the head, neck and face. In addition to her early disease onset at age 14, multiple family members of this patient also had a history of head and neck tumors [8], which strongly implied a potential underlying genetic cause of this rare disease. Over a century later in 1995, Biggs et al. discovered the locus of the susceptibility gene on chromosome 16q12-q13 by linkage analysis of the members of two affected families, revealing the potential loss of a likely tumor suppressive gene associated with this rare syndrome [9]. The following year, Biggs et al. provided further evidence to suggest that *CYLD* (referred to as *Cyld1*) may be the only tumor suppressor gene involved in the *CYLD* cutaneous syndrome [10]. A subsequent larger study with 21 affected families ultimately helped to identify the gene associated with this syndrome to be the *CYLD* gene on chromosome 16q12 and detected, for the first time, germline and somatic mutations of *CYLD* in affected patients [1]. The gene was cloned by fine-mapping and positional cloning and it was confirmed that *CYLD* germline mutations are associated with and are the underlying cause of this cutaneous syndrome in humans [1].

The term, *CYLD* cutaneous syndrome, was proposed recently by Rajan et al. [11] to describe this rare inheritable condition that is known to be caused by germline mutations of the *CYLD* gene based on genetic evidence [9]. The occurrence rate of *CYLD* germline defects is ~1:100,000 based on the UK data [12]. Patients with this syndrome are clinically characterized with multiple tumors of the skin appendages often in the head and neck region (i.e. skin lesions derived from the epidermal appendages, hair follicles, sweat apparatus, etc.). The *CYLD* syndrome encompasses three previously known appendageal tumor predisposition syndromes: familial cylindromatosis (FC, or Turban tumor syndrome; OMIM 132700), multiple familial trichoepithelioma 1 (MFT1; also called epithelioma adenoides cysticum, EAC, or Brooke-Fordyce trichoepitheliomas; OMIM 601606), and Brooke-Spiegler syndrome (BSS or BRSS; OMIM 605041), which are believed to be allelic disorders with overlapping phenotypes associated with *CYLD* mutations. The clinical manifestations of these *CYLD*-associated syndromes as well as the images for the head and neck, and facial manifestations have been recently reviewed [13]. All three tumor predisposition syndromes are autosomal dominant disorders, in which a germline *CYLD* mutation was inherited, and a second, non-inherited

CYLD mutation or loss of heterozygosity (LOH) occurs in cells for tumor formation. FC is typically presented with multiple cylindromas (i.e. benign tumors with differentiation towards apocrine sweat glands that increase in number and size over age). These multiple cylindromas growing in the scalp may coalesce and cover the entire scalp like a turban (thus FC is also called the Turban tumor syndrome). MFT1 is characterized by multiple trichoepitheliomas (i.e. skin tumors on the face with histologic dermal aggregates of basaloid cells with connection to or differentiation toward hair follicles), which can turn into basal cell carcinoma [14]. BSS, mostly with early adulthood onset, is classically characterized by multiple skin appendage tumors including cylindroma, trichoepithelioma, and spiradenoma (eccrine spiradenomas or cystic epitheliomas of the sweat gland, usually solitary, deep-seated dermal nodule typically located in the head and neck region [15]). Since members of a single family can manifest as FC, MFT1 or BSS with CYLD aberrations, many consider these three diseases as a phenotypic spectrum of a single disease entity with underlying CYLD mutation. These tumors can be painful, itchy and irritating, and in some cases, turn to malignancies. Due to the very disfiguring nature of these head and neck, facial tumors, surgical removal and often repeated surgeries are performed on these individuals to limit tumor growth over their life-time. The psychological impacts due to the disfiguring appearance of affected individuals may lead to depression and social withdrawal [16].

To date, the CYLD cutaneous syndrome has been reported in various ethnic backgrounds, with age onset as early as 5, to 40 years old. The average age onset is around teenage (~16 years old) [11]. Such an early age onset of multiple tumor formation distinctly in the head and neck region strongly imply a potential critical role of CYLD mutations in promoting head and neck tumorigenesis.

CYLD Germline and somatic mutations in individuals with the CYLD cutaneous syndrome

As of today, a total of 107 germline CYLD mutations have been reported in patients developing FC, BSS and MFT1 (Table 1). Most reported mutations reside between exons 9 and 20 of the CYLD gene. The current data revealed several hotspot mutation sites of CYLD: 1112C > A (S371*), 2272C > T (R758*) and 2806C > T (R936*) in 14, 10 and 13 independent families, respectively [17–19] (Fig. 1). Note that all three hotspot mutations are nonsense mutations, which are likely to produce truncated forms of the CYLD protein, potentially representing loss-of-function of the CYLD protein. In fact, the majority of CYLD germline mutations are deleterious mutations, including frameshift (44 %), splice-site (11 %), nonsense mutations (25 %), germline deletions (2.7 %) followed by missense mutations (11 %) and silent mutations (1 %) (Table 1). Note that a few

studies reported the absence of detectable CYLD germline mutation in a small number of affected individuals [20, 21]. It is possible that some CYLD alterations may have been missed as these previous studies examined only certain exons/regions CYLD using direct sequencing, or probe-based fluorescence in-situ hybridization (FISH) or linkage analysis. Thus far, no single study has sequenced the entire CYLD gene including the regulatory and intronic regions, which can also be potentially altered but missed by targeted sequencing. Note that sporadic occurrences of the syndrome have also been reported. In those cases, only the affected individual, but not their family members, will carry a germline CYLD mutation and present with the syndrome phenotype [22, 23].

Theoretically, it is possible that other genetic events, besides CYLD, may be involved. Candidates like Patched 1 (PTCH1) has been proposed earlier, but later disputed to be a potential candidate for the CYLD cutaneous syndrome [21, 24, 25]. As next-generation sequencing (NGS) can now be easily employed to study various diseases, it is likely that whole-exome or even whole-genome studies of these head and neck tumors from affected individuals can reveal previously unidentified genetic changes associated with the disease, in addition to CYLD.

Patients with the CYLD cutaneous syndrome inherit one copy of the mutated CYLD gene, while LOH or mutation of the second copy of the CYLD gene occur somatically for tumor formation. Several studies investigated the actual genetic change of CYLD in the developed tumors versus that of the germline aberrations in affected individuals. A total of 15 such cases have been reported thus far. As shown in Table 2, tumors from each of the 15 cases all harbored additional CYLD aberration(s) different from the original germline CYLD mutation. In some cases, somatic CYLD changes among different tumors of the same individual can also be different. In general, nonsense CYLD mutations seem to be the most common germline event, while LOH or loss-of function CYLD mutations (nonsense, or frameshift mutations) were frequently detected as somatic events (Table 2). This genetic pattern is supportive of the 2-hit hypothesis of tumorigenesis, similar to that of the retinoblastoma 1 (RB1) gene alterations for the development of retinoblastoma. Not only genetic heterogeneity was observed among tumors from the same individual, the pathologies of these tumors can also vary from benign to malignant in some cases. It is likely that CYLD alteration is an early event for head and neck tumorigenesis, and potentially supportive of later malignant transformation over time.

CYLD aberrations with benign tumor formation or malignant transformation?

Most clinical reports on the CYLD cutaneous syndrome indicate that the majority of tumors developed in the

Table 1 Germline *CYLD* mutations reported in patients with the *CYLD* cutaneous syndrome

Exon	Germline *CYLD* mutations		No. of families	Reference
	DNA	Protein		
5	561-562dupT	Q188Sfs	1	[23]
9	1027dupA	T343Nfs	1	[20]
9	1096_1097delCA	Q366Tfs	2	[20, 81]
9	1112C > A	S371[a]	14	[1, 17, 20, 21, 81–85]
9	1135G > T	E379[a]	1	[86, 87]
10	1139-1148A > G	splice site mutation	1	[20]
10	1178_1179delCA	T393Rfs	1	[88]
10	1207C > T	Q403[a]	1	[86, 87]
10	1364_1365delAA	Q455Rfs	1	[89]
10	1392_1393dupT	G465Wfs	1	[23]
10	1455 T > G	Y485[a]	1	[90]
10	1455 T > A	Y485[a]	2	[1, 20]
10	1462delA	I488Sfs	1	[25]
10	1473C > T	I491I	unavailable	[91]
10	1518 + 2 T > C	splice site mutation	1	[92]
11	1569 T > G	Y523[a]	1	[1]
11	1628del2	S543[a]	1	[81]
11	1681_1682del	L561Sfs	1	[1]
11	1682 T > A	L561[a]	1	[85]
11	1684 + 1G > A	splice site mutation	2	[20, 93]
12	1758insGATA	M587Dfs	2	[20, 82]
12	1758ins2	M587fs	1	[81]
12	1776delA	G593Afs	1	[1]
12	1783C > T	Q595[a]	1	[94]
12	1787G > A	G596D	1	[95]
12	1821_1826 + 1del-insCT	splice site mutation	1	[96]
12	1826 + 1G > A	splice site mutation	1	[97]
12	1826 + 1G > T	splice site mutation	2	[20, 21]
13	1830-1831insA	F611Ifs	1	[1]
13	1843delT	S615Lfs	1	[98]
13	1859_1860delTG	V620fs	2	[1, 81]
13	1863insA	L622Tfs	1	[81]
13	1893_1906delATATTATAGTGAAA	E631Dfs	1	[23]
13	1925delC	T642Kfs	1	[108]
13	1935dupT	N646[a]	1	[1]
14	1950-2A > T	splice site mutation	1	[23]
14	1950_1953-1delGATA	splice site mutation	1	[23]
14	1961 T > A	V654E	2	[26]
14	2012-2021del10	A671Dfs	1	[99]
14	2032G > T	E678[a]	unavailable	[91]
15	2041 + 1G > T	splice site	1	[100]
15	2042-1G > C	splice site	1	[109]
15	2042A > G	D681G	1	[86, 87]

Table 1 Germline *CYLD* mutations reported in patients with the *CYLD* cutaneous syndrome *(Continued)*

15	2065_2066delCT	*L689Vfs*	1	[85]
15	2068_2069delTTinsC	*F690Lfs*	1	[85]
15	2070delT	*H691Ifs*	1	[110]
15	2081delT	L694[a]	1	[86, 87]
15	2104delA	I702[a]	2	[20, 90]
15	2104_2105insA	I702Nfs	1	[24]
15	2108G > A	R703K	1	[111]
15	2108G > C	R703T	2	[20, 90]
16	2116_2117insATTAG	G706Dfs	1	[112]
16	2119C > T	Q707[a]	3	[20, 90]
16	2128C > T	*Q710*[a]	2	[25, 108]
16	2138delA	Y713Sfs	1	[1]
16	2146C > A	*Q716K*	1	[85]
16	2154insT	*M719Yfs*	1	[81]
16	2155dupA	M719Nfs	1	[20]
16	2170_2172insTC	K724Ifs	3	[20, 90]
16	2172delA	V725Lfs	3	[1, 15, 81]
16	2214delT	F738Lfs	1	[81]
16	2240A > G	E747G	2	[81, 101]
16	2240_2241delAG	E747fs	1	[102]
17	2252delG	C751Ffs	1	[103]
17	2255delT	*L752Rfs*	1	[83]
17	2259dupT	I754Yfs	2	[20, 21]
17	2272C > T	R758[a]	10	[1, 18, 20, 21, 85, 104, 113]
17	2288_2289delTT	F763[a]	1	[20]
17	2290_2294del	K764Ifs	1	[81]
17	2291_2295delAACTA	K764Ifs	2	[20]
17	2299A > T	K767[a]	5	[20, 83, 90]
17	2305_2306insC	I769Tfs	1	[1]
17	2305delA	I769Ffs	4	[82]
17	2330_2331delTA	I777Nfs	2	[20, 105]
17	2339 T > G	L780[a]	2	[81, 82]
18	2350 + 5G > A	Splice Site Mutation	2	[1, 85]
18	2355_2358delCAGA	R786Sfs	1	[106]
18	2409C > G	Y803[a]	1	[89]
18	2449delT	C817Vfs	1	[114]
18	2460delC	*C820*[a]	2	[1, 11]
18	2465insAACA	*T822Tfs*	1	[107]
18	2467C > T	Q823[a]	1	[1]
18	2469 + 26G > A	splice site mutation	1	[99]
18	2469 + 1G > A	splice site mutation	2	[1, 11]
19	2546G > A	W849[a]	1	[86, 87]
19	2552_2553insA	*H851Qfs*	1	[115]
19	2569C > T	Q857[a]	1	[1]

Table 1 Germline *CYLD* mutations reported in patients with the *CYLD* cutaneous syndrome *(Continued)*

19	2602G > T	E868[a]	2	[1, 116]
19	2613C > G	H871Q[#]	2	[91, 117]
19	2641delG	D881Tfs	1	[20]
19	2655G > A	*W885[a]*	1	[85]
19	2662_2664delTTT	*F888del*	1	[85]
19	2666A > T	D889V	1	[96]
20	2687G > C	G896A	1	[118]
20	2709dupT	*P904Sfs*	1	[119]
20	2711C > T	P904L	1	[83]
20	2712delT	*Q905Kfs*	1	[96]
20	2713C > T	Q905[a]	1	[20]
20	2729dupC	E911Rfs	3	[20, 90]
20	2806C > T	R936[a]	13	[1, 19, 20, 22, 26, 81, 82, 91, 120]
20	2814_2817delGCTT	L939Vfs	3	[20, 90]
20	2822A > T	D941V	1	[25]
-	2686 + 60_[a]3340del5632[b]	germline deletion	1	[85]
-	34111_[a]297858del378779[c]	germline deletion	1	[121]
-	914-6398_1769del13642ins20[d]	germline deletion	1	[121]

A total of 107 germline mutations of *CYLD* have been reported in the literature thus far. This table summarizes the reported DNA changes, protein changes, frequency and original report of 105 germline *CYLD* mutations. Two additional germline mutations of *CYLD* were originally reported as 1862 + 2 T > G (splice site mutation) [102] and 2317G > A [122], however, the protein change cannot be interpreted by sequence analysis and are therefore not included in this table. Based on the nucleotide sequences provided by the original articles, we predicted the mutational changes on the CYLD protein using the Integrated Genomic Viewer (IGV) software (Broad Institute, USA) as *italicized*- based on the reference GenBank number NM_015247 for *CYLD*. Abbreviations: *del* deletion, *ins* insertion, *dup* duplicate, [a] = introduction of stop codon. Notes: [b]Large deletion (~5.3kB) in the catalytic domain UCH region of *CYLD*. [c]Large deletion (~13.6kB) from intron 6 to exon 12 affecting the 3rd CAP domain and beginning of the UCH domain, additionally, a 20 bp insertion was detected. [d]Large deletion (0.4 MB) of entire *CYLD* gene and some surrounding regions

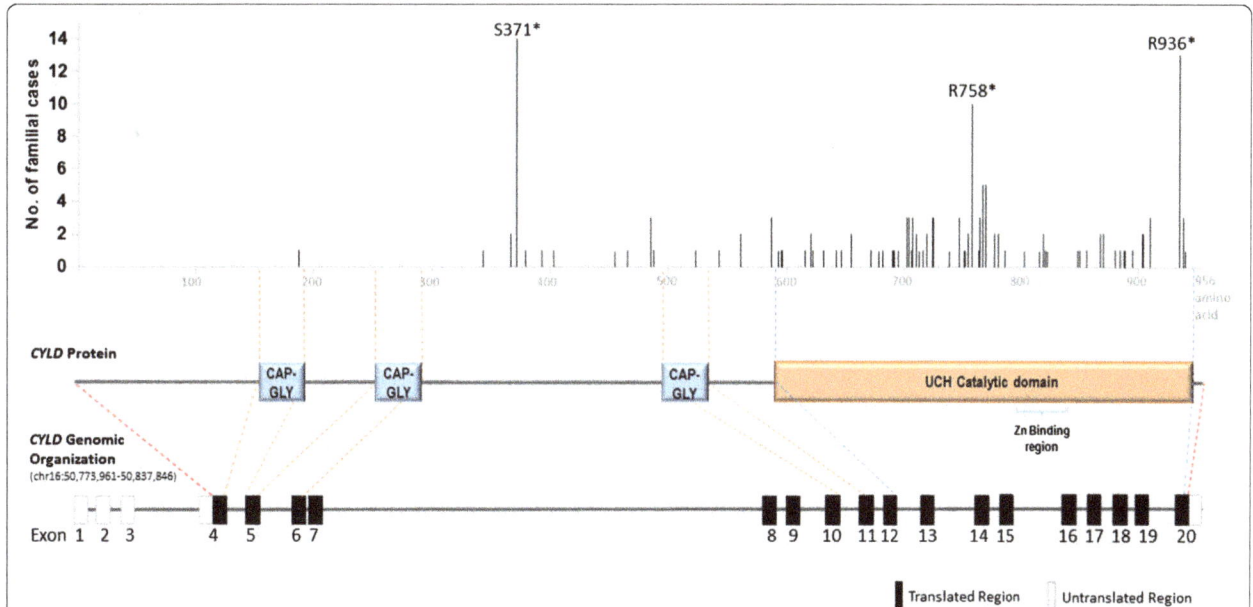

Fig. 1 Reported *CYLD* germline mutations in patients with the *CYLD* cutaneous syndrome [1, 11, 17, 19–23, 25, 26, 81, 120]. The frequency of familial cases of *CYLD* cutaneous syndrome with germline *CYLD* mutations, and the corresponding amino acid positions affected by these mutations are indicated (as detailed in Table 1 and predicted using the Integrative Genomics Viewer (IGV) software, the Broad Institute, USA). The CYLD protein contains three CAP-GLY domains (aa 155–198, 253–286, 492–535), a UCH catalytic domain (aa 591–950) and a Zinc binding region (aa 778–842) within in the catalytic domain based on the NCBI number NP_056062.1

Table 2 Reported paired germline and somatic CYLD mutations in patients with the CYLD cutaneous syndrome

Age of onset, Gender	Severity	Germline Mutation DNA	Germline Mutation Protein		Somatic Mutation DNA	Somatic Mutation Protein	Malignancy	Sequencing method and reference
35, F	Md	2070delT	F690fs	T1	n.s., n.s.	I645V, R936c	Benign	PCR. Sequenced (exons 4 GenBank#NT010498.15 [
				T2	n.s.	Q731c	Benign	
				T3	undetectable	undetectable	Benign	
24, F	S-VS	2806C > T	R936c	T1	n.s., n.s.	R936c, D889N	Benign	PCR. All
teens, F	S	2012-2021del 10, 2469 + 26G > A	A671fs, splice site mutation	T1	LOH	-	BCC	PCR. Sequenced and splice sites. GenBank#: NT010505. Tumor LOH analysis using markers: D16S3044, D16S308, D16S503 [
n.s., M	Md	2104_2105insA	I702fs	T1	2541G > A	W847c	Benign	PCR. Sequenced (exons 4 AJ250014. Tumor LOH analysis using markers: D9S925, D9S171 & D9S169- (chr.9p2), D9S15, D9S252, D9S303, and D9S287 (chr.9q22.3) and D16S 769, D16S 753, CDRP 28, CDRP 23, D16S 416, D16S 771, D16S 673 (chr.16) [
n.s., F (Family1 mother)	S	1455 T > G	Y458c	T1	1736_1739dupTGGA	E580Dfs	n.s.	Sequenced regions (exons 1
				T2	LOH	-		
				T3	1794C > A	Y598c		
n.s., F (Family1 daughter)	S	1455 T > G	Y458c	T1	LOH	-	n.s.	GenBank#AC007728. Tumor LOH analysis using markers: D16S304, D16S308, D16S419, D16S476, and D16S541 (chr.16q) and D16S407 (chr.16p) [
				T2	LOH	-	n.s.	
				T3	1540dupA	T514Nfs	n.s.	
n.s., F (Family2 mother)	S	2104delA	I702c	T1	1112C > A	S371c	n.s.	
n.s., F (Family2 daughter)	Md-S	2104delA	I702c	T1	2467C > T	Q823c	n.s.	
n.s., M	S	2108G > C	R703T	T1	2806C > T	R936c	n.s.	
				T2	LOH	-	n.s.	
n.s., F	Md-S	2119C > T	Q707c	T1	LOH	Q905c	n.s.	
				T2	2713C > T		n.s.	
46, F	Md	2170_2171insTC	K724lfs	T1	2046_2047ins AGATCCG	E683Rfs	n.s.	
18, F	S	2299A > T	K767c	T1	LOH	-	n.s.	
		2279dupC	E911Rfs	T2	LOH	-		
		2279dupC	E911Rfs	T3	2107A > T	R703c		
n.s., F	Md-S	2729dup C	E911Ffs	T1	LOH	-	n.s.	

Table 2 Reported paired germline and somatic CYLD mutations in patients with the CYLD cutaneous syndrome (Continued)

n.s., M	Md-S	2814_2817delGCTT	L939Vfs	T1	LOH	-		n.s.	Sequencing regions were not reported. Tumor LOH analysis was performed (markers not specified) [
~26, M	S	1684+1G>A	splice site mutation	T1T2	LOH	-		Benign	
				T3	LOH	-		Benign	
				T4	LOH	-		BCC	
				T5	LOH	2322delA	E774Dfs	BCC	
								CCD /	

The CYLD cutaneous syndrome patient cases reported with paired germline and somatic CYLD mutations; and including disease severity information and reported sequencing methods. Severity was defined as mild (Md), severe (S) or very severe (VS) using the following criteria: Md = few, small tumors, not painful or overgrowing. S = Multiple large growths, painful/ulcerating and resulting in tumor excision. VS = Multiple large tumors, often disfiguring, painful/ulcerating, resulting in multiple tumor excisions and/or complete scalp removal. Abbreviations: *del* deletion, *ins* insertion, *dup* duplicate, ^{c} = introduction of stop codon, carcinoma, *LOH* Loss of heterozygosity, *n.s.* not stated, *CCD* clear cell differentiation, *T* individual tumor used for analysis

Notes: [a]Cases from related members of a family (mother and daughter), [b]Cases from another family (mother and daughter)

head and neck region are benign in nature, with progressive growth in size and number over one's lifetime. However, emerging evidence is supportive of malignant transformation of these usually benign tumors into malignancies in some affected individuals, perhaps even in situ, arising from the original benign tumors [26]. In fact, the very first case report of such cutaneous syndrome (though with unclear genetics), had extensively documented multiple tumor formation in the patient's peritoneum, reminiscent of the patient's head and neck tumors. The patient who later manifested a state of cachexia did suggest a "malignancy" as indicated in the report [8]. Yet, it remains unclear if these tumors in the peritoneum were originated in situ or were actually metastatic lesions from the head and neck tumors.

Due to the rarity of the syndrome, and repeated surgeries for most patients (for cosmetic reasons), documentation of malignant transformation of these seemingly benign tumors is scarce. Recently, Kazakov et al. reported multiple cases with histological evidences suggesting that the malignant lesions seemed to develop or transform in situ at the original "benign" tumors of the cutaneous syndrome patients [26]. A histological study showed that in an invasive carcinoma, the basal cell adenocarcinoma (BCAC) of the salivary gland that was developed in the affected individual, there remained a residuum of spiradenoma which merged with the invasive carcinoma by histology. Similar findings in another affected individual showed that the benign tumor had developed into an invasive lesion in the skull with a BCAC histology. Invasive adenomas of various histologies have been identified in several affected individuals as well. How did these malignant transformations occur in situ? Did the tumors acquire additional genetic aberrations that caused or supported malignant transformation? Or were the *CYLD* genetic aberrations (two copies of *CYLD* mutated or loss) sufficient to drive such a malignant transformation over time if the tumors had not been excised early enough by surgery?

As demonstrated by chemically-induced colon and liver cancer models with $CYLD^{-/-}$ mice [16, 27], it seems that phenotypically invasive or potentially metastatic tumors can develop with a *CYLD* deficient background in vivo. This may imply that *CYLD* loss, together with a strong cancer inducing agent or DNA mutagen, can turn normal cells to tumors with the potential to further transform into malignancies. This notion is further supported by findings from Alameda et al. that expression of a catalytically inactive form of CYLD in a Ha-*ras*-mutated tumorigenic epidermal cell line (PDVC57) significantly promoted in vitro cell proliferation, migration (with changes to a mesenchymal phenotype), anchorage-independent growth, as well as pronounced in vivo tumor growth and angiogenesis with upregulation of

vascular endothelial growth factor-A (VEGF-A) expression [28]. Using a subcutaneous tumor model, the authors demonstrated that the *CYLD* mutant tumors not only grew faster and larger in size, but also showed a more aggressive, poorly differentiated phenotype when compared to the control tumors which bore a less aggressive, differentiated phenotype. It was hypothesized that the presence of Ha-*ras* mutation in this cell model, PDVC57, together with *CYLD* mutation, may be responsible for such an aggressive phenotype, which is in contrast with the observed benign skin tumors developed in $CYLD^{-/-}$ mice as previously reported by Massoumi et al. [29]. These findings may suggest that CYLD may cooperate with other oncogenic events, in this case Ha-*ras* mutation, to promote malignant transformation. Thus, future investigations on *CYLD* gene interaction may further define the biological importance of *CYLD* in head and neck carcinogenesis and progression.

CYLD Mutations in head and neck cancers, and other human malignancies

CYLD has been suggested to be a tumor suppressor gene, as supported by evidences from the first genetic susceptibility study for the *CYLD* cutaneous syndrome [1]. It is known that deleterious loss of an important tumor suppressor gene in germline settings can confer cancer predisposition in an inherited manner. A well-known comparable example is the Li–Fraumeni syndrome, a rare cancer predisposition hereditary disease caused by germline tumor protein 53 (*TP53*) mutations and the affected individuals often develop various cancers at young age. Although our current understanding of CYLD is insufficient, the very first reported case of such a cutaneous syndrome in Frances Massenger (1842) who first developed multiple scalp and face tumors, and later, multiple abdominal/peritoneal tumors reminiscent of the ones in her head and neck, and subsequently died with symptoms of cancer cachexia did suggest a potential link of the cutaneous syndrome to malignant conditions [8]. Several female family members also had a history of head and neck tumors (grandmother, mother, and sister), and breast tumors (sister), suggesting the inheritable nature of the syndrome linked to human malignancies. In fact, a recent study by Kazakov et al. reported a total of 5 patients with BSS, who were found to develop malignancies arising from pre-existing tumors in the head and neck region [26]. Further microscopic analyses of the tumors confirmed the presence of "residuum of a pre-existing benign neoplasm" indicative of in situ development of malignancies from the apparently benign lesions. A handful of malignant cases developed in patients with BSS have also been reported by others [30–49]. These malignancies included salivary gland type basal cell adenocarcinoma-like pattern, low-grade (BCAC-LG), and high grade (BCAC-HG), invasive adenocarcinomas (IACs), squamous cell carcinomas (SCCs), anaplastic neoplasms and sarcomatoid (metaplastic) carcinomas [34, 50–59].

Although it remains unclear how CYLD genomic aberrations precisely drive multiple head and neck tumor formation, and potentially, malignant progression, CYLD somatic mutations have been reported in a subset of head and neck squamous cell carcinoma (HNSCC) patients as revealed by recent WES efforts of The Cancer Genome Atlas (TCGA, USA). HNSCC is the most common type of head and neck cancer, ranking the sixth most common cancer worldwide. A total of 8 CYLD somatic mutations (8/279 patient cases) have been identified in primary HNSCC tumors by WES [60]. These include: F110L, V180Cfs*23, N300S, S361Lfs*47, S371*, T575S, D618A, and K680*. Among which, the S371* mutation has been found to be a hotspot germline mutation in patients with the CYLD cutaneous syndrome as mentioned above. Yet, the functional role of these CYLD mutations in HNSCC development remains unknown. Among the 8 CYLD-mutated HNSCC tumors, 4 were Human Papilloma virus (HPV)-negative (all smokers; age onset is 71.75 ± 3.77 years old) and the remaining 4 were HPV-positive (with 1 smoker only; age onset is 54.00 ± 6.82 years old). All HPV-negative CYLD-mutated tumors were also TP53 mutated, while as expected, the HPV-positive counterparts were all TP53 wildtype. Although all patients carrying the CYLD-mutated HNSCC tumors had advanced disease at the time of diagnosis [Stage III (2/8 cases) and Stage IV (6/8 cases)], the published TCGA cohort with only 8 CYLD-mutated cases was not able to reveal any CYLD-mutation and overall patient survival correlation (data not shown).

Besides the published HNSCC TCGA dataset, a recent study has identified a high incidence of CYLD aberrations in a rare salivary gland tumor, namely the dermal analogue tumor, which can be of sporadic or familial origins. Dermal analogue tumor is a subtype of basal cell monomorphic adenoma with remarkable histological and clinical resemblance to cylindromas. Choi et al. reported that as high as 80.9 % (17/21) of the sporadic cases, and 75 % of familial cases (9/12 tumors from two sisters) harbored LOH near the CYLD gene locus (16q12-13) [51]. These findings suggest that both skin adnexal tumors, which are commonly associated with the CYLD cutaneous syndrome, and dermal analogue tumors may share a common genetic basis, namely CYLD genetic alteration.

Besides HNSCC, the TCGA WES efforts also revealed other human cancers with a ≥3 % mutation rate of CYLD. These include (arranged in descending order of percent cases mutated in each cohort and the actual number shown in the legend; Additional file 1: Figure S1): uterine corpus endometrial carcinoma (5.2 %; 13/248 cases), lung squamous cell carcinoma (4.5 %; 8/177 cases), stomach adenocarcinoma (3.8 %; 15/395 cases) and lung adenocarcinoma (3 %; 7/230 cases). An additional 15 cancer types harbor somatic CYLD mutations at ~1-3 % rates. These are cancers of the skin, esophagus, colon, glioma, pancreas, liver and cervix, as well as intrahepatic cholangiocarcinoma, small cell lung cancer, large B cell lymphoma, thymoma, chromophobe renal cell carcinoma, multiple myeloma, uveal melanoma, glioblastoma (TCGA, USA; www.cbioportal.org; [61, 62]). Interestingly, two of the germline CYLD hotspot mutations (S371* and R758*) in CYLD cutaneous syndrome patients are also found in primary tumors of HNSCC, lung and stomach. Yet, the roles of these CYLD mutations in these solid tumors remain undetermined. It is possible that CYLD alterations may be involved in the tumorigenesis of many other cancers, in addition to head and neck cancers.

CYLD signaling

Important cellular processes are known to be regulated by ubiquitination and deubiquitination of cellular proteins. Ubiquitination of a protein can determine and regulate its stability, and even its signaling functions [63]. Ubiquitins (Ubs) are small proteins (8.5 kDa) with seven lysine (K) residues (K6, K11, K27, K29, K33, K48 and K63). Ubiquitination of different K residues can serve different biological functions. For instance, K48-linked ubiquitin chains on a target protein directs the protein for proteosome degradation, while K63 links can promote protein-protein interactions and signaling activation [2].

The CYLD protein has three cytoskeletal-associated protein-glycine-conserved (CAP-GLY) domains and a UCH catalytic domain with a zinc-motif [1] (Fig. 1). The CAP-GLY domains combined with proline-rich regions are responsible for microtubule and target protein binding, while the UCH domain mediates deubiquitination, and the zinc-motif allows for CYLD folding and domain interaction [1]. CYLD is highly specific for K63 ubiquitin chains [64], however has also been demonstrated to mediate K48 deubiquitination of target proteins [65]. Target proteins of CYLD include B-cell lymphoma 3 (Bcl-3), Histone-deacetylase 6 (HDAC6), Transient receptor potential cation channel A1 (TRPA1), NF-kB essential modulator (NEMO), TRAF interacting protein (TRIP), transforming growth factor-β-activated kinase 1 (TAK1), receptor-interacting protein 1 (RIP1), retinoic acid-inducible gene-1 (RIG1) and TNF-receptor associated factor (TRAF) proteins, etc. [66]. Through deubiquitination of these signaling proteins, CYLD has been shown to regulate major signaling pathways including the NF-kappaB (NF-kB) (canonical and non-canonical), Wnt/β-catenin and c-Jun NH(2)-terminal kinase (JNK) pathways (Fig. 2) [5–7, 67]. Several studies showed that the tumor suppressor CYLD inhibits NF-kB as well as

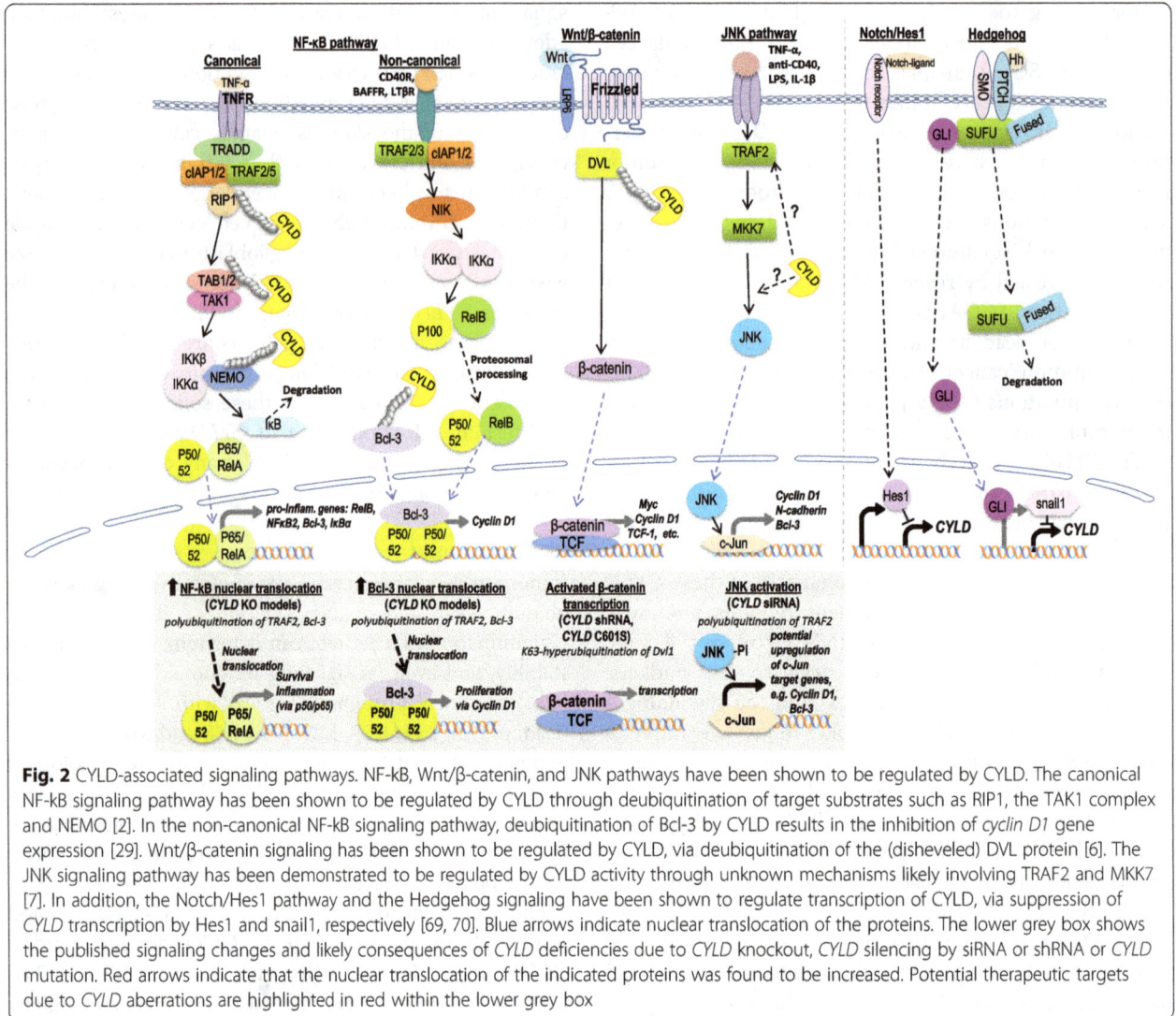

Fig. 2 CYLD-associated signaling pathways. NF-kB, Wnt/β-catenin, and JNK pathways have been shown to be regulated by CYLD. The canonical NF-kB signaling pathway has been shown to be regulated by CYLD through deubiquitination of target substrates such as RIP1, the TAK1 complex and NEMO [2]. In the non-canonical NF-kB signaling pathway, deubiquitination of Bcl-3 by CYLD results in the inhibition of *cyclin D1* gene expression [29]. Wnt/β-catenin signaling has been shown to be regulated by CYLD, via deubiquitination of the (disheveled) DVL protein [6]. The JNK signaling pathway has been demonstrated to be regulated by CYLD activity through unknown mechanisms likely involving TRAF2 and MKK7 [7]. In addition, the Notch/Hes1 pathway and the Hedgehog signaling have been shown to regulate transcription of CYLD, via suppression of *CYLD* transcription by Hes1 and snail1, respectively [69, 70]. Blue arrows indicate nuclear translocation of the proteins. The lower grey box shows the published signaling changes and likely consequences of *CYLD* deficiencies due to *CYLD* knockout, *CYLD* silencing by siRNA or shRNA or *CYLD* mutation. Red arrows indicate that the nuclear translocation of the indicated proteins was found to be increased. Potential therapeutic targets due to *CYLD* aberrations are highlighted in red within the lower grey box

the p38 MAPK pathway activation by deubiquitinating several upstream regulatory signaling molecules of these pathways, thus suppressing these signaling pathways [68]. Alternatively, CYLD has been shown to be negatively regulated by the Notch [69] and Sonic Hedgehog (Shh) [70] signaling pathways in T-cell leukemia and skin cancer, respectively (Fig. 2). As of today, among all currently identified target proteins of CYLD, many are signaling regulators of the NF-kB pathway (e.g. the TRAF proteins, NEMO, TRIP, RIP1, TAK1 and Bcl-3). Therefore, it is believed that genomic aberrations of *CYLD* may alter NF-kB signaling activity, which may also contribute to the pathophysiology of the *CYLD* cutaneous syndrome and tumor formation.

Although it is unclear if other non-NF-kB signaling pathways are potentially involved, recent evidences revealed such a possibility. *CYLD* has recently been shown to promote ciliogenesis, a process that is plausibly associated with tumorigenesis. The primary cilium is a cell surface antenna-like structure sensing chemical and mechanical signals from the environment on almost all mammalian cells. Since the formation of the primary cilium is coordinately regulated with the cell cycle progression via its connection with the centrosome, it has been hypothesized that regulators of ciliogenesis may also control cell proliferation and tissue homeostasis, and defects in primary cilium formation or function may contribute to tumorigenesis due to "non-communicative and unrestrained growth" [71–73]. In fact, in addition to this *CYLD* tumor suppressor, several key tumor suppressors and oncogenes such as the *VHL*, *PDGFR-α*, and *Shh/Patched 1* (*Shh/Ptch1*) were recently identified to regulate ciliogenesis [3, 4, 74]. Eguether et al. demonstrated that both the centrosomal localization (via interaction with a centrosomal protein CAP350) and deubiquitination activity of CYLD were required for its ciliogenic activity, independent of NF-kB [3]. Note that another NF-kB-independent and ciliogenic signaling pathway, the Shh/Ptch1 pathway, which is the most critical signaling pathway regulating cell proliferation and differentiation of basal cell carcinoma (a type of skin cancer arising from epidermal stem cell of the hair follicles) [75], has been recently identified as an upstream regulator of CYLD expression (Fig. 2). It remains to be investigated if this Shh/Ptch1-CYLD link is relevant for ciliogenesis as well as tumorigenesis of the skin, which can be pathologically related to this CYLD Cutaneous syndrome.

CYLD and potential mechanisms of multiple head and neck tumor development

Although the genetic link between CYLD defects and the CYLD cutaneous syndrome has been identified, there remain many interesting questions to be answered regarding this peculiar syndrome. How do CYLD germline mutations give rise to "multiple" tumor formation, in particular, in the head and neck region in these patients? Furthermore, what are the molecular mechanisms underlying the progression of benign tumor lesions to malignancies in some patients?

Loss of CYLD links to multiple tumor development?

Almost all CYLD cutaneous syndrome patients do carry a germline mutation of CYLD which is inheritable. Interestingly, CYLD somatic mutations have also been identified in sporadic cases of cylindroma [1] and spiradenoma patients [76]. This evidence suggests that CYLD aberration is associated with the disease phenotype of multiple head and neck tumors. Thus far, CYLD is the only tumor suppressor gene identified to be linked with the disease. Genetically-engineered mouse models have been generated to study the function of CYLD in mammalian settings. A study by Massoumi et al. demonstrated that CYLD knockout mice (with disruption of ATG start codon) were much more susceptible to chemically-induced cutaneous squamous papilloma formation upon a single dose of 7,12-dimethybenza(a)anthracene (DMBA) followed by 12-Otetradecanoylphorbol-13-acetate (TPA) treatment [29]. All $CYLD^{-/-}$ mice developed skin tumors (papillomas) after 11 weeks vs. only 50–60 % of tumor incidence in $CYLD^{+/+}$ mice at a later time of 16 weeks. Importantly, mice with homozygous as well as heterozygous loss of CYLD (i.e. $CYLD^{-/-}$ and $CYLD^{+/-}$ mice) both developed multiple tumor phenotype on the skin much earlier than the $CYLD^{+/+}$ mice. By week 16, $CYLD^{-/-}$ and $CYLD^{+/-}$ mice harbored ~30 and 15 tumors/mouse, as compared to only 5 tumors per mouse in the $CYLD^{+/+}$ group. These results indicated that the loss of a single copy of CYLD gene was sufficient to confer a "multiple tumor phenotype" upon chemical insults in mice (although the tumor-bearing phenotype is more severe when both copies of CYLD were lost). Further, the average

tumor size of papilloma developed in the $CYLD^{-/-}$ mice were >2.8 times of those found in the $CYLD^{+/+}$ mice, implicating a potential CYLD gene dose effect on tumor cell proliferation. Despite the fact that spontaneous tumor development was not observed in the $CYLD^{-/-}$ mice, loss of CYLD (either one or both copies) did confer a "tumor susceptible phenotype" reminiscent of patients with the CYLD cutaneous syndrome. It was further noted that the tumor number and size in $CYLD^{-/-}$ and $CYLD^{+/-}$ mice did grow over time after the initial DMBA/TPA insult, which is also reminiscent of the tumor characteristics reported in patients with the syndrome [1, 29]. Yet, all the tumors developed in the $CYLD^{-/-}$ and $CYLD^{+/-}$ backgrounds were hyperplastic lesions with no signs of malignancy [29]. It is likely that the loss of this CYLD tumor suppressor gene makes the entire epithelium of the skin highly prone to tumor initiation by chemicals or environmental insults in the "affected site", skin in this model, thus multiple tumors can develop in this "primed soil".

This is further supported by another CYLD knockout mice study, in which multiple tumors were developed in the colon of the $CYLD^{-/-}$ mice in a chemical-induced colitis-associated cancer (CAC) model [27], with which a DNA mutagen (azoxymethane; AOM) and an inflammation-inducing chemical (dextran sulphate sodium; DSS) were used in the drinking water to target the colon epithelium of the animals. The study demonstrated that as early as second round of DSS treatment, the $CYLD^{-/-}$ mice developed multiple measurable broad-based adenocarcinomas (i.e. flattened, or called sessile) in the colonic epithelium, as compared to almost no tumor in the $CYLD^{+/+}$ mice. In humans, it is noted that sessile polys or adenomas are pre-cancerous lesions in the colon [77]. Further investigation demonstrated that CYLD could limit inflammation and tumorigenesis by regulating ubiquitination [27]. Similar multi-tumor phenotype was also observed in a diethylnitrosamine (DEN)-induced carcinogenic liver injury model, in which significantly more, larger and multiple tumors with invasive or metastatic potential (displaying trabecular sinusoidal structures related to initial stage of invasion and metastasis in human hepatocellular carcinoma) were observed in the livers of the $CYLD^{-/-}$ mice as compared to that of the $CYLD^{+/+}$ mice [68]. The observation that multiple papillomas, colon adenocarcinomas, and liver tumors were easily induced upon treatment with chemical insults or DNA mutagens in CYLD knockout mice did strongly imply a generalized tumor susceptibility nature of the affected epithelium or tissue due to CYLD mutation or CYLD loss. However, it remains unclear as to why some tissues seem to develop potentially malignant tumors (e.g. liver, and colon), while some tissues tend to develop more benign tumors (e.g. skin papilloma) in vivo. Thus, it is important to determine if

CYLD aberrations do confer any tissue-specific oncogenic activity in various human cancer types.

Why do these tumors develop predominantly in the head and neck region?

The next question is why these tumors mostly developed in the head and neck, and face of the affected individuals? The possible reason(s) may lie in the fact that these areas are always exposed to strong chemical or DNA-damaging insults. It is possible that frequent exposure to UV, a strong DNA-damaging insult can serve as a tumor inducer or potentiating agent for tumor development in the epithelium of the head and neck, and the face. It has been shown by Massoumi et al. that UV light could trigger cellular proliferation of *CYLD*$^{-/-}$ keratinocytes, as well as cyclin D1 expression [29]. The study proposed a model that in the presence of UV light and in conjunction with *CYLD* loss, Bcl-3 will translocate into the nucleus, complexed with p50 to induce cyclin D1 expression, thus cellular proliferation, while the presence of intact CYLD will inhibit Bcl-3 nuclear translocation and growth.

Another equally important possibility is the likely origin(s) of tumor from the hair stem cells as previously suggested for cylindromas [78]. As the region of head and neck, and the face harbor many stem cell -containing hair follicles in the sebaceous and sweat glands, *CYLD* genetic aberrations may affect the proliferation control, or inflammatory status of the stem cell niches, thus resulting in predominant head and neck tumor formation. Evidence for this can be noted as these tumors never grow from the hair-less parts of the body (e.g. the palms and soles), but only in the hairy parts of the body. It is also possible that hair follicle stem cells that harbor *CYLD* alterations may acquire additional genetic changes over one's lifetime thus resulting in tumor formation. However, since the origin of these tumors of the *CYLD* cutaneous syndrome patients is still of debate, this hypothesis remains to be proven. Another possibility that remains to be proven is that, maybe, CYLD is specifically and functionally associated with developmental control or growth regulation of the head and neck or hair follicles in humans. Thus, germline defects of *CYLD* in patients with the *CYLD* cutaneous syndrome are mainly presented with head and neck tumors or tumors in regions with lots of hair follicles.

As *CYLD* somatic mutations occur in HNSCC tumors, and *CYLD* aberrations seem to be the key genetic driver for multiple head and neck tumor formation in patients with this cutaneous syndrome, an unanswered question is whether *CYLD* aberration alone is sufficient to directly drive head and neck tumor formation. Do additional genetic or chemical insults associated with head and neck carcinogenesis, such as smoking, drinking, or HPV infection, promote tumorigenesis in *CYLD*-mutated head and neck cancers? Is the immune system involved as well, since CYLD is also implicated in the regulation of immunity? All these questions remain to be addressed.

Conclusions

The genetics of the *CYLD* cutaneous syndrome underlies the formation of multiple tumors in the head and neck epithelium. Current treatments are limited, except for repeated surgical removal of the tumors when needed. Inhibition of NF-kB signaling can potentially be a treatment option. Yet, a prior clinical trial on the topical use of salicylic acid showed some efficacies in some affected individuals only (2/12 cases) [79]. A recent study showed that *CYLD* mutations can cause activation of the tropomyosin kinase (TRK) signaling in tumors of affected individuals [80]. Further, inhibition of TRK signaling in *CYLD*-mutant tumor models demonstrated the potential efficacies of TRK targeting. Thus TRK inhibitors can be a potential treatment strategy for these patients. It is important to understand more about the genetics and biology of these *CYLD*-mutant tumors, which may point to new treatment or prevention of these disfiguring tumors. Further understanding of the role of CYLD in head and neck epithelial biology may also identify mechanisms of tumorigenesis and progression of head and neck cancers, as well as other human malignancies.

Additional file

Additional file 1: Figure S1. Graph showing the mutation frequencies of *CYLD* gene in major cancer types. Data were extracted from the cBioPortal database (www.cbioportal.org; dated 3rd August, 2016). The *CYLD* mutation frequencies of 15 most updated TCGA Provisional cancer cohorts, and five other important cancer types with *CYLD* mutation rates of >1–3 % rates were shown, with actual number of mutated cases shown in this legend. *Abbreviations:* Uterine (TCGA Provisional): Uterine Corpus Endometrial Carcinoma 13/248 cases (5.2 %), Lung squ (TCGA Provisional): Lung Squamous Cell Carcinoma 8/177 cases (4.5 %), Stomach (TCGA Provisional): Stomach Adenocarcinoma 15/395 cases (3.8 %), Lung adeno (TCGA Provisional): Lung Adenocarcinoma 7/230 cases (3 %), Head & neck (TCGA Provisional): Head and Neck Squamous Cell Carcinoma 15/512 cases (2.9 %), Cholangiocarcinoma (JHU, 2013): Intrahepatic Cholangiocarcinoma 1/40 (2.5 %), Small Cell Lung (JHU, 2012): Small Cell Lung Cancer 1/42 (2.4 %), Melanoma (TCGA Provisional): Skin Cutaneous Melanoma 8/368 cases (2.2 %), Esophagus (TCGA Provisional): Esophageal Carcinoma 4/185 cases (2.2 %), DLBC (TCGA Provisional): Lymphoid Neoplasm Diffuse Large B-cell Lymphoma 1/48 case (2.1 %), Colorectal (TCGA Provisional): Colorectal Adenocarcinoma 4/223 cases (1.8 %), Glioma (UCSF, 2014): Low-Grade Gliomas 1/61 (1.6 %), Thymoma (TCGA Provisional): Thymoma 2/123 cases (1.6 %), chRCC (TCGA Provisional): Kidney Chromophobe 1/66 case (1.5 %), MM (Broad, 2014): Multiple Myeloma 3/205 (1.5 %), Pancreas (TCGA Provisional): Pancreatic Adenocarcinoma 2/150 cases (1.3 %), Uveal melanoma (TCGA Provisional): Uveal melanoma 1/80 case (1.3 %), GBM (TCGA, 2008): Glioblastoma 1/91 (1.1 %), Liver (TCGA Provisional): Liver Hepatocellular Carcinoma 4/373 cases (1.1 %), Cervical (TCGA Provisional): Cervical Squamous Cell Carcinoma & Endocervical Adenocarcinoma 2/194 cases (1 %). (PPTX 77 kb)

Acknowledgements
Not applicable.

Funding
VWYL was supported by the School of Biomedical Sciences Start-up Fund, Faculty of Medicine, Chinese University of Hong Kong, the Theme-based Research Grant (T12-401/13-R) and General Research Fund (#17114874), Research Grants Council (RGC), Hong Kong Government, Hong Kong. KRV and HLN were supported by the Hong Kong PhD Fellowship Scheme, RGC, Hong Kong Government, and HKU SPACE Research Fund, University of Hong Kong, respectively. There is no other source of funding directly related to this manuscript.

Authors' contributions
KRV contributed to manuscript writing. HLN did *CYLD* mutational analyses. VWYL conceived the idea, and contributed to the writing. All authors read and approved the final manuscript.

Competing interests
VWYL served as a Consultant for Novartis Pharmaceuticals (HK) Ltd. All other authors declare no conflict of interest.

Author details
[1]Department of Clinical Oncology, Li-Ka Shing Faculty of Medicine, the University of Hong Kong, Hongkong, SAR, Hong Kong. [2]School of Biomedical Sciences, Li-Ka Shing Faculty of Medicine, the University of Hong Kong, Hongkong, SAR, Hong Kong. [3]School of Biomedical Sciences, Faculty of Medicine, the Chinese University of Hong Kong, Hongkong, SAR, Hong Kong.

References
1. Bignell GR, et al. Identification of the familial cylindromatosis tumour-suppressor gene. Nat Genet. 2000;25(2):160–5.
2. Sun SC. CYLD: a tumor suppressor deubiquitinase regulating NF-kappaB activation and diverse biological processes. Cell Death Differ. 2010;17(1):25–34.
3. Eguether T, et al. The deubiquitinating enzyme CYLD controls apical docking of basal bodies in ciliated epithelial cells. Nat Commun. 2014;5:4585.
4. Yang Y, et al. CYLD mediates ciliogenesis in multiple organs by deubiquitinating Cep70 and inactivating HDAC6. Cell Res. 2014;24(11):1342–53.
5. Kovalenko A, et al. The tumour suppressor CYLD negatively regulates NF-kappaB signalling by deubiquitination. Nature. 2003;424(6950):801–5.
6. Tauriello DV, et al. Loss of the tumor suppressor CYLD enhances Wnt/beta-catenin signaling through K63-linked ubiquitination of Dvl. Mol Cell. 2010;37(5):607–19.
7. Reiley W, Zhang M, Sun SC. Negative regulation of JNK signaling by the tumor suppressor CYLD. J Biol Chem. 2004;279(53):55161–7.
8. Ancell H. History of a remarkable case of tumours, developed on the head and face; accompanied with a similar disease in the abdomen. Med Chir Trans. 1842;25:227–306. 11.
9. Biggs PJ, et al. Familial cylindromatosis (turban tumour syndrome) gene localised to chromosome 16q12-q13: evidence for its role as a tumour suppressor gene. Nat Genet. 1995;11(4):441–3.
10. Biggs PJ, et al. The cylindromatosis gene (cyld1) on chromosome 16q may be the only tumour suppressor gene involved in the development of cylindromas. Oncogene. 1996;12(6):1375–7.
11. Rajan N, et al. Tumor mapping in 2 large multigenerational families with CYLD mutations: implications for disease management and tumor induction. Arch Dermatol. 2009;145(11):1277–84.
12. Dubois A, et al. CYLD GeneticTesting for Brooke-Spiegler Syndrome, Familial Cylindromatosis and Multiple Familial Trichoepitheliomas. PLoS Curr, 2015. 7
13. Rajan N, Ashworth A. Inherited cylindromas: lessons from a rare tumour. Lancet Oncol. 2015;16(9):e460–9.
14. Johnson SC, Bennett RG. Occurrence of basal cell carcinoma among multiple trichoepitheliomas. J Am Acad Dermatol. 1993;28(2 Pt 2):322–6.
15. Scheinfeld N, et al. Identification of a recurrent mutation in the CYLD gene in Brooke-Spiegler syndrome. Clin Exp Dermatol. 2003;28(5):539–41.
16. Parren LJ, et al. A novel therapeutic strategy for turban tumor: scalp excision and combined reconstruction with artificial dermis and split skin graft. Int J Dermatol. 2014;53(2):246–9.
17. Li ZL, et al. Germline mutation analysis in the CYLD gene in Chinese patients with multiple trichoepitheliomas. Genet Mol Res. 2014;13(4):9650–5.
18. Farkas K, et al. The CYLD p.R758X worldwide recurrent nonsense mutation detected in patients with multiple familial trichoepithelioma type 1, Brooke-Spiegler syndrome and familial cylindromatosis represents a mutational hotspot in the gene. BMC Genet. 2016;17(1):36.
19. Nagy N, et al. A mutational hotspot in CYLD causing cylindromas: a comparison of phenotypes arising in different genetic backgrounds. Acta Derm Venereol. 2013;93(6):743–5.
20. Grossmann P, et al. Novel and recurrent germline and somatic mutations in a cohort of 67 patients from 48 families with Brooke-Spiegler syndrome including the phenotypic variant of multiple familial trichoepitheliomas and correlation with the histopathologic findings in 379 biopsy specimens. Am J Dermatopathol. 2013;35(1):34–44.
21. Kazakov DV, et al. Multiple (familial) trichoepitheliomas: a clinicopathological and molecular biological study, including CYLD and PTCH gene analysis, of a series of 16 patients. Am J Dermatopathol. 2011;33(3):251–65.
22. Ponti G, et al. Brooke-Spiegler syndrome tumor spectrum beyond the skin: a patient carrying germline R936X CYLD mutation and a somatic CYLD mutation in Brenner tumor. Future Oncol. 2014;10(3):345–50.
23. Nasti S, et al. Five novel germline function-impairing mutations of CYLD in Italian patients with multiple cylindromas. Clin Genet. 2009;76(5):481–5.
24. Salhi A, et al. Multiple familial trichoepithelioma caused by mutations in the cylindromatosis tumor suppressor gene. Cancer Res. 2004;64(15):5113–7.
25. Zheng G, et al. CYLD mutation causes multiple familial trichoepithelioma in three Chinese families. Hum Mutat. 2004;23(4):400.
26. Kazakov DV, et al. Morphologic diversity of malignant neoplasms arising in preexisting spiradenoma, cylindroma, and spiradenocylindroma based on the study of 24 cases, sporadic or occurring in the setting of Brooke-Spiegler syndrome. Am J Surg Pathol. 2009;33(5):705–19.
27. Zhang J, et al. Impaired regulation of NF-kappaB and increased susceptibility to colitis-associated tumorigenesis in CYLD-deficient mice. J Clin Invest. 2006;116(11):3042–9.
28. Alameda JP, et al. An inactivating CYLD mutation promotes skin tumor progression by conferring enhanced proliferative, survival and angiogenic properties to epidermal cancer cells. Oncogene. 2010;29(50):6522–32.
29. Massoumi R, et al. Cyld inhibits tumor cell proliferation by blocking Bcl-3-dependent NF-kappaB signaling. Cell. 2006;125(4):665–77.
30. Antonescu CR, Terzakis JA. Multiple malignant cylindromas of skin in association with basal cell adenocarcinoma with adenoid cystic features of minor salivary gland. J Cutan Pathol. 1997;24(7):449–53.
31. Gerretsen AL, et al. Cutaneous cylindroma with malignant transformation. Cancer. 1993;72(5):1618–23.
32. Beideck M, Kuhn A. Malignant transformation of cutaneous cylindromas. 2 case reports and a review of the literature. Z Hautkr. 1985;60(1–2):73–8.
33. Braun-Falco M, Hein R, Ring J. Cylindrospiradenomas in Brooke-Spiegler syndrome. Hautarzt. 2001;52(11):1021–5.
34. De Francesco V, et al. Carcinosarcoma arising in a patient with multiple cylindromas. Am J Dermatopathol. 2005;27(1):21–6.
35. Durani BK, et al. Malignant transformation of multiple dermal cylindromas. Br J Dermatol. 2001;145(4):653–6.
36. Hammond DC, Grant KF, Simpson WD. Malignant degeneration of dermal cylindroma. Ann Plast Surg. 1990;24(2):176–8.
37. Iyer PV, Leong AS. Malignant dermal cylindromas. Do they exist? A morphological and immunohistochemical study and review of the literature. Pathology. 1989;21(4):269–74.
38. Korting GW, Hoede N, Gebhardt R. Malignant degeneration of Spiegler's tumor. Dermatol Monatsschr. 1970;156(3):141–7.
39. Kostler E, et al. Psoriasis and Brooke-Spiegler syndrome with multiple malignancies. J Eur Acad Dermatol Venereol. 2005;19(3):380–1.

40. Lausecker H. Beitrag zu den Naevo-epitheliomen. Arch Dermatol Syph. 1952;194(6):639–62.

41. Lotem M, et al. Multiple dermal cylindroma undergoing a malignant transformation. Int J Dermatol. 1992;31(9):642–4.

42. Lyon JB, Rouillard LM. Malignant degeneration of turban tumour of scalp. Trans St Johns Hosp Dermatol Soc. 1961;46:74–7.

43. Pierard-Franchimont C, Pierard GE. Development and neoplastic progression of benign and malignant cutaneous cylindroma. Ann Dermatol Venereol. 1984;111(12):1093–8.

44. Pingitore R, Campani D. Salivary gland involvement in a case of dermal eccrine cylindroma of the scalp (turban tumor). Report of a case with lung metastases. Tumori. 1984;70(4):385–8.

45. Pizinger K, Michal M. Malignant cylindroma in Brooke-Spiegler syndrome. Dermatology. 2000;201(3):255–7.

46. Rockerbie N, et al. Malignant dermal cylindroma in a patient with multiple dermal cylindromas, trichoepitheliomas, and bilateral dermal analogue tumors of the parotid gland. Am J Dermatopathol. 1989;11(4):353–9.

47. Tsambaos D, Greither A, Orfanos CE. Multiple malignant Spiegler tumors with brachydactyly and racket-nails. Light and electron microscopic study. J Cutan Pathol. 1979;6(1):31–41.

48. Volter C, et al. Cylindrocarcinoma in a patient with Brooke-Spiegler syndrome. Laryngorhinootologie. 2002;81(3):243–6.

49. Zontschew P. Cylindroma capitis mit maligner Entartung. Zentralbl Chir. 1961;86:1875–9.

50. Chou SC, Lin SL, Tseng HH. Malignant eccrine spiradenoma: a case report with pulmonary metastasis. Pathol Int. 2004;54(3):208–12.

51. Dabska M. Malignant transformation of eccrine spiradenoma. Pol Med J. 1972;11(2):388–96.

52. Engel CJ, et al. Eccrine spiradenoma: a report of malignant transformation. Can J Surg. 1991;34(5):477–80.

53. Fernandez-Acenero MJ, et al. p53 expression in two cases of spiradenocarcinomas. Am J Dermatopathol. 2000;22(2):104–7.

54. Galadari E, Mehregan AH, Lee KC. Malignant transformation of eccrine tumors. J Cutan Pathol. 1987;14(1):15–22.

55. Ishikawa M, et al. Malignant eccrine spiradenoma: a case report and review of the literature. Dermatol Surg. 2001;27(1):67–70.

56. Leonard N, Smith D, McNamara P. Low-grade malignant eccrine spiradenoma with systemic metastases. Am J Dermatopathol. 2003;25(3):253–5.

57. McCluggage WG, et al. Malignant eccrine spiradenoma with carcinomatous and sarcomatous elements. J Clin Pathol. 1997;50(10):871–3.

58. McKee PH, et al. Carcinosarcoma arising in eccrine spiradenoma. A clinicopathologic and immunohistochemical study of two cases. Am J Dermatopathol. 1990;12(4):335–43.

59. Swanson PE, et al. Eccrine sweat gland carcinoma: an histologic and immunohistochemical study of 32 cases. J Cutan Pathol. 1987;14(2):65–86.

60. Cancer Genome Atlas, N. Comprehensive genomic characterization of head and neck squamous cell carcinomas. Nature. 2015;517(7536):576–82.

61. Cerami E, et al. The cBio cancer genomics portal: an open platform for exploring multidimensional cancer genomics data. Cancer Discov. 2012;2(5):401–4.

62. Gao J, et al. Integrative analysis of complex cancer genomics and clinical profiles using the cBioPortal. Sci Signal. 2013;6(269):pl1.

63. Hershko A, Ciechanover A. The ubiquitin system for protein degradation. Annu Rev Biochem. 1992;61:761–807.

64. Komander D, et al. The structure of the CYLD USP domain explains its specificity for Lys63-linked polyubiquitin and reveals a B box module. Mol Cell. 2008;29(4):451–64.

65. Reiley WW, et al. Regulation of T cell development by the deubiquitinating enzyme CYLD. Nat Immunol. 2006;7(4):411–7.

66. Massoumi R. Ubiquitin chain cleavage: CYLD at work. Trends Biochem Sci. 2010;35(7):392–9.

67. Ke H, et al. CYLD inhibits melanoma growth and progression through suppression of the JNK/AP-1 and beta1-integrin signaling pathways. J Invest Dermatol. 2013;133(1):221–9.

68. Reiley WW, et al. Deubiquitinating enzyme CYLD negatively regulates the ubiquitin-dependent kinase Tak1 and prevents abnormal T cell responses. J Exp Med. 2007;204(6):1475–85.

69. Espinosa L, et al. The Notch/Hes1 pathway sustains NF-kappaB activation through CYLD repression in T cell leukemia. Cancer Cell. 2010;18(3):268–81.

70. Massoumi R. CYLD: a deubiquitination enzyme with multiple roles in cancer. Future Oncol. 2011;7(2):285–97.

71. Castresana, JS. Cancer as a Ciliopathy: The Primary Cilium as a New Therapeutic Target. Carcinogenesis & Mutagenesis, 2015. 6(6).

72. Moser JJ, Fritzler MJ, Rattner JB. Primary ciliogenesis defects are associated with human astrocytoma/glioblastoma cells. BMC Cancer. 2009;9:448.

73. Michaud EJ, Yoder BK. The primary cilium in cell signaling and cancer. Cancer Res. 2006;66(13):6463–7.

74. Yang Y, Zhou J. CYLD - a deubiquitylase that acts to fine-tune microtubule properties and functions. J Cell Sci. 2016;129(12):2289–95.

75. Bonilla X, et al. Genomic analysis identifies new drivers and progression pathways in skin basal cell carcinoma. Nat Genet. 2016;48(4):398–406.

76. Dijkhuizen T, et al. Cytogenetics of a case of eccrine spiradenoma. Hum Pathol. 1992;23(9):1085–7.

77. Deutsch, J., Sessile Serrated Adenomas and Melanosis Coli Visible Human Journal of Endoscopy, 2014. 13(1)

78. Massoumi R, et al. Cylindroma as tumor of hair follicle origin. J Invest Dermatol. 2006;126(5):1182–4.

79. Oosterkamp HM, et al. An evaluation of the efficacy of topical application of salicylic acid for the treatment of familial cylindromatosis. Br J Dermatol. 2006;155(1):182–5.

80. Rajan N, et al. Dysregulated TRK signalling is a therapeutic target in CYLD defective tumours. Oncogene. 2011;30(41):4243–60.

81. Saggar S, et al. CYLD mutations in familial skin appendage tumours. J Med Genet. 2008;45(5):298–302.

82. Bowen S, et al. Mutations in the CYLD gene in Brooke-Spiegler syndrome, familial cylindromatosis, and multiple familial trichoepithelioma: lack of genotype-phenotype correlation. J Invest Dermatol. 2005;124(5):919–20.

83. Lv H, et al. Three mutations of CYLD gene in Chinese families with multiple familial trichoepithelioma. Am J Dermatopathol. 2014;36(7):605–7.

84. Linos K, et al. Recurrent CYLD nonsense mutation associated with a severe, disfiguring phenotype in an African American family with multiple familial trichoepithelioma. Am J Dermatopathol. 2011;33(6):640–2.

85. van den Ouweland AM, et al. Identification of a large rearrangement in CYLD as a cause of familial cylindromatosis. Fam Cancer. 2011;10(1):127–32.

86. Almeida S, et al. Five new CYLD mutations in skin appendage tumors and evidence that aspartic acid 681 in CYLD is essential for deubiquitinase activity. J Invest Dermatol. 2008;128(3):587–93.

87. Blake PW, Toro JR. Update of cylindromatosis gene (CYLD) mutations in Brooke-Spiegler syndrome: novel insights into the role of deubiquitination in cell signaling. Hum Mutat. 2009;30(7):1025–36.

88. Ying ZX, et al. A novel mutation of CYLD in a Chinese family with multiple familial trichoepithelioma. J Eur Acad Dermatol Venereol. 2012;26(11):1420–3.

89. Liang YH, et al. Novel substitution and frameshift mutations of CYLD in two Chinese families with multiple familial trichoepithelioma. Br J Dermatol. 2008;158(5):1156–8.

90. Sima R, et al. Brooke-Spiegler syndrome: report of 10 patients from 8 families with novel germline mutations: evidence of diverse somatic mutations in the same patient regardless of tumor type. Diagn Mol Pathol. 2010;19(2):83–91.

91. Nagy N, et al. Phenotype-genotype correlations for clinical variants caused by CYLD mutations. Eur J Med Genet. 2015;58(5):271–8.

92. Ly H, Black MM, Robson A. Case of the Brooke-Spiegler syndrome. Australas J Dermatol. 2004;45(4):220–2.

93. Kazakov DV, et al. Brooke-Spiegler syndrome: report of a case with a novel mutation in the CYLD gene and different types of somatic mutations in benign and malignant tumors. J Cutan Pathol. 2010;37(8):886–90.

94. Pinho AC, et al. Brooke-Spiegler Syndrome - an underrecognized cause of multiple familial scalp tumors: report of a new germline mutation. J Dermatol Case Rep. 2015;9(3):67–70.

95. Zuo YG, et al. A novel mutation of CYLD in a Chinese family with multiple familial trichoepithelioma and no CYLD protein expression in the tumour tissue. Br J Dermatol. 2007;157(4):818–21.

96. Tantcheva-Poor I, et al. Report of Three Novel Germline CYLD Mutations in Unrelated Patients with Brooke-Spiegler Syndrome, Including Classic Phenotype, Multiple Familial Trichoepitheliomas and Malignant Transformation. Dermatology. 2016;232(1):30–7.

97. Huang TM, Chao SC, Lee JY. A novel splicing mutation of the CYLD gene in a Taiwanese family with multiple familial trichoepithelioma. Clin Exp Dermatol. 2009;34(1):77–80.

98. Reuven B, et al. Multiple trichoepitheliomas associated with a novel heterozygous mutation in the CYLD gene as an adjunct to the histopathological diagnosis. Am J Dermatopathol. 2013;35(4):445–7.

99. Heinritz W, et al. A case of Brooke-Spiegler syndrome with a new mutation in the CYLD gene. Br J Dermatol. 2006;154(5):992–4.

100. Kacerovska D, et al. A novel germline mutation in the CYLD gene in a Slovak patient with Brooke-Spiegler syndrome. Cesk Patol. 2013;49(2):89–92.

101. Hu G, et al. A novel missense mutation in CYLD in a family with Brooke-Spiegler syndrome. J Invest Dermatol. 2003;121(4):732–4.

102. Liang YH, et al. Two novel CYLD gene mutations in Chinese families with trichoepithelioma and a literature review of 16 families with trichoepithelioma reported in China. Br J Dermatol. 2005;153(6):1213–5.

103. Poblete Gutierrez P, et al. Phenotype diversity in familial cylindromatosis: a frameshift mutation in the tumor suppressor gene CYLD underlies different tumors of skin appendages. J Invest Dermatol. 2002;119(2):527–31.

104. Oiso N, et al. Mild phenotype of familial cylindromatosis associated with an R758X nonsense mutation in the CYLD tumour suppressor gene. Br J Dermatol. 2004;151(5):1084–6.

105. Hester CC, et al. A new Cylindromatosis (CYLD) gene mutation in a case of Brooke-Spiegler syndrome masquerading as basal cell carcinoma of the eyelids. Ophthal Plast Reconstr Surg. 2013;29(1):e10–1.

106. Zhang XJ, et al. Identification of the cylindromatosis tumor-suppressor gene responsible for multiple familial trichoepithelioma. J Invest Dermatol. 2004; 122(3):658–64.

107. Hunstig F, et al. A case of Brooke-Spiegler syndrome with a novel mutation in the CYLD gene in a patient with aggressive non-Hodgkin's lymphoma. J Cancer Res Clin Oncol. 2016;142(4):845–8.

108. Chen M, et al. Mutation analysis of the CYLD gene in two Chinese families with multiple familial Trichoepithelioma. Australas J Dermatol. 2011;52(2):146–7.

109. Malzone MG, et al. Brooke-Spiegler syndrome presenting multiple concurrent cutaneous and parotid gland neoplasms: cytologic findings on fine-needle sample and description of a novel mutation of the CYLD gene. Diagn Cytopathol. 2015;43(8):654–8.

110. Guardoli D, et al. A novel CYLD germline mutation in Brooke-Spiegler syndrome. J Eur Acad Dermatol Venereol. 2015;29(3):457–62.

111. Shiver M, et al. A novel CYLD gene mutation and multiple basal cell carcinomas in a patient with Brooke-Spiegler syndrome. Clin Exp Dermatol. 2016;41(1):98–100.

112. Melly L, Lawton G, Rajan N. Basal cell carcinoma arising in association with trichoepithelioma in a case of Brooke-Spiegler syndrome with a novel genetic mutation in CYLD. J Cutan Pathol. 2012;39(10):977–8.

113. Zhang G, et al. Diverse phenotype of Brooke-Spiegler syndrome associated with a nonsense mutation in the CYLD tumor suppressor gene. Exp Dermatol. 2006;15(12):966–70.

114. Amaro C, et al. Multiple trichoepitheliomas–a novel mutation in the CYLD gene. J Eur Acad Dermatol Venereol. 2010;24(7):844–6.

115. Scholz IM, et al. New mutation in the CYLD gene within a family with Brooke-Spiegler syndrome. J Dtsch Dermatol Ges. 2010;8(2):99–101.

116. Oranje AP, et al. Multiple familial trichoepithelioma and familial cylindroma: one cause! J Eur Acad Dermatol Venereol. 2008;22(11):1395–6.

117. Nagy N, et al. A novel missense mutation of the CYLD gene identified in a Hungarian family with Brooke-Spiegler syndrome. Exp Dermatol. 2012;21(12):967–9.

118. Espana A, et al. A novel missense mutation in the CYLD gene in a Spanish family with multiple familial trichoepithelioma. Arch Dermatol. 2007;143(9):1209–10.

119. Furuichi M, et al. Blaschkoid distribution of cylindromas in a germline CYLD mutation carrier. Br J Dermatol. 2012;166(6):1376–8.

120. Young AL, et al. CYLD mutations underlie Brooke-Spiegler, familial cylindromatosis, and multiple familial trichoepithelioma syndromes. Clin Genet. 2006;70(3):246–9.

121. Vanecek T, et al. Large germline deletions of the CYLD gene in patients with Brooke-Spiegler syndrome and multiple familial trichoepithelioma. Am J Dermatopathol. 2014;36(11):868–74.

122. Wang FX, et al. A novel missense mutation of CYLD gene in a Chinese family with multiple familial trichoepithelioma. Arch Dermatol Res. 2010; 302(1):67–70.

4

Oral and dental health in head and neck cancer survivors

Firoozeh Samim[1*], Joel B. Epstein[2], Zachary S. Zumsteg[3], Allen S. Ho[4] and Andrei Barasch[5]

Abstract

Therapeutic improvements and epidemiologic changes in head and neck cancer (HNC) over the last three decades have led to increased numbers of survivors, resulting in greater need for continuing management of oral and dental health in this population. Generally, the HNC patient oral health needs are complex, requiring multidisciplinary collaboration among oncologists and dental professionals with special knowledge and training in the field of oral oncology. In this review, we focus on the impact of cancer treatment on oral health, and the oral care protocols recommended prior to, during and after cancer therapy. The management of oral complications such as mucositis, pain, infection, salivary function, taste and dental needs are briefly reviewed. Other complications and their management, including osteonecrosis of the jaw and recurrent/new primary malignancies are also described. This review offers clinical protocols and information for medical providers to assist in understanding oral complications and their management in HNC patients and survivors, and their oral and dental health care needs. Oral and dental care is impacted by the patient's initial oral and dental status, as well as the specific cancer location, type, and its treatment; thus, close communication between the dental professional and the oncology team is required for appropriate therapy.

Keywords: Cancer treatment protocol, Cancer pre-treatment protocol, Oral hygiene, Oral complication management, Head and neck cancer survivors

Background

More than 600,000 cases of HNC are diagnosed each year worldwide. With evolving etiologies and advances in treatment, HNC survival has improved in recent decades and the population of HNC survivors continues to grow [1]. This increasing number of survivors raises additional challenges, particularly in the management of those patients who have complex medical, oral/dental, and psychosocial needs. Management of the oral complications in this population typically requires multidisciplinary collaboration among different professionals and healthcare providers, including head and neck surgeons, medical oncologists, radiation oncologists, and dental professionals with special knowledge and training in the field of oral oncology.

HNC may present with oral manifestations, which necessitates recognition and appropriate referral/treatment [2, 3]. Generally, therapy for malignant diseases affects the mouth both directly through cytotoxicity, and indirectly through the effects on immune function or other systemic side effects. Common oral complications include pain, mucositis, salivary gland dysfunction, taste loss/change, infections, dysphagia, fibrosis, soft tissue and/or bone necrosis, exacerbation of dental and periodontal diseases, and recurrent or secondary malignancy [4]. The incidence and severity of oral complications are affected by cancer treatment modality(s) used, anatomic location and stage of the cancer, extent of oral or dental diseases prior to treatment, comorbidities and genetic risk, oral hygiene and nutrition [5]. To effectively prevent as well as treat oral complications, dental professionals play important roles prior to, during and following active cancer treatment [6].

For HNC survivors, it is generally recognized that trained/experienced dental professionals serve as integral components of the multidisciplinary oncology team. These dental professionals can play a role in prevention of oral complications through patient education (improve oral

* Correspondence: f.samim@alumni.ubc.ca
[1]Department of Oral Medicine Oral Pathology, University of British Columbia, Vancouver, BC, Canada
Full list of author information is available at the end of the article

hygiene, maintain nutrition, reduce alcohol and tobacco use), treatment of dental disease, prophylactic strategies and treatment of oral complications, and early detection of oral malignancy in high-risk patients [7]. The related referral pathways are through dental and medical specialists with oncology experience [8]. This review focuses on the role of dental health care providers, and protocols of oral care in HNC patients.

Head and neck cancer treatment and its impact on the oral cavity

All treatment modalities for HNC produce oral complications, including surgery (e.g. mutilation and physiologic changes), radiation therapy (e.g. mucositis, dysphagia, hyposalivation, osteoradionecrosis), and neoadjuvant, adjuvant and/or concurrent chemotherapy (e.g. mucositis, taste changes, immune suppression) [9]. Additionally, newer targeted therapies may also result in oral mucosal complications [10, 11]. These medications include epidermal growth factor inhibitors, which cause erythematous mucosal reactions; tyrosine kinase inhibitors and mammalian target of rapamycin (mTOR) inhibitors, both of which may cause isolated aphthous-like lesions; and emerging immunotherapies, which may induce lichenoid reactions [12]. Given the commonality of oral complications of therapy, pre-treatment oral conditions may affect therapeutic options selected for some patients [2]. Additionally, the long-term oral sequelae of these treatments require oral and dental follow-up and fastidious long-term oral care.

Oncologists need to recognize the importance of pre-treatment dental care, and use available resources to effectively address oral needs [13]. For improved outcomes, it is imperative that a thorough oral assessment, implementation of basic oral care protocols, management of pre-existing dental conditions, and prevention and management of emerging oral complications be completed before HNC treatment. This is best accomplished by integrated teams with oncology-trained/experienced dental providers who provide timely dental treatment and preventive protocols that do not disrupt cancer therapy.

The following sections provide a summary of evidence-based guidelines related to oral/dental management in HNC patients, with the goal of improving health outcomes and enhancing long-term quality of life.

Before HNC therapy

It is important to be aware that some practicing dentists may have limited experience in care of the oncology patient, and that dental professionals with oncology experience may be required to identify and manage oral conditions and diseases in HNC patients [14]. According to the Multinational Association of Supportive Care in Cancer/ International Society of Oral Oncology (MASCC/ISOO) guidelines, thorough basic oral care is recommended to all

cancer patients for control of bacterial flora and reduction of inflammatory and/or infectious complications [15, 16]. Oral hygiene recommendations are shown in Table 1.

HNC patients should receive a comprehensive oral assessment prior to any cancer treatment, as soon as possible after diagnosis, and ideally, within 2 to 3 weeks prior to beginning cytotoxic therapy, in order to allow time for healing if surgical dental procedures are indicated [17–19]. The assessment should include full periodontal examination, radiographic examination, salivary gland functional assessment, and jaw range of motion measurement. Other treatments, such as non-surgical dental needs and stabilizing dental conditions can be completed as needed, or postponed until after cancer therapy, if deemed elective [20, 21].

Individual HNC patients should be managed according to cancer therapy-specific pre-treatment dental protocols [22]. Absence of symptomatic and occult oral disease is the desired goal, and elimination of acute and chronic infections that may require future surgical care is indicated prior to cancer therapy. Oral tissues within the high dose radiation fields must receive particular attention, as post-radiation surgery in this region may be risky. Custom oral devices (positioning/opening devices, midline blocks or anti-scatter trays) may be prescribed to minimize radiation exposure to oral structures unaffected by cancer and to assist in tissue positioning in order to support radiation exposure to movable tissues on a repeated basis. Compromises in timing and extent of dental treatment may be necessary, particularly when tumor burden is excessive, but generally, the healthier the mouth, the better the odds for good outcomes [21, 22].

During HNC treatment

It is essential that oncologists and other physicians involved in cancer care communicate with trained dental professionals in complex and unique cancer cases [23] so that necessary treatment is provided in timely fashion, unnecessary treatment is avoided, and preventive protocols are instituted. Even though cancer patients may be inclined to discontinue oral hygiene due to discomfort, the avoidance of basic hygiene results in increased microbial loads, gingival/oral inflammation and risk of infections. Thus, maintenance of oral hygiene should be encouraged. If oral hygiene is compromised during cancer treatment, the daily use of aqueous chlorhexidine 0.12 % solution can control the overall microbial load, including fungal and yeast overgrowth [24]. Devices built for prophylactic purposes (midline blocks, custom trays, etc.), must be used according to protocol.

Oral pain, predominantly due to mucositis, is one of the major symptoms in radiation therapy with or without chemotherapy. The biology of mucositis has been described and is leading to study of interventions based on the

Table 1 Oral care prior to and post cancer treatment in head and neck cancer survivors

Pre – Cancer Treatment	o Pre-treatment assessment 2–3 weeks prior to cancer therapy o Comprehensive head and neck, oral mucosa, dental and periodontal examination o Radiographs to assess dental and periodontal status o Baseline jaw range of motion (interincisal opening), baseline resting and stimulated saliva o Advanced caries, advanced periodontal disease: definitive treatment may require surgery with goal of 1–2 weeks of healing time o Periodontal debridement maintenance; oral hygiene instruction o Custom fluoride carriers, custom oral positioning devices
During Cancer Treatment	o Individual treatment as cancer type and planned treatment indications o Oral hygiene reinforced o Small carious lesions may be treated with fluoride and/or sealants; daily fluoride applications o Symptom management: Pain: topical analgesic and anesthetic agents; systemic analgesics; dry mouth: hydration, oral rinses and coating agents; lip management o Mucositis reduction: Patient education: o Regular brushing, flossing; prosthesis cleaning o Bland oral rinses, water based/wax or lanolin lip lubricant o Fluoridated toothpaste; or home fluoride trays daily in high risk patients o Soft toothbrushes; Electric or ultrasonic brushes for tolerated patients o Super-soft brush for severe mucositis or foam brush with chlorhexidine if brushing not possible o Dietary instruction; nutritional guidance, tobacco and alcohol avoidance
Post – Cancer Treatment	o Monitoring, prevention and management of oral complications (mucositis, dry mouth, mucosal pain, taste change, infection, dental demineralization, dental caries, periodontal disease, soft tissue/osteonecrosis etc.) o Checking for cancer recurrence or secondary primary cancer o Dental caries prevention, periodontal maintenance o Determine frequency of dental hygiene follow-up interval based on level of hyposalivation, demineralization/caries rate and patient's oral hygiene post-radiotherapy; patients with dry mouth, may require hygiene and recall every 3–4 months o Patient education o Fluoridated toothpaste; in high risk patients home fluoride trays daily o Good oral hygiene, soft toothbrushes or electric or ultrasonic brushes, flossing o Maintain lubrication of mouth and lips o Encourage non-cariogenic diet and cessation of tobacco & alcohol

pathogenesis of the condition [25]. For pain management due to mucositis, MASCC/ISOO recommends topical analgesic/anesthetic agents (e.g., lidocaine, benzocaine, diphenhydramine), or in severe cases, patient-controlled analgesia (parenteral morphine sulphate). Study of potential prevention of mucositis is ongoing, with recent suggestion for use of low-energy laser (LLLT), which may significantly reduce the severity and duration of mucositis [2, 14]. Medications that affect neuropathic pain such as gabaminergic agents (e.g. gabapentin), or tricyclic antidepressants (e.g. imipramine, amitriptyline) should be considered in addition to systemic analgesics [26]. Pain management strategies for this group of patients are summarized in Table 2. In

Table 2 Pain management Techniques in oncology (modified from Epstein et al.; Orofacial pain in Cancer; Part II- Clinical Perspective and Management; J Dent Res 86(6)2007

Palliative Radiation Therapy
Topical Analgesics/topical anesthetics
Systemic analgesics
Adjunctive medications (eg: Anxiolytics, Anticonvulsants, Antidepressant)
Physical and rehabilitative therapy: (massage/Physiotherapy; Cold/moist heat compresses)
Photobiomodulation/acupuncture
Psychologist support (Cognitive behavioral therapy, hypnosis)

addition, dietary instruction, frequent use of saline/bicarbonate rinses, and good oral hygiene should be addressed. Finally, a number of medical devices typically described as mucosal coating agents (eg: Biotene ®, Gelclair®, Mugard ®, Gelclair ® and others), has been cleared by the FDA but data supporting impact on mucositis are limited and no guidelines have been developed by MASSC/ISOO to date. Nevertheless, these over-the-counter coating agents may be soothing and promote temporary oral comfort.

In addition to mucositis, acute oral/dental infection during radiation therapy may be a cause for cancer treatment interruptions and excess morbidity. Extractions or other surgical procedures are not indicated during cytoreductive therapy. Hence, the alternative to surgical treatment is medical management, using antibiotics and analgesics that may control, but not resolve the infection, and create additional issues for the patient. Dental disease prevention must include regular daily fluoride applications, best applied via custom-made fluoride trays; when not able to be used (e.g. if severe mucositis develops), application by brushing on teeth or rinse application can be substituted. Fluoride application must be continued on a daily basis as long as dry mouth persists. In these patients, it is also important to provide a topical calcium source for the teeth in addition to fluoride. Special toothpastes (e.g. Enamelon ®) have been designed for this purpose.

Patient education is an integral part of dental treatment in order to support nutrition, reduce alcohol and tobacco use, and receive optimal oral care, which are important for both oral health and effective completion of cancer therapy [27, 28]. In addition, other factors such as taste changes, mucosal sensitivity, and xerostomia may negatively impact diet and nutritional intake, which may affect oral and general health. As a consequence, oral symptoms need attention from both oncologists and dental professionals in order to ensure timely diagnosis and appropriate treatment, as well as patient compliance with treatment recommendations.

Post HNC treatment

Cytotoxic treatment-induced oral complications can be severe, and impact not only the quality of life, but also cancer therapy outcomes. This can be challenging, as patients are known to under-report oral complications to their medical providers during and following cancer therapy. HNC patients should be monitored closely to reinforce prevention, early diagnosis and management of late complications, and optimal oral care to prevent these complications. Timely identification of cancer recurrence and/or metastasis, leading to early referral is also indicated [29]. Effective management of oral infection, residual mucositis, sensory changes (mucosal pain, taste change/loss), reduced/altered salivation, dental and periodontal disease, soft tissue/bone necrosis, and temporomandibular joint disorders must be integral part of post-cancer therapy care [30]. Follow-up dental visits should be tailored and individualized based on patient conditions. At least twice per year check-ups are recommended, although an every 2–3 month schedule may be indicated for some cases (Table 1).

Patients should be instructed in daily atraumatic tooth brushing, bland oral rinses, flossing and fluoride gel applications, as well as management of mucositis and other residual sequelae, based on the MASCC/ISOO evidence-based guidelines [2, 11]. Ultrasonic or electric brushes may be recommended, although soft or supersoft manual toothbrushes are standard [31]. Prescription toothpaste/gel with 5000 ppm fluoride are recommended for dentate patients, but if the patient cannot tolerate due to mucositis, fluoride rinses may be substituted for short periods; return to brushing with prescription toothpaste should be conducted as soon as possible and maintained for the duration of the patient's dentate life.

Patients skilled at dental flossing should be instructed to continue, avoiding trauma to the gingival tissue. Other interdental cleaning aids may be chosen if they are effective, and can be used atraumatically [32, 33]. Diet and supplements that are rich in carbohydrates, as well as sucrose-sweetened medications should be avoided, or when needed to support energy intake,

should be taken with meals, and may be best after oral hygiene is performed [34].

Management of specific oral complications related to HNC
Mucositis

Mucositis is recognized as a critical, dose-limiting toxicity of current HNC cytotoxic therapy and its prevalence approaches 100 %. Acute signs and symptoms typically develop during second or third week of therapy and may continue for weeks to months following completion of treatment, particularly in those patients treated with chemoradiation [35]. Chronic mucosal sensitivity may be increased in those who experienced severe acute mucosal damage [33]. Radiation-induced loss of stem cells in the basal layer interferes with the replacement of cells in the superficial mucosal layers when they are lost through normal physiologic sloughing. The subsequent denuding of the epithelium results in mucositis, which can be painful and interfere with oral intake and nutrition. Chemotherapy can have a similar effect on the mucosa. Patient education includes frequent use of non-medicated bland oral rinses, possible use of film forming, lubricating mucosal coating agents, and topical analgesics/anesthetics as needed. Mouthwashes with alcohol, foods with acidic or spicy qualities, and coarse or abrasive foods should be avoided [36, 37]. Thorough and consistent oral hygiene is recommended.

Active research continues to evaluate novel prevention and treatment approaches to mucositis for future clinical application. Current management is focused on palliation of symptoms with topical and systemic analgesics. It is also important to recognize that pain due to mucositis is related to tissue damage and inflammation, resulting in nociceptive pain, but also due to neuropathic sensitization (neuropathic pain), which can be treated with neurologically active medications such as gabapentin and doxepin [37–41].

Oral mucosal infections – viral, bacterial and fungal infections

Patient monitoring is critical in diagnosis of viral, bacterial and fungal infections. Diagnosis can be challenging during the period of mucositis, as there may be considerable overlap in signs and symptoms of mucositis and infection. Viral infections such as Herpes simplex virus (HSV), and other herpes viruses are common in patients treated with chemotherapy, while HSV reactivation is uncommon in HNC patients treated with radiation alone. Acyclovir and valcyclovir are considered equally effective in HSV prevention and treatment [42, 43]. Oral manifestations of viral infection may be more severe, with altered presentation and a more protracted course in cancer survivors. The more severe reactivation of

Varicella-Zoster virus (shingles) requires larger doses of antiviral agents, which may be combined with systemic corticosteroids.

Bacterial infection occurs most commonly in association with dental or periodontal infection that may worsen during cancer treatment. For suitable selections of antibiotics (begin on an empiric basis for oral and dental infection), bacterial culture and antibacterial sensitivity tests may be required due to potential shifts in oral colonization, particularly in hospitalized patients, and in patients not responding to therapy as expected [34].

Oral yeast infection, most commonly due to *Candida albicans* is found in 7.5, 39.1 and 32.6 % prior to, during and post HNC therapy, respectively [44]. Clinical presentation of oropharyngeal candidiasis may be variable and not easily recognized, presenting as white patches, erythematous patches or plaques, as hyperplastic candidiasis or mixed presentation [44]. Recognition of infection may be challenging due to multiple presentations and overlap with other mucosal changes such as mucositis. Other symptoms such as coated sensation in the mouth, burning sensation and taste change can be associated with candidiasis and should raise attention.

Topical therapy for local disease is always preferable, but systemic antifungals may be necessary in the setting of immune deficiency or loss of mucosal integrity. Oncologists need to be aware that topical antifungal agents have had inconsistent efficacy and some are high in sugar, which reduces efficacy and increases dental caries risk in dry mouth dentate patients. Antifungals that are not sugar sweetened (e.g. vaginal suppositories), and oral systemic agents are more effective [45, 46]. Furthermore, additional fungal species with increased resistance to antifungal agents are observed in cancer patients, and therefore the principles of culture and identification of the fungal species may be important to guide therapy, particularly in non-responding cases [44].

Other oral complications and their management

Other oral complications in HNC survivors are common. The key is to identify risk factors and early onset symptoms, and to offer referral for expert care. For example, HNC patients receiving cytotoxic chemotherapy and radiotherapy can have dry mouth or xerostomia that continues indefinitely due to reduced saliva production (hyposalivation) [47, 48]. Dry mouth is a common and significant chronic complication and drives late oral complications; some patients may accommodate to ongoing hyposalivation over time and may report reduced or even no symptoms. However, effects of reduced saliva on the health of oral tissues continue. Hyposalivation management includes assessment of saliva production, with first approach to treatment being stimulation of any residual function (chewing and taste stimulation, systemic sialagogues such as pilocarpine, civemiline, or bethanechol), and palliative topical products [49]. In addition to reduced production of saliva, changes in the quality of saliva, with thickened or viscous secretions can be challenging to manage, and trials of mucolytic agents may be considered (guaifenesin, acetyl-cysteine). Encouraging good daily oral hygiene, frequent dental visits, and dental fluoride and remineralization supplementation can help counteract the changes induced by insufficient salivation. For those patients with persisting hyposalivation, wetting of oral surfaces, and replacement of calcium, phosphate, and use of antimicrobial rinses have been shown to be safe and effective in relieving symptoms of dry mouth and minimizing infection potential. Dry mouth-associated taste change, gastrointestinal upset, mucosal sensitivity, inflammation and ulceration [50] significantly limit food intake, and may lead to dietary compromise that complicates nutrition and general health. Dry mouth increases risk of dental demineralization and tooth cavitation that can lead to rampant dental damage, increase risk for progression of periodontal disease and increase risk of osteoradionecrosis of the jaw (ORN). Dental sensitivity to temperature is also associated with lower saliva secretion and lower salivary pH. Oral burning sensation due to mucosal sensitivity is associated with hyposalivation and arises from peripheral neuropathy [2, 51]. In addition, 50–75 % of HNC patients have dysgeusia, which contributes to the reduction in quality of life. Radiation- and chemotherapy-induced neuropathies are associated with inflammation, neurotoxicity, oxidative stress, and ischemia, which may persist long after clinical mucositis resolved [52, 53].

Among other complications, ORN is a known risk following head and neck radiotherapy. It is associated with dental disease and dental procedures, but can occur spontaneously, without identified stimulus. This risk may be increased in people on medications such as bisphosphonates or denosumab for osteoporosis, people with diabetes, on immunosuppressives, and in tobacco users [54]. Prevention of ORN is the key concept and it reinforces the need for dental stabilization before cancer therapy, and continuing good oral/dental health in survivors. Management of ORN after onset must be individualized in coordinated dental and medical care.

Current treatment strategies are based on limited research and clinical anecdotes and thus, should be undertaken by experienced healthcare providers due to the complexity of care. Hyperbaric oxygen (HBO) therapy and use of antiseptic oral rinses, and sometimes antibiotics when secondary infection is diagnosed, has been the medical approach to therapy [55]. However, the use of HBO is expensive and controversial and no good evidence for or against it has been published. More recently medical management with local infection management and pentoxifylline and Vitamin E has been supported in phase II clinical trials [51]. If necrosis develops, continuation of these medications is recommended with the addition of clodronate to stimulate new bone formation [56]. As necrotic bone cannot be regained, the goal of treatment is prevention of progression, pain control, and management of secondary infection in hard and soft tissues (osteomyelitis, cellulitis). Surgical management with local sequestrectomy or vascularized tissue transfer may be needed [57].

Post treatment fibrosis is best managed by early recognition and physical therapy. Pentoxifylline and vitamin E has been suggested [58].

Recurrent or second primary oral malignancy is a known risk and people with prior upper aerodigestive tract cancer are the highest risk population for a post-treatment malignant lesion. Post-radiation mucosal changes can make detection of early changes difficult, and the potentially delayed healing in the high dose radiation fields make determination to biopsy more challenging.

Speech and swallow therapists and nutrition/dietary instruction are important aspects of care in the HNC patient, and these professionals are important part of the multidisciplinary HNC team.

Conclusion

The number of HNC survivors has increased, due mostly to change in risk factors for cancer (HPV), and advances in cancer therapeutics and supportive care. This growing population requires specialized oral care by personnel trained in managing the intricacies of these complex patients. Oncologists and dentists must collaborate to optimize care, as well as to increase knowledge of preventive and therapeutic options for oral health maintenance, oral cancer detection and suitable referral conditions with pathways. The oncology team should include dental professionals specialized in head and neck cancer survivor management, which will contribute to better oral complication prevention, detection, and treatment, and an improved quality of life.

Abbreviations
HNC: Head and neck cancer; HPV: Human papilloma virus; HSV: Herpes simplex virus; LLLT: Low-energy laser; MASCC/ISOO: Multinational Association of Supportive Care in Cancer/International Society of Oral Oncology; mTOR: Mammalian target of rapamycin; ONJ: Osteoradionecrosis of the jaw

Funding
Not applicable. There was no funding for this review paper.

Authors' contribution
FS and JE initiated the review paper, each author contributed to writing and review of the entire review paper. All authors edited, read and reviewed the paper prior to submission.

Competing interests
The authors declare that they have no competing interests.

Author details
[1]Department of Oral Medicine Oral Pathology, University of British Columbia, Vancouver, BC, Canada. [2]Samuel Oschin Comprehensive Cancer Institute, Cedars-Sinai Medical Center, Los Angeles, CA, USA. [3]Radiation Oncology, Samuel Oschin Comprehensive Cancer Institute, Cedars-Sinai Medical Center, Los Angeles, CA, USA. [4]Department of Surgery, Samuel Oschin Comprehensive Cancer Institute, Cedars-Sinai Medical Center, Los Angeles, CA, USA. [5]Department of Medicine, Weill Cornell Medical College, New York, NY, USA.

References
1. Baxi SS, Pinheiro LC, Pati SM, Pfister DG, Oeffinger KC, Elkin EB. Causes of death in long term survivors of head and neck cancer. Cancer. 2014;120:1507–13.
2. Epstein JB, Thariat J, Bensadoun RJ, Barasch A, Murphy BA, Kolnick L, Popplewell L, Maghami E. Oral complications of cancer and cancer therapy: from cancer treatment to survivorship. CA Cancer J Clin. 2012;62(6):400–22.
3. Islam NM, Bhattacharyya I, Cohen DM. Common oral manifestations of systemic disease. Otolaryngol Clin North Am. 2011;44(1):161–82.
4. Epstein JB, Raber-Drulacher J, Wilkins A, et al. Advances in hematologic stem cell transplant: an update for oral health care providers. Oral Surg Oral Med Oral Pathol Oral Radiol Endod. 2009;107:301–12.
5. Bethesda MD. Oral Complications of Chemotherapy and Head/Neck Radiation. National Cancer Institute. 2013. https://www.cancer.gov/about-cancer/treatment/side-effects/mouth-throat/oral-complications-hp-pdq#section/_13. Accessed 5 Oct 2016.
6. Sankaranarayanan R, Ramadas K, Thomas G, et al. Trivandrum Oral Cancer Screening Study Group. Effect of screening on oral cancer mortality in Kerala, India: A cluster-randomised controlled trial. Lancet. 2005;365(9475):1927–33.
7. American Dental Hygienists' Association. Access to care position paper. Chicago: American Dental Hygienists' Association; 2001. https://www.cdha.ca/pdfs/Profession/Resources/position_paper_access_angst.pdf. Accessed 5 Oct 2016.
8. Epstein JB, Güneri P, Barasch A. Appropriate and necessary oral care for people with cancer: guidance to obtain the right oral and dental care at the right time. Support Care Cancer. 2014;22(7):1981–8.
9. Perterson DE, Jensen SB. Oral complications of nonsurgical cancer therapies: diagnosis and treatment. In: Glick M, editor. Burket's Oral Medicine. 12th ed. Shelton: PMPH-USA, Ltd; 2014. p. 201–18.
10. Thariat J, Vignot S, Lapierre A, et al. Integrating genomics in head and neck cancer treatment: Promises and pitfalls. Crit Rev Oncol Hematol. 2015;95(3):397–406.
11. Jackson LK, Johnson DB, Sosman JA, Murphy BA, Epstein JB. Oral health in oncology: impact of immunotherapy. Support Care Cancer. 2015;23(1):1–3.
12. Ackson LK, Johnson DB, Sosman JA, Murphy BA, Epstein JB. Oral health in oncology: impact of immunotherapy. Support Care Cancer. 2015;23:1–3. doi:10.1007/s00520-014-2434-6.
13. Ganzer H, Epstein JB, Touger-Decker R, et al. Nutrition management of the cancer patient. In: Touger-Decker R, Mobley C, Epstein JB, editors. Nutrition and Oral Medicine. New York: Human Press, Springer; 2014. p. 235–53. https://www.youtube.com/embed/MnignqBw4CY. Accessed 5 Oct 2016.
14. Oral Complications of Chemotherapy and Head/Neck Radiation–for health professionals (PDQ®) https://www.cancer.gov/about-cancer/treatment/side-effects/mouth-throat/oral-complications-pdq. Accessed 5 Oct 2016
15. Lalla RV, Bowen J, Barasch A, Elting L, Epstein J, et al. Mucositis Guidelines Leadership Group of the Multinational Association of Supportive Care in Cancer and International Society of Oral Oncology (MASCC/ISOO). MASCC/ISOO clinical practice guidelines for the management of mucositis secondary to cancer therapy. Cancer. 2014;120(10):1453–61.
16. Elad S, Raber-Durlacher JE, Brennan MT. Basic oral care for hematology-oncology patients and hematopoietic stem cell transplantation recipients: a position paper from the joint task force of the Multinational Association of Supportive Care in Cancer/International Society of Oral Oncology (MASCC/ISOO) and the European Society for Blood and Marrow Transplantation (EBMT). Support Care Cancer. 2015;23(1):223–36.
17. National Institute of dental and craniofacial research; Oral Complications of Cancer Treatment: What the Dental Team Can Do. http://www.nidcr.nih.gov/oralhealth/Topics/CancerTreatment/OralComplicationsCancerOral.htm. Accessed 5 Oct 2016.

18. Epstein JB, Ransier A, Sherlock CH. Acyclovir prophylaxis of oral herpes virus during bone marrow transplantation. Eur J Cancer B Oral Oncol. 1996;32:158–62.

19. Jackson LK, Epstein JB, Migliorati CA, et al. Development of tools for the oral health and panoramic evaluation of the head and neck cancer patient: A methodological study. Spec Care Dentist. 2015. doi:10.1111/scd.12125. [Epub ahead of print].

20. Rankin K, Jones D, Redding S, et al. Oral Health in Cancer Therapy: A Guide for Health Care Professionals; third edition. 2008. http://www.exodontia.info/files/Oral_Health_in_Cancer_Therapy_-_A_Guide_for_Health_Care_Professionals_3rd_edition.pdf. Accessed 5 Oct 2016.

21. Schubert MM, Peterson DE. Oral complications of hema-topoietic cell transplantation. In: Appelbaum RF, Forman SJ, Negrin RS, Blume KG, editors. Thomas' Hematopoietic Cell Transplantation: Stem Cell Transplantation. 4th ed. Oxford: Wiley-Blackwell; 2009. p. 1589–607.

22. Lalla RV, Brennan MT, Schubert MM. Oral complications of cancer therapy. In: Yagiela JA, Dowd FJ, Johnson BS, Marrioti AJ, Neidle EA, editors. Pharmacology and Therapeutics for Dentistry. 6th ed. St. Louis: Mosby-Elsevier; 2011. p. 782–98.

23. Joshi VK. Dental treatment planning and management for the mouth cancer patient. Oral Oncol. 2010;46(6):475–9.

24. Elad S, Epstein JB, von Bultzingslowen I, Drucker S, Tzach R, Yarom N. Topical immunomodulators for management of oral mucosal conditions, a systematic review; Part II: miscellaneous agents. Expert Opin Emerg Drugs. 2011;16:183–202.

25. Villa A, Sonis ST. Mucositis: pathobiology and management. Curr Opin Oncol. 2015;27:159–64.

26. Epstein JB, Elod S, Eliav E, Jurevic R, Benoliel R. Orofacial pain in cancer: Part II-Clinical Perspective and Management. J Dent Res. 2007;86:6–506.

27. National Cancer Institute. Oral Complications of Chemotherapy and Head/Neck Radiation. Bethesda: National Cancer Institute; 2013. http://www.webmd.com/cancer/tc/oral-complications-of-chemotherapy-and-headneck-radiation-pdq-supportive-care—health-professional-information-nci-about-this-pdq-summary?page=2. Accessed 5 Oct 2016.

28. Ganzer H, Touger-Decker R, Parrott JS, Murphy BA, Epstein JB, Huhmann MB. Symptom burden in head and neck cancer: impact upon oral energy and protein intake. Support Care Cancer. 2013;21(2):495–503.

29. Kasperts N, Slotman B, Leemans CR, Langendijk JA. A review on re-irradiation for recurrent and second primary head and neck cancer. Oral Oncol. 2005; 41(3):225–43.

30. Bensinger W, Schubert M, Ang KK, et al. NCCN Task Force Report, Prevention and management of mucositis in cancer care. J Natl Compr Canc Netw. 2008;6(Suppl 1):S1–21.

31. Hong CH, daFonseca M. Considerations in the pediatric population with cancer. Dent Clin N Am. 2008;52(1):155–81.

32. Ransier A, Epstein JB, Lunn R, Spinelli J. A combined analysis of a toothbrush, foam brush, and a chlorhexidine-soaked foam brush in maintaining oral hygiene. Canc Nurs. 1995;18(5):393–6.

33. Keefe DM, Schubert MM, Elting LS, et al. Updated clinical practice guidelines for the prevention and treatment of mucositis. Cancer. 2007;109(5):820–31.

34. Hong CH, Napeñas JJ, Hodgson BD, et al. A systematic review of dental disease in patients undergoing cancer therapy. Support Care Cancer. 2010;18(8):1007–21.

35. Elting LS, Cooksley CD, Chambers MS, Garden AS. Risk, outcomes and costs of Radiation induced oral mucositis among patients with head and neck malignancies. Int J Radiat Oncol Biol Phys. 2007;68(4):1110.

36. Lalla RV, Sonis ST, Peterson D. Management of oral mucositis in patient with cancer. Dent Clin North Am. 2008;52(1):61.

37. Sonis ST. Pathobiology of oral mucositis: novel insights and opportunities. J Support Oncol. 2007;5(9 Suppl 4):3–11.

38. Epstein JB, Saunders DP. Managing Oral Mucositis Cancer Therapy. 2015. http://www.oralhealthgroup.com/features/managing-oral-mucositis-cancer-therapy/. Accessed 5 Oct 2016.

39. Epstein JB, Epstein JD, Epstein MS, Oien H, Truelove EL. Doxepin rinse for management of mucositis pain in patients with cancer: one week follow-up of topical therapy. Spec Care Dentist. 2008;28(2):73–7.

40. Saunders DP, Epstein JB, Elad S, Allemano J, Bossi P, et al. Systematic review of antimicrobials, mucosal coating agents, anesthetics and analgesics for the management of oral mucositis in cancer patients. Support Care Cancer. 2013; 21:3191–207.

41. Kataoka T, Kiyoita N, Shimada T, Funakoshi Y, Charahara N, et al. Randomized trial of standard pain control with or without gabapentin for pain related to radiation-induced mucositis in head and neck cancer. Auris Nasus larynx. 2016;43(6):677–84.

42. Reusser P. Management of viral infections in immunocompromised cancer patients. Swiss Med Wkly. 2002;132(27–28):374–8.

43. Arduino PG, Porter SR. Oral and perioral herpes sim- plex virus type 1 (HSV-1) infection: review of its management. Oral Dis. 2006;12(3):254–70.

44. Lalla RV, Latortue MC, Hong CH, et al. A systematic review of oral fungal infections in patients receiving cancer therapy. Support Care Cancer. 2010; 18(8):985–92.

45. Worthington HV, Clarkson JE, Khalid T, et al. Interventions for treating oral candidiasis for patients with cancer receiving treatment. Cochrane Database Syst Rev. 2010;7:CD001972.

46. Gøtzche PC, Johansen HK. Nystatin prophylaxis and treatment in severely immunocompromised patients. Cochrane Database Syst Rev. 2002;2:CD002033.

47. Nieuw Amerongen AV, Veerman EC. Current therapies for xerostomia and salivary gland hypofunction associated with cancer therapies. Support Care Cancer. 2003;11(4):226–31.

48. Epstein JB, Beier Jensen S. Management of Hyposalivation and Xerostomia: Criteria for Treatment Strategies. Compend Contin Educ Dent. 2015;36(8):600–3.

49. Turner MD, Ship JA. Dry mouth and its effects on the oral health of elderly people. J Am Dent Assoc. 2007;138(Suppl):15S–20.

50. Watters AL, Epstein JB, Agulnik M. Oral complications of targeted cancer therapies: a narrative literature review. Oral Oncol. 2011;47(6):441–8.

51. Saunders DP, Epstein JB, Elad SA, et al. For The Mucositis Study Group of the Multinational Association of Supportive Care in Cancer/International Society of Oral Oncology (MASCC/ISOO). Systematic review of antimicrobials, mucosal coating agents, anesthetics, and analgesics for the management of oral mucositis in cancer patients. Support Care Cancer. 2013;21(11):3191–207.

52. Dropcho EJ. Neurotoxicity of radiation therapy. Neurol Clin. 2010;28(1):217–34.

53. Cooperstein E, Gilbert J, Epstein JB, et al. Vanderbilt Head and Neck Symptom Survey version 2.0: report of the development and initial testing of a subscale for assessment of oral health. Head Neck. 2012;34:797–804.

54. Ruggiero SL, Dodson TB, Fantasia J, et al. American Association of Oral and Maxillofacial Surgeons Position Paper on Medication-Related Osteonecrosis of the Jaw—2014 Update. J Oral Maxillofac Surg. 2014;72:1938–56.

55. Bennett MH, Feldmeier J, Hampson N, Smee R, Milross C. Hyperbaric oxygen therapy for late radiation tissue injury. Cochrane Database Syst Rev. 2012;(5): CD005005.

56. Robard L, Louis MY, Blanchard D, Babin E, Delanian S. Medical treatment of osteoradionecrosis of the mandible by PENTOCLO: preliminary results. Eur Ann Otorhinolaryngol Head Neck Dis. 2014;131:333–8.

57. Gal T, Futran NC. Influence of prior hyperbaric oxygen therapy in complications following microvascular reconstruction for advanced osteoradionecrosis. Arch Otol Head Neck Surg. 2003;129:72–6.

58. Zecha JA, Raber-Durlacher JE, Nair RG, Epstein JB, et al. Low-level laser therapy/photobiomodulation in the management of side effects of chemoradiation therapy in head and neck cancer: part 1: proposed applications and treatment protocols. Support Care Cancer. 2016;24:2793–805.

Human papillomavirus-related small cell carcinoma of the oropharynx

Marcelo Bonomi[1], Tamjeed Ahmed[1*], David Warner[2], Joshua Waltonen[3], Christopher Sullivan[3], Mercedes Porosnicu[1], Katharine Batt[1], Jimmy Ruiz[1] and James Cappellari[4]

Abstract

Background: Small cell carcinoma (SCC) is a rare variant of head and neck cancer characterized by a high-grade neuroendocrine cancer with similar features to small cell lung carcinoma (SCLC). Human papillomavirus (HPV) is an increasingly recognized cause of head and neck cancer but usually associated squamous cell carcinoma of the oropharynx. In this report, we present the clinical presentation, diagnosis, and management of a patient with HPV-related SCC of the oropharynx that responded favorably to chemotherapy with cisplatin plus etoposide and concomitant radiation therapy, a regimen typically used in SCLC.

Case presentation: We present a rare case of a 56-year-old man who presented with a three-month history of an enlarging left-sided neck mass. Imaging was consistent with a soft tissue density at the left tongue base, left level IIB nodal conglomerate, and multiple bilateral cervical lymph nodes, without evidence of distant metastasis. The patient underwent a core biopsy of the left neck level II node which read as a poorly differentiated neuroendocrine carcinoma consistent with small cell carcinoma. Polymerase chain reaction revealed that the tumor was positive for HPV16. The tumor was staged T1N2cM0 (stage IVA). He went on to receive four cycles of cisplatin and etoposide. On cycle two, he started radiotherapy to the oropharynx and involved neck nodes. He received a dose of 70 Gray (2 Gy/fraction) over a seven week-period. During the concomitant phase of chemo-radiation, the patient experienced grade IV mucositis, grade II nausea, and dehydration for which he received additional outpatient fluid and electrolyte replacement. Three months after completion of therapy, a PET/CT showed complete resolution of the tumor and metastatic lymph nodes along with no evidence of distant metastasis.

Conclusion: Patients with HPV-related cancer of the oropharynx require identification of the small cell variant to optimize therapy and improve outcomes.

Keywords: Head and neck, Oropharynx, Chemotherapy, Radiation therapy

Background

Small cell carcinoma (SCC) is a rare variant of head and neck cancer characterized by a high-grade neuroendocrine cancer with similar features to small cell lung carcinoma (SCLC). The most common location of head and neck SCC is the larynx, but it has also been reported in the sinonasal tract, salivary glands, trachea, oral cavity, and oropharynx [1]. Human papillomavirus (HPV) is an increasingly recognized cause of head and neck cancer with HPV-associated oropharyngeal squamous cell carcinoma (OPSqCC) being the most common variant. Although HPV positivity is a favorable prognostic factor in OPSqCC, HPV-related SCC of the oropharynx may share the same aggressive clinical features of SCLC [2]. In this report, we present a case of HPV-related SCC of the oropharynx that responded favorably to chemotherapy with cisplatin plus etoposide and concomitant radiation therapy, a regimen typically used in SCLC.

* Correspondence: tahmed@wakehealth.edu
[1]Section on Hematology and Oncology, Wake Forest School of Medicine, Winston-Salem, NC 27157, USA
Full list of author information is available at the end of the article

Case presentation

A 56-year-old man with no history of tobacco use or alcohol consumption presented with a three-month history of an enlarging left-sided neck mass and worsening headaches. A positron emission tomography/computed tomography (PET/CT) showed an [18 F]fluorodeoxyglucose FDG-avid soft tissue density at the left tongue base measuring approximately 1.8 × 2 cm, a centrally hypodense hypermetabolic left level IIB nodal conglomerate measuring 3.6 × 4 cm, and multiple bilateral hypermetabolic cervical lymph nodes, without evidence of distant metastasis. Brain MRI was negative for brain metastasis.

The patient underwent a core biopsy of the left neck level II node which read as a poorly differentiated neuroendocrine carcinoma consistent with small cell carcinoma.

Core biopsy of the left neck level II node revealed sheets of malignant cells with small to intermediate-sized nuclei, indistinct nucleoli, and scant cytoplasm consistent with SCC. The tumor exhibited areas of necrosis as well as abundant mitotic figures and apoptotic bodies. The neoplastic cells were positive for cytokeratin AE1/AE3, synaptophysin, p16, and TTF-1 with a nuclear staining pattern; they were negative for cytokeratin 5/6, CAM 5.2, p63, chromogranin, CD56, and EBV (by in-situ hybridization) (Fig. 1).

The tumor was positive for p16, but the combined morphologic and immunophenotypic features argued against conventional HPV-associated OPSqCC. Polymerase chain reaction demonstrated that the tumor was positive for HPV16, negative for HPV18, 31, 33, 35, 39, 45, 51, 52, 56, 59, 66, and 68.

The tumor was staged T1N2cM0 (stage IVA). A percutaneous endoscopic gastrostomy tube (PEG) was placed before the beginning of treatment to meet his nutritional and hydration needs during treatment. He received four cycles of chemotherapy at 21 day-intervals. The chemotherapy regimen consisted of cisplatin 75 mg/m2 on day one and etoposide 80 mg/m2 on days one to three. On cycle two, day eight, he started radiotherapy to the oropharynx and involved neck nodes. He received a dose of 70 Gray (2 Gy/fraction) over a seven week-period. During the concomitant phase of chemoradiation, the patient experienced grade IV mucositis, grade II nausea, and dehydration for which he received

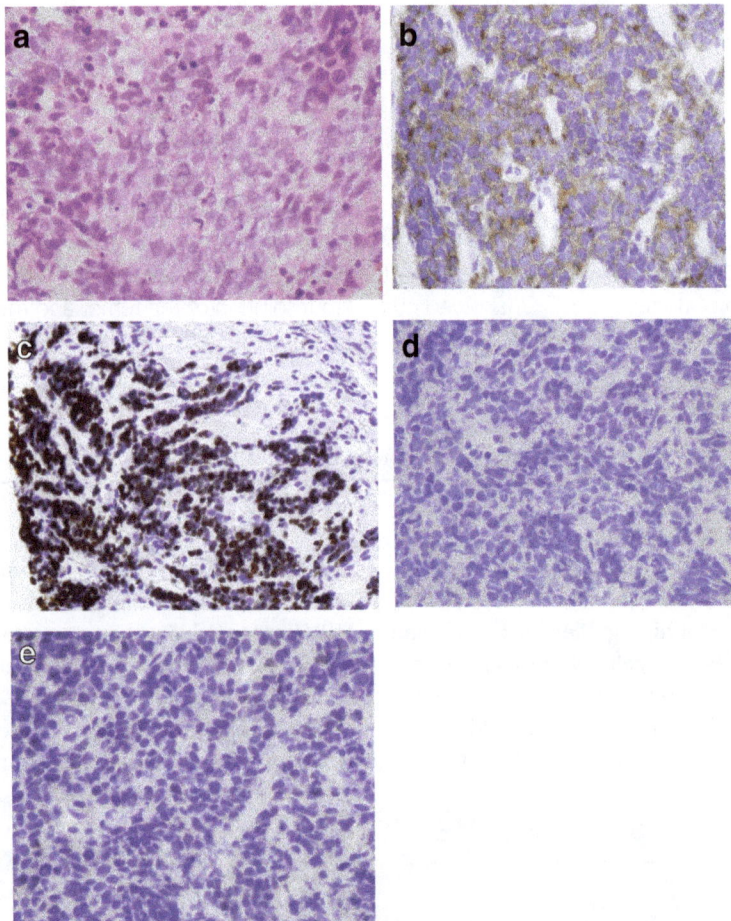

Fig. 1 a Hematoxylin and Eosin tumor stain. **b** Synaptophysin tumor stain. **c** TTF-1 tumor stain. **d** Cytokeratin 5/6 stain. **e** P63 tumor stain

additional outpatient fluid and electrolyte replacement. Due to grade III neutropenia, the dose of cisplatin and etoposide was reduced by 25% during the last cycle of chemotherapy.

Three months after completion of therapy, a PET/CT showed complete resolution of the tumor and metastatic lymph nodes along with and no evidence of distant metastasis (Fig. 2). He also had complete resolution of his mucositis and was able to resume a full oral diet resulting in removal of the PEG tube.

Discussion and conclusions

Small cell lung cancer is distinguished by its rapid doubling time, high growth fraction, and early development of widespread metastases. Although highly responsive to chemotherapy and radiation initially, the majority of patients will eventually relapse with broadly resistant disease a few months to a year from initial therapy. SCLC occurs almost exclusively in smokers and appears to be most common in heavy smokers. Historically, SCLC has been rare in non-smokers, representing just 2.9% of lung cancer cases in women and none in men as reported in a case control series [3].

High risk HPV, particularly the 16 type, has been established as a causative agent for a significant proportion of OPSqCC. These tumors typically originate from the tonsillar crypts and have a characteristic appearance described as infiltration of the lymphoid stroma as lobules of immature basaloid cells with minimal cytoplasmic keratinization [4].

Routine HPV testing of OPSqCC has expanded the morphologic spectrum of HPV-related cases. These histologic variants include papillary, lymphoepithelial-like, basaloid squamous, and adenosquamous. Although these phenotypic variations may be diagnostically relevant, they do not appear to impact prognosis. The presence of HPV consistently imparts a favorable prognosis, even when detected in more aggressive phenotypes such as the basaloid squamous cell carcinoma [5].

For patients with HPV-related cancer of the oropharynx, recognition of the small cell variant and its distinction from HPV-related squamous cell carcinoma is important although not straightforward. Both tumor types share morphologic features that include small hyperchromatic cells with scant cytoplasm and comedonecrosis [6]. Absence of p63 is often used to differentiate SCLC from squamous cell carcinoma of the lung [7, 8] yet in one case series 4 of 8 tested oropharyngeal SCCs were p63 positive suggesting poor reliability of this biomarker. Cytokeratin 5/6 on the other hand, seems to be a more reliable distinguishing marker [2]. In contrast to OPSqCCs that are consistently cytokeratin 5/6 positive, all SCCs are cytokeratin 5/6 negative. A minority of oropharyngeal SCC is TTF-1 positive which seems to signify high specificity for SCC in this setting [9]. In general, all SCCs demonstrate immunohistochemical evidence of neuroendocrine differentiation namely synaptophysin and chromogranin positivity [2]. In the case of SCCs of the oropharynx, p16 positivity may not be a reliable surrogate marker for HPV infection given that in one study, 2 of 4 SCCs were p16 positive but HPV negative by insitu hybridization. This is likely consistent with the finding of p16 positivity in many sites of SCC due to mechanisms unrelated to HPV infection [2, 10].

In SCLC, the most frequently used chemotherapy regimen is a platinum (either cisplatin or carboplatin) with etoposide based upon the clinical activity and toxicity profile of the platinum agent. Because both agents possess little mucosal toxicity, limited risk for interstitial pneumonitis, and modest hematologic toxicity, platinum plus etoposide is the regimen of choice to use with concurrent chest radiation therapy in patients with limited

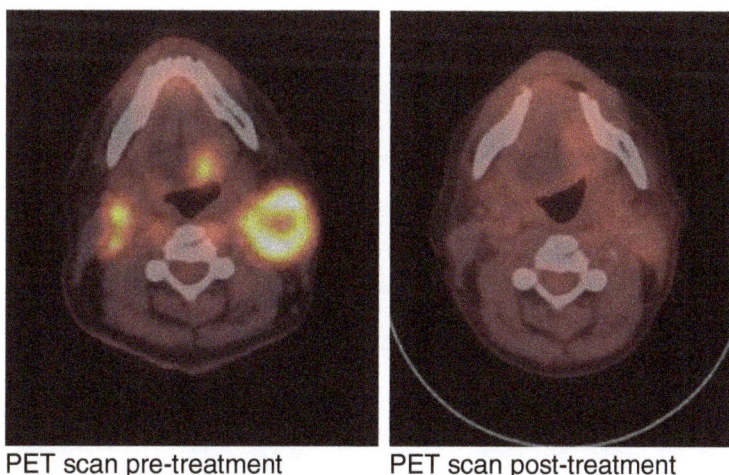

PET scan pre-treatment   PET scan post-treatment

Fig. 2 *Left* PET scan pre-treatment. *Right* PET scan post-treatment

stage SCLC. Due to its proven activity in SCLC and its favorable toxicity profile when used in combination with external radiation therapy, we decided to use this regimen for four cycles with concomitant definitive radiation. The patient's HPV status did not influence our treatment decision. We hope that HPV positivity portends a favorable prognosis in this case but from reviewing the few cases in the literature, it appears that these patients clinically behave similar to the aggressive nature of SCLC [11]. Further studies are needed to determine the pathophysiology of how HPV results in SCC, only then can potential molecular targets be discovered which will lead to the development of targeted treatments. In this patient, the regimen was proven to be active with manageable toxicities, but longer follow-up will be needed to determine true efficacy.

In conclusion, patients with HPV-associated cancer of the oropharynx require an accurate diagnosis to distinguish the more common squamous cell carcinoma from the rare small cell variant. This identification is vital in order to optimize therapy and improve treatment outcomes.

Abbreviations
HPV: Human papillomavirus; OPSqCC: Oropharyngeal squamous cell carcinoma; PET/CT: Positron emission tomography/computed tomography; SCC: Small cell carcinoma; SCLC: Small cell lung cancer

Acknowledgments
Not applicable.

Funding
This study had no funding.

Authors' contributions
MB, MP, and JR provided direct medical care of the patient and provided chemotherapy. TA, DW and KB contributed to manuscript. CS and JW provided radiation therapy to patient. JC assisted with the pathologic diagnosis and provided the figures. All authors read and approved the final manuscript.

Authors' information
Not applicable.

Competing interests
The authors declare that they have no competing interests.

Author details
[1]Section on Hematology and Oncology, Wake Forest School of Medicine, Winston-Salem, NC 27157, USA. [2]Internal Medicine, Wake Forest School of Medicine, Winston-Salem, NC 27157, USA. [3]Department of Otolaryngology, Wake Forest School of Medicine, Winston-Salem, NC 27157, USA. [4]Department of Pathology, Wake Forest School of Medicine, Winston-Salem, NC 27157, USA.

References
1. Renner G. Small cell carcinoma of the head and neck: a review. Semin Oncol. 2007;34(1):3–14.
2. Bishop JA, Westra WH. Human papillomavirus-related small cell carcinoma of the oropharynx. Am J Surg Pathol. 2011;35(11):1679–84.
3. Muscat JE, Wynder EL. Lung cancer pathology in smokers, ex-smokers and never smokers. Cancer Lett. 1995;88(1):1–5.
4. Westra WH. The changing face of head and neck cancer in the 21st century: the impact of HPV on the epidemiology and pathology of oral cancer. Head Neck Pathol. 2009;3(1):78–81.
5. Begum S, Westra WH. Basaloid squamous cell carcinoma of the head and neck is a mixed variant that can be further resolved by HPV status. Am J Surg Pathol. 2008;32(7):1044–50.
6. Serrano MF, El-Mofty SK, Gnepp DR, Lewis Jr JS. Utility of high molecular weight cytokeratins, but not p63, in the differential diagnosis of neuroendocrine and basaloid carcinomas of the head and neck. Hum Pathol. 2008;39(4):591–8.
7. Kalhor N, Zander DS, Liu J. TTF-1 and p63 for distinguishing pulmonary small-cell carcinoma from poorly differentiated squamous cell carcinoma in previously pap-stained cytologic material. Mod Pathol. 2006;19(8):1117–23.
8. Zhang H, Liu J, Cagle PT, Allen TC, Laga AC, Zander DS. Distinction of pulmonary small cell carcinoma from poorly differentiated squamous cell carcinoma: an immunohistochemical approach. Mod Pathol. 2005;18(1):111–8.
9. BM W, P D, SB K. World Health Organization Classification of Tumours Pathology and Genetics of Head and Neck Tumors. In: L B, JW E, P R, D S, editors. Neuroectodermal tumours. Lyon France: IARC Press; 2005. p. 66–75.
10. Yuan J, Knorr J, Altmannsberger M, et al. Expression of p16 and lack of pRB in primary small cell lung cancer. J Pathol. 1999;189(3):358–62.
11. Kraft S, Faquin W, Krane J. HPV-associated neuroendocrine carcinoma of the oropharynx: a rare new entity with potentially aggressive clinical behavior. Am J Surg Pathol. 2012;36(3):321–30.

6

Disparities in radiation therapy delivery: current evidence and future directions in head and neck cancer

Henry S. Park and Roy H. Decker[*]

Abstract

Background: Though treatments for head and neck cancer have improved in recent years, significant variation persists in the delivery of surgery, radiation therapy, and systemic therapy to patients throughout the United States.

Body: In this review, we explore the current evidence regarding radiation therapy utilization inequities across the spectra of race, socioeconomic status, and age. We also discuss hypothesized mechanisms for how non-clinical factors may influence shared clinical decisions between patients and providers. Finally, we suggest future directions for research in treatment disparities.

Conclusions: Radiation therapy continues to be delivered inequitably among certain subpopulations with head and neck cancer and other cancers. More research into the drivers of these disparities and interventions designed to address them are necessary.

Keywords: Disparities, Inequity, Race, Age, Insurance, Socioeconomic, Delivery, Radiation therapy, Radiotherapy, Head and neck cancer

Background

The multidisciplinary management of head and neck cancer (HNC) has advanced rapidly in recent years. Sophisticated conformal radiation therapy techniques like intensity-modulated radiation therapy and proton beam radiation therapy, surgical approaches like transoral robotic surgery, and targeted biologic agents like cetuximab have been increasingly utilized in combination with each other to maximize tumor control while minimizing toxicities. In the setting of the rising prevalence of HPV-associated HNC, much research is devoted to optimizing management strategies for every patient subgroup.

However, not all patients may have equal access to such advancements in cancer therapy, specifically radiation therapy. In this review, we explore the current evidence demonstrating radiation therapy utilization inequities across the spectra of race, socioeconomic status, and age. We first focus on HNC before expanding to evidence from other more common malignancies in

order to allow for a broader context. We also discuss hypothesized mechanisms for how sociodemographic factors may influence shared clinical decisions between patients and providers. Finally, we suggest potential future directions for research and interventions in this area.

Main text

Evidence of radiation therapy delivery disparities in HNC

One of the most heavily studied subjects in cancer treatment delivery disparity research has revolved around race. Two recent manuscripts have indicated differences in definitive treatment receipt by racial group for patients with HNC. First, Mahal et al. used Surveillance, Epidemiology, and End Results (SEER) database to determine that African-American patients with non-metastatic HNC were less likely to receive definitive treatment (surgery, radiation therapy, or both per National Comprehensive Cancer Network guidelines) than those who were not African-American (adjusted odds ratio 0.63, 95 % confidence interval 0.55–0.72) [1]. These results persisted in subsets of patients with cancers of the oral cavity, hypopharynx, nasopharynx, and larynx, but not oropharynx. In

* Correspondence: roy.decker@yale.edu
Department of Therapeutic Radiology, Yale University School of Medicine, 15 York St, New Haven, CT 06519, USA

a sensitivity analysis in which other-cause mortality was used as a proxy for comorbidity in multivariable logistic regression, the results did not change significantly. Second, Subramanian et al. also examined the effect of race on treatment receipt among Medicaid patients in California and Georgia with HNC [2]. After adjustment for demographics, stage at diagnosis, and tumor site, black race was not associated with differences in radiotherapy utilization, though it was associated with a lower likelihood of receiving surgery.

Medicaid insurance and lack of insurance have also been associated with disparities in treatment delivery in HNC. Inverso et al. reported that after adjustment for patient demographic data, socioeconomic factors, and tumor characteristics, uninsured patients with nonmetastatic HNC in the SEER database were more likely to not receive definitive treatment than those with any type of insurance (adjusted odds ratio 1.64, 95 % CI 1.37–1.96) [3]. Sensitivity analyses further categorizing insurance status found that patients with no insurance or Medicaid insurance were more likely to not receive definitive treatment than those with private insurance.

Appropriate receipt vs. inappropriate omission of radiation therapy is not the only factor affecting optimal treatment delivery. Prolonged time from cancer diagnosis to treatment initiation may have an impact on tumor control and mortality [4–6]. Murphy et al. noted significant variation in time to treatment initiation by race, Hispanic ethnicity, insurance status, zip-code-level income, zip-code-level education, and age among patients with HNC in the NCDB [6].

Another source of disparities in high-quality radiation therapy delivery may be access to advanced techniques like intensity-modulated radiation therapy or proton beam radiation therapy. Both modalities have been associated with significant improvements in toxicities and quality-of-life [7–9], with one retrospective study even suggesting a cancer-specific survival benefit to intensity-modulated radiation therapy over 3D-conformal radiation therapy [10]. Using the SEER-Medicare linked database, Sher et al. found that patients living in a census tract with higher median income were significantly more likely to be treated with intensity-modulated radiation therapy [11]. No difference in intensity-modulated radiation therapy utilization by race, sex, or age was noted in any of the three published SEER-Medicare studies on this subject [10–12]. The value of proton beam radiation therapy for HNC is currently under active investigation. Though there are no publications available regarding disparities in proton beam radiation therapy utilization in HNC to our knowledge, this is potentially a promising field of study in the future.

An increasing amount of data supports the hypothesis that radiation therapy by high-volume providers is associated with improved outcomes in HNC [13, 14] and multiple non-HNC malignancies like lung, cervical, and prostate cancers [15–18]. In HNC, two recent large national database analyses have noted disparities in access to high-volume providers, which may serve as another proxy for access to high-quality cancer care. First, Boero et al. found that in the SEER-Medicare linked database, white patients receiving 3D-conformal radiation therapy and intensity-modulated radiation therapy for HNC were more significantly likely to be treated by high-volume radiation oncologists than non-white patients [13]. Second, Wuthrick et al. reported that patients with private insurance were more likely to receive HNC treatment at high-accruing facilities into Radiation Therapy Oncology Group trials than those without private insurance [14].

Table 1 summarizes the primary themes of the disparities observed in HNC.

Evidence of radiation therapy delivery disparities in non-HNC malignancies

It should be noted that racial, socioeconomic, and age disparities in radiation therapy delivery are well-documented in non-HNC cancers, such as prostate cancer [19]. Based on SEER data, African-American patients were less likely to receive curative-intent therapy (adjusted odds ratio 0.82, 95 % confidence interval 0.79–0.86), especially among patients with NCCN high-risk disease (adjusted odds ratio 0.60, 95 % confidence interval 0.56–0.64) [20]. Filipino men were also less likely to receive definitive treatment in localized prostate cancer in a SEER study of Asian-Americans [21]. Among patients receiving definitive therapy, African-American men are more likely to receive radiation therapy but less likely to undergo surgery [20, 22].

In addition, Bledsoe et al. examined the effect of insurance status on treatment selection among nonelderly patients with prostate cancer in the NCDB [23]. Even after adjustment for race and other sociodemographic and clinical factors, Medicaid patients were less than half as likely to receive minimally invasive surgery and instead

Table 1 Summary of major themes associated with disparities in radiation therapy delivery

Disparity Theme	Evidence for Disparities in Head & Neck Cancer
1) Underutilization of Definitive Radiation Therapy and/or Surgery	Race [1, 2]; Insurance [3]
2) Delayed Time from Diagnosis to Radiation Therapy Initiation	Race, Ethnicity, Insurance, Age, Income, Education [6]
3) Underutilization of Advanced Radiation Therapy Techniques (i.e. Intensity-Modulated Radiation Therapy)	Income [11]
4) Limited Access to High-Volume Radiation Therapy Providers	Race [13]; Insurance [14]

were more than twice as likely to receive external beam radiation therapy compared to patients with private insurance. There were no differences in minimally invasive surgery and external beam radiation therapy utilization rates between patients with Medicaid insurance compared to no insurance at all. For prostate cancer patients who do receive radiation therapy in the National Cancer Data Base (NCDB) database, black and Hispanic patients were found to be significantly less likely to receive proton beam radiation therapy than white patients [24].

There is also evidence of disparities in treatment delivery beyond external beam radiation therapy in HNC and prostate cancer. Grant et al. examined patients in the SEER database to determine the association between insurance status and brachytherapy receipt [25]. The study showed that patients who received radiation therapy definitively for prostate and cervical cancer or postoperatively for breast cancer were less likely to receive brachytherapy if they had Medicaid coverage (odds ratio 0.57, 95 % CI 0.53–0.61) or no insurance coverage (odds ratio 0.50, 95 % CI 0.45–0.56) compared to those with non-Medicaid insurance. A SEER study of 3,851 black patients and 44,010 white patients with rectal cancer showed that black patients were significantly more likely to receive no radiation therapy for stage II to III disease (adjusted odds ratio 1.30, 95 % confidence interval 1.15–1.47) [26]. Older patients were less likely to receive the standard-of-care combination of radiation therapy with fluorouracil-based chemotherapy among 1,807 Medicare beneficiaries with stage II to III rectal cancer in the SEER-Medicare database [27]. Similar trends were noted in stage I to II breast cancer, as older women were less likely to receive optimal local treatment with radiation therapy and surgery [28, 29].

Potential mechanisms

We have now shown that sociodemographic factors may play a significant role in contributing to gaps in radiation therapy delivery. Disparities in radiation therapy delivery may be at least partially related to differences in referral patterns to radiation oncologists. The lung cancer literature has studied this feature most extensively. Goulart et al. analyzed data from 28,977 patients with stage III and IV non-small cell lung cancer diagnosed in 2000–2005 from the SEER-Medicare database linked with the American Medical Association Masterfile database [30]. On multivariable analysis, older age, black race, and female sex were associated with a lower likelihood of seeing all cancer specialists (medical oncologists, radiation oncologists, and thoracic or general surgeons). Seeing all three types of cancer specialists was predictive of a significantly higher likelihood of receiving National Comprehensive Cancer Network (NCCN) guideline-based therapies. Although these numbers were not explicitly

reported in the manuscript, our calculations reveal that the likelihood of receiving guideline-based therapies for patients with vs. without radiation oncologist referral was 64.1 % vs. 20.1 % for stage IIIA disease and 56.3 % vs. 6.3 % for stage IIIB disease.

Australian data by Vinod et al. also show disparities in radiation oncologist referrals [31]. Based on questionnaire data from diagnosing and treating clinicians for 1,812 lung cancer patients from New South Wales, the authors found significant underutilization of curative-intent radiation therapy to the primary site (20 % actual vs. 50 % optimal), especially in patients with limited-stage small cell lung cancer (46 % actual vs. 94 % optimal). Older patients were again less likely to be referred to radiation oncologists, as were patients who lived in areas that were not highly accessible by distance to major service centers based on the Accessibility and Remoteness Index for Australia. Patient sex did not impact referral patterns, while race and income level were not analyzed in this study.

Other reasons for disparities in radiation therapy delivery can be considered within a framework involving three broad categories: poverty, culture, and social injustice [32]. Barriers related to poverty and low socioeconomic status include the lack of a primary care physician, who would conduct screening and diagnostic follow-up; limited access to healthcare based on geographical inconveniences; competing survival priorities such as obtaining food, shelter, and safety; medical comorbidities; lack of adequate health insurance; lack of information and knowledge; and risk-promoting lifestyles, like poor nutrition and physical inactivity [33, 34].

Cultural factors, which reflect a set of learned and shared beliefs, values, traditions, world views, communication styles, and behavior common to a particular social group, can also play a large role in racial disparities in treatment delivery. Factors like spirituality, perceived susceptibility to cancer, cultural beliefs about cancer, and medical mistrust can be major barriers for certain cultural groups [33]. For instance, black women often consider themselves at lower risk for developing breast cancer than white women, even among those with a family history of breast cancer, which may translate into low perceived need for mammography or delays in seeking treatment for a breast abnormality [35]. There may also be a more fatalistic attitude regarding breast cancer treatment, less confidence in Western medicine, more confidence that spirituality and divine intervention are more effective in promoting cure, and a cultural norm against discussing breast cancer among certain cultural groups [36–39]. Traditional practices like Ayurvedic and Traditional Chinese medicine or Mexican herbal mixtures may or may not have beneficial or harmful effects on cancer treatment, especially regarding interactions with radiation therapy or chemotherapy. However, disclosure of this information by patients may be hindered by fear of receiving judgmental or dismissive comments from oncology providers, thereby excluding the potential of communication about these issues [34]. Patient-provider communication is also critical when addressing medical truth-telling at the end-of-life in certain family and community-centered societies, where practices of nondisclosure often persist due to cancer-related social stigma [34].

Social injustice, including factors like racial prejudice and discrimination, may also factor into racial disparities, but this relationship does not appear to have been as well studied as socioeconomic status or culture [32]. Provider perceptions of racial minority patients may affect quality of care, as physicians rated black patients with coronary artery disease as less educated and less likely to comply with treatment, even after adjusting for socioeconomic status [40]. In addition, black women were more likely to report a lack of physician recommendation as a reason for not undergoing mammography [41]. While it is certainly debatable whether or not these findings due to racial prejudice or other factors, perceived racial discrimination by patients may also play a role in differences in cancer incidence as well as treatment and satisfaction with care [42]. For instance, black women younger than 50 years who reported higher levels of racial discrimination in "everyday" experiences were at greater risk of subsequently developing breast cancer, since perceived racism could act as a chronic stressor that alters immune functioning and/or endogenous hormone levels [43].

Conclusions

Radiation therapy continues to be delivered inequitably among certain subpopulations with head and neck cancer and other cancers. Ultimately, it appears that the key to future research on treatment disparities in cancer lies upon disentangling apparent effects of race, poverty, age, education, and discrimination. It is also important to improve the measurement accuracy of specific indicators of socioeconomic status beyond broad measures of household income in a given zip code or census tract. In order to close these gaps, we must evaluate various communication practices in the way treatments are decided and patient autonomy is upheld.

We must also venture well beyond medical care itself. Patient education regarding high-risk behavior like smoking, obesity, and environmental hazards; programs facilitating travel to healthcare organizations; legislative action to improve access to healthcare; and general improvements in housing, schooling, and neighborhood safety must all be addressed before disparities caused by these factors can be minimized. However, it is still unclear if and how interventions addressing these areas could make a measurable difference.

With improving awareness of the complexity of this problem, there will hopefully be a growth in research infrastructure capturing this necessary data. More sophisticated analyses that account for these covariates will help clarify the most critical determinants of these disparities and to create and evaluate interventions on individual, locoregional, national, and international levels to address and eliminate them.

Abbreviations

HNC: head and neck cancer; NCDB: National Cancer Data Base; SEER: Surveillance, Epidemiology, and End Results.

Authors' contributions

HP drafted the manuscript. All authors (HP and RD) read and approved the final manuscript.

Competing interests

Neither Dr. Park nor Dr. Decker have any competing interests to report.

Disclosures

Dr. Park has received honoraria and travel expenses from Varian Medical Systems, Inc. (past). Dr. Decker receives research funding from 21st Century Oncology (ongoing) and Merck & Co., Inc. (ongoing), and has consulted for AMAG Pharmaceuticals, Inc. (past) and Leidos Biomedical Research, Inc. (ongoing). These funding sources had no involvement in the design, analysis, or preparation of the manuscript. The authors have no relevant competing interests to disclose.

References

1. Mahal BA, Inverso G, Aizer AA, et al. Impact of African-American race on presentation, treatment, and survival of head and neck cancer. Oral Oncol. 2014;50:1177–81.
2. Subramanian S, Chen A. Treatment patterns and survival among low-income medicaid patients with head and neck cancer. JAMA Otolaryngol Head Neck Surg. 2013;139:489–95.
3. Inverso G, Mahal BA, Aizer AA, et al. Health Insurance Affects Head and Neck Cancer Treatment Patterns and Outcomes. J Oral Maxillofac Surg. 2016; Epub ahead of print. doi:10.1016/j.joms.2015.12.023.
4. Neal RD, Tharmanathan P, France B, et al. Is increased time to diagnosis and treatment in symptomatic cancer associated with poorer outcomes? Systematic review. Br J Cancer. 2015;112 Suppl 1:S92–107.
5. McLaughlin JM, Anderson RT, Ferketich AK, et al. Effect on survival of longer intervals between confirmed diagnosis and treatment initiation among low-income women with breast cancer. J Clin Oncol. 2012;30:4493–500.
6. Murphy CT, Galloway TJ, Handorf EA, et al. Survival Impact of Increasing Time to Treatment Initiation for Patients With Head and Neck Cancer in the United States. J Clin Oncol. 2016;34:169–78.
7. Kam MK, Leung SF, Zee B, et al. Prospective randomized study of intensity-modulated radiotherapy on salivary gland function in early-stage nasopharyngeal carcinoma patients. J Clin Oncol. 2007;25:4873–9.
8. Nutting CM, Morden JP, Harrington KJ, et al. Parotid-sparing intensity modulated versus conventional radiotherapy in head and neck cancer (PARSPORT): a phase 3 multicentre randomised controlled trial. Lancet Oncol. 2011;12:127–36.
9. Romesser PB, Cahlon O, Scher E, et al. Proton beam radiation therapy results in significantly reduced toxicity compared with intensity-modulated radiation therapy for head and neck tumors that require ipsilateral radiation. Radiother Oncol. 2016;118:286–92.

10. Beadle BM, Liao KP, Elting LS, et al. Improved survival using intensity-modulated radiation therapy in head and neck cancers: a SEER-Medicare analysis. Cancer. 2014;120:702–10.

11. Sher DJ, Neville BA, Chen AB, et al. Predictors of IMRT and conformal radiotherapy use in head and neck squamous cell carcinoma: a SEER-Medicare analysis. Int J Radiat Oncol Biol Phys. 2011;81:e197–206.

12. Yu JB, Soulos PR, Sharma R, et al. Patterns of care and outcomes associated with intensity-modulated radiation therapy versus conventional radiation therapy for older patients with head-and-neck cancer. Int J Radiat Oncol Biol Phys. 2012;83:e101–7.

13. Boero IJ, Paravati AJ, Xu B, et al. Importance of Radiation Oncologist Experience Among Patients With Head-and-Neck Cancer Treated With Intensity-Modulated Radiation Therapy. J Clin Oncol. 2016;34:684–90.

14. Wuthrick EJ, Zhang Q, Machtay M, et al. Institutional clinical trial accrual volume and survival of patients with head and neck cancer. J Clin Oncol. 2015;33:156–64.

15. Chen AB, D'Amico AV, Neville BA, et al. Provider case volume and outcomes following prostate brachytherapy. J Urol. 2009;181:113–8. discussion 118.

16. Chen YW, Mahal BA, Muralidhar V, et al. Association Between Treatment at a High-Volume Facility and Improved Survival for Radiation-Treated Men With High-Risk Prostate Cancer. Int J Radiat Oncol Biol Phys. 2016;94:683–90.

17. Wang EH, Rutter CE, Corso CD, et al. Patients Selected for Definitive Concurrent Chemoradiation at High-volume Facilities Achieve Improved Survival in Stage III Non-Small-Cell Lung Cancer. J Thorac Oncol. 2015;10:937–43.

18. Lin JF, Berger JL, Krivak TC, et al. Impact of facility volume on therapy and survival for locally advanced cervical cancer. Gynecol Oncol. 2014;132:416–22.

19. McGinley KF, Tay KJ, Moul JW. Prostate cancer in men of African origin. Nat Rev Urol. 2016;13:99–107.

20. Mahal BA, Aizer AA, Ziehr DR, et al. Trends in disparate treatment of African American men with localized prostate cancer across National Comprehensive Cancer Network risk groups. Urology. 2014;84:386–92.

21. Chao GF, Krishna N, Aizer AA, et al. Asian Americans and prostate cancer: A nationwide population-based analysis. Urol Oncol. 2016;34:233.e7–233.e15.

22. Moses KA, Paciorek AT, Penson DF, et al. Impact of ethnicity on primary treatment choice and mortality in men with prostate cancer: data from CaPSURE. J Clin Oncol. 2010;28:1069–74.

23. Bledsoe TJ, Park HS, Rutter CE, et al. Minimally invasive surgery and external beam radiation therapy selection for prostate cancer varies significantly by health insurance status. Int J Radiat Oncol Biol Phys. 2015;93:e358–59.

24. Mahal BA, Chen YW, Efstathiou JA, et al. National trends and determinants of proton therapy use for prostate cancer: A National Cancer Data Base study. Cancer. 2016;122:1505–12.

25. Grant SR, Walker GV, Koshy M, et al. Impact of Insurance Status on Radiation Treatment Modality Selection Among Potential Candidates for Prostate, Breast, or Gynecologic Brachytherapy. Int J Radiat Oncol Biol Phys. 2015;93:968–75.

26. Morris AM, Billingsley KG, Baxter NN, et al. Racial disparities in rectal cancer treatment: a population-based analysis. Arch Surg. 2004;139:151–5. discussion 156.

27. Neugut AI, Fleischauer AT, Sundararajan V, et al. Use of adjuvant chemotherapy and radiation therapy for rectal cancer among the elderly: a population-based study. J Clin Oncol. 2002;20:2643–50.

28. August DA, Rea T, Sondak VK. Age-related differences in breast cancer treatment. Ann Surg Oncol. 1994;1:45–52.

29. Ayanian JZ, Guadagnoli E. Variations in breast cancer treatment by patient and provider characteristics. Breast Cancer Res Treat. 1996;40:65–74.

30. Goulart BH, Reyes CM, Fedorenko CR, et al. Referral and treatment patterns among patients with stages III and IV non-small-cell lung cancer. J Oncol Pract. 2013;9:42–50.

31. Vinod SK, Simonella L, Goldsbury D, et al. Underutilization of radiotherapy for lung cancer in New South Wales, Australia. Cancer. 2010;116:686–94.

32. Freeman HP, Chu KC. Determinants of cancer disparities: barriers to cancer screening, diagnosis, and treatment. Surg Oncol Clin N Am. 2005;14:655–69.

33. Gerend MA, Pai M. Social determinants of Black-White disparities in breast cancer mortality: a review. Cancer Epidemiol Biomarkers Prev. 2008;17:2913–23.

34. Kagawa-Singer M, Dadia AV, Yu MC, et al. Cancer, culture, and health disparities: time to chart a new course? CA Cancer J Clin. 2010;60:12–39.

35. Lannin DR, Mathews HF, Mitchell J, et al. Influence of socioeconomic and cultural factors on racial differences in late-stage presentation of breast cancer. JAMA. 1998;279:1801–7.

36. Lannin DR, Mathews HF, Mitchell J, et al. Impacting cultural attitudes in African-American women to decrease breast cancer mortality. Am J Surg. 2002;184:418–23.

37. Phillips JM, Cohen MZ, Tarzian AJ. African American women's experiences with breast cancer screening. J Nurs Scholarsh. 2001;33:135–40.

38. Johnson KS, Elbert-Avila KI, Tulsky JA. The influence of spiritual beliefs and practices on the treatment preferences of African Americans: a review of the literature. J Am Geriatr Soc. 2005;53:711–9.

39. George M, Margolis ML. Race and lung cancer surgery–a qualitative analysis of relevant beliefs and management preferences. Oncol Nurs Forum. 2010;37:740–8.

40. van Ryn M, Burke J. The effect of patient race and socio-economic status on physicians' perceptions of patients. Soc Sci Med. 2000;50:813–28.

41. Vernon SW, Vogel VG, Halabi S, et al. Factors associated with perceived risk of breast cancer among women attending a screening program. Breast Cancer Res Treat. 1993;28:137–44.

42. Mandelblatt JS, Edge SB, Meropol NJ, et al. Predictors of long-term outcomes in older breast cancer survivors: perceptions versus patterns of care. J Clin Oncol. 2003;21:855–63.

43. Taylor TR, Williams CD, Makambi KH, et al. Racial discrimination and breast cancer incidence in US Black women: the Black Women's Health Study. Am J Epidemiol. 2007;166:46–54.

7

Outcomes for patients with head and neck squamous cell carcinoma presenting with N3 nodal disease

Matthew E. Witek[1]* (iD), Aaron M. Wieland[2], Shuai Chen[3], Tabassum A. Kennedy[4], Craig R. Hullett[1], Evan Liang[5], Gregory K. Hartig[2], Randy J. Kimple[1] and Paul M. Harari[1]

Abstract

Background: The present study evaluated clinical outcomes for patients with head and neck squamous cell carcinoma presenting with N3 nodal disease.

Methods: A retrospective analysis of N3 head and neck squamous cell carcinoma patients was performed. Pearson chi-square and Wilcoxon signed-rank tests were used to analyze patient demographics, disease characteristics, and treatment variables. Survival was evaluated using Kaplan-Meier curves with the log-rank test. Univariate analysis using Cox proportional hazards models was used to define factors associated with overall survival. Patient and tumor characteristics associated with treatment assignments were analyzed by univariate multinomial logistic regression.

Results: We identified 36 patients with radiographically-defined N3 disease. For the entire cohort, median follow-up was 23.6 (range 2.8–135.0) months, and overall survival was 60% at 2 years and 30% at 5 years. Overall survival was similar between patients receiving primary surgery, radiotherapy, or chemoradiotherapy ($p = 0.10$). Primary, regional, and distant control at 5 years was 71%, 66%, and 53%, respectively. There was a trend towards improved regional control with primary surgery ($p = 0.07$). Planned neck dissection following primary chemoradiotherapy did not improve regional control ($p = 0.55$). Patients with p16-positive tumors exhibited improved overall ($p = 0.05$) and metastatic recurrence-free survival ($p < 0.05$). There were no factors predictive of treatment assignment nor factors associated with overall survival, local and regional control, or distant metastases free-survival on univariate analysis.

Conclusions: Patients with N3 head and neck squamous cell carcinoma exhibit 5-year overall survival rates of approximately 30% regardless of treatment modality. Planned neck dissection does not improve regional control in patients undergoing definitive chemoradiotherapy. p16-positive patients represent a favorable cohort. Distant failure comprises the major failure pattern and should be the focus of future studies in improving the outcome of this patient cohort.

Keywords: Head and neck cancer, N3 nodal staging, Surgery, Radiation, Chemotherapy

* Correspondence: mattewitek@gmail.com
[1]Department of Human Oncology, University of Wisconsin, 600 Highland Avenue, K4/B100-0600, Madison, WI, Madison, WI 53792, USA
Full list of author information is available at the end of the article

Background

There is controversy regarding the optimum treatment of patients with head and neck squamous cell carcinoma and N3 nodal disease (N3 HNSCC). The variability in treatment approaches reflects the paucity of level one data to guide decision making as limited numbers of patients with N3 disease are included in randomized controlled trials meant to establish standards of care [1–6]. The rarity of inclusion of patients with N3 disease is notable in a recently completed randomized controlled trial in which only 11% of patients enrolled had N3 disease despite this being a stated goal of study accrual [3]. Clinical management of N3 HNSCC patients is typically influenced by case series that may reflect institutional bias, patient selection, and disease characteristics. Despite these confounders, the majority of data suggests that favorable rates of locoregional control can be achieved although there remains a high rate of distant metastatic disease approaching 40% [7–11].

The current study evaluates the long-term outcomes of patients with N3 HNSCC treated with either primary surgery, radiotherapy, or chemoradiotherapy approaches, compares treatment-specific toxicities, and evaluates the clinical impact of p16 status on N3 oropharyngeal squamous cell primary tumors.

Methods

Study population

Data collection for this retrospective analysis was approved by the University of Wisconsin-Madison Institutional Review Board. Patients included in the head and neck data base gave approval and written consent for usage of their information for research purposes. We identified 74 patients with N3 HNSCC treated at the University of Wisconsin-Madison from 1991 to 2015. Thirteen patients were excluded for having non-squamous cell histology, 3 for having distant metastatic disease at presentation, 3 for undergoing palliative intent treatment, 2 for having N2b disease, and 17 for not having cross-sectional imaging available for review. The final cohort consisted of 36 patients with either oral cavity, oropharyngeal, hypopharyngeal, laryngeal, or unknown primary squamous cell carcinoma with N3 disease (> 6 cm) as determined by radiographic assessment. Clinical records were reviewed in order to obtain patient characteristics, TNM classification, primary tumor site, radiographic nodal characteristics, p16 status (used as a surrogate for high-risk human papillomavirus (HPV) infection), primary and adjuvant treatment modalities, time to local, regional, and distant failures, and death.

Statistical analysis

Standard descriptive statistics were used to analyze the distribution of covariates throughout the patient cohort. All of the baseline patient demographics and characteristics were analyzed using Pearson chi-square tests, and the Wilcoxon signed-rank test was used to test the continuous variables age, radiation dose, fraction size, and nodal volume. Survival was evaluated using Kaplan-Meier curves. The log-rank test was used to compare overall survival among the different treatment groups. Univariate analysis using Cox proportional hazards models was utilized to determine factors associated with overall survival. Univariate multinomial logistic regression was applied to patient and tumor characteristics to examine factors associated with treatment assignments. Statistical analyses were performed using SAS 9.4 (SAS Institute Inc., Cary, NC). All p-values were two-sided, and a $p \leq 0.05$ was considered statistically significant for all analyses.

Radiographic analysis

The computed tomographic images of each patient were retrospectively analyzed by a board certified neuroradiologist (TK) specializing in head and neck imaging. The largest abnormal nodal mass was identified in each patient and was measured in craniocaudal, anterior-posterior and transverse planes. Nodal volume was estimated by the ellipsoid calculation with which volume is approximated as half the product of the maximum dimensions in each axis (volume $\approx \frac{1}{2} x X y X z$).

Therapy

All patients included in this analysis had a performance status that permitted curative therapy. Treatment recommendations were made through group consensus at a Head and Neck tumor board attended by Head and Neck Surgery, Radiation Oncology, Medical Oncology, Radiology, and Pathology. Patients treated prior to 2001 received definitive radiotherapy (RT) given the standard of care of the time. Following 2001 patients typically received concurrent chemoradiotherapy (CRT) given randomized data supporting its superiority to RT alone [12]. RT was delivered by either Tomotherapy-based intensity modulated radiotherapy (IMRT) or 3D conformal technique using lateral photon fields supplemented with a matched low neck anterior-posterior photon field and nodal boosting with posterior neck electron fields. When given concurrently with chemotherapy, approximately 67% of patients received 70 Gy in 33 fractions of 2.12 Gy while the remaining 33% received 70 Gy in 35 fractions of 2 Gy. If chemotherapy was not utilized, radiotherapy was often given in BID (twice per day) fractions of 1.2–1.53 Gy to a total dose of 69.9–74.6 Gy. Varying low and intermediate risk dose and fractionation schemes approximating 54 Gy and 60 Gy, respectively, were used at the treating radiation oncologist's discretion. Treatment volumes included gross disease and nodal volumes II, III, IV, and at the treating radiation oncologist's discretion, lateral retropharyngeal lymph nodes, levels IB and V. The majority of patients received weekly concurrent cisplatin chemotherapy at 30 mg/m^2. Cetuximab or cisplatin-docetaxel doublet were used occasionally. Radical, modified radical, or selective neck dissections were performed at the head and neck surgeon's discretion.

Results

Patient, tumor, and treatment characteristics

We identified 36 patients with N3 HNSCC treated definitively from 1991 to 2015 at the University of Wisconsin-Madison that were followed for a median of 23.6 (range 2.8–135.0) months. Patient, tumor, and treatment characteristics are detailed in Table 1. Oropharyngeal tumors comprised 67% of the cohort representing the most common primary site. Of the 68% of oropharyngeal primaries that were stained for p16, 67% were positive. Unknown primary (11%), hypopharynx (11%), larynx (8%), and oral cavity (3%) were less common. Primary tumor stages were well represented. Median nodal volume was 42.7 (range 15.9–194.8) cm^3 and was similar between all treatment cohorts ($p = 0.88$). Fifty-six percent of patients underwent primary CRT and 22% received either primary surgery or RT. Planned neck dissections were performed in 55% and 62% of patients receiving primary CRT or RT, respectively ($p = 0.27$).

Treatment assignments

We evaluated patient and disease factors associated with receipt of treatment. Using surgery as the dependent variable, odds ratios were created and are shown in Table 2. In comparing RT with surgery and CRT with surgery, we were unable to identify any specific factor including age, T-stage, p16-status, and nodal volume that significantly predicted for treatment receipt.

Treatment outcomes

Clinical outcomes for the entire cohort are shown in Fig. 1. Overall survival at 2 and 5 years for the entire cohort was 60% and 30%, respectively. Local control was 86% and 71% and regional control was 77% and 66% at 2 and 5 years, respectively. Distant metastases disease free survival at 5 years was 53% (Fig. 1a-d).

Clinical outcomes were next evaluated in context of the primary treatment modality for either surgery, RT, or CRT. There were no statistically significant differences in overall survival, local-, regional-, and metastases-free survival ($p = 0.10$, $p = 0.60$, $p = 0.07$, $p = 0.90$, respectively) (Fig. 2a-d). Planned neck dissection did not impact

regional recurrence-free survival following definitive CRT with approximately 70% being regionally controlled at 5 years ($p = 0.55$) (Fig. 3). Within the subset of patients with oropharyngeal primary tumors, p16 positivity conferred a survival advantage with 2-year overall survivals of 65% and 20% for p16-positive and p16-negative disease, respectively ($p < 0.05$) (Fig. 4a). Metastatic recurrence-free survival was also significantly different between patients with p16-positive and p16-negative oropharyngeal primaries (p < 0.05) (Fig. 4b).

The median time to the development of local, regional, and distant disease recurrences was 7.4 months (range 5.0–49.7), 9.7 months (range 3.1–40.0), and 13.8 (range 3.5–38.4) months, respectively. The majority of failures were distant metastases with lung and bone metastases being most common. Distant metastases were the most common cause of death (Table 3).

Salvage surgery was not performed for progressive nodal disease given unresectability in all cases. Salvage surgery for recurrent primary disease was performed on 2 patients. The remaining patients with locoregional or distant disease progression received palliative chemotherapy.

Toxicity

Acute toxicities were similar between patients undergoing either primary surgery or radiotherapy except for grade 3 or higher mucositis, which was higher in patients treated with radiotherapy compared to surgery (81.3% versus 30.0%; $p < 0.05$). Sixty-eight percent of patients in the surgical and radiotherapy (68.4% v 68.0%; $p = 0.98$) groups required a feeding tube for a median of 6 months (range 2–42 months versus 3–33 months; $p = 0.59$). Neither treatment group had a patient with a permanent feeding tube requirement. Unplanned hospitalization within 6 months from diagnosis was similar between primary surgery and radiation groups (27.8% versus 36.0%; $p = 0.57$). There was no difference in weight loss between the groups with a median of approximately 12.5 kg measured from the beginning of the first treatment whether that being surgery, RT, or CRT to the end of treatment. Patients undergoing surgery as part of their care had various cranial nerves sacrificed with CN XI being most common occurring in 40% of patients.

Discussion

Patients with N3 HNSCC disease comprise approximately 10% of subjects enrolled on randomized clinical trials. The applicability of the outcomes of these trials to patients with N3 HNSCC is therefore unclear. As such, the majority of data regarding management and outcomes of N3 HNSCC patients is derived from single institution studies. Along these lines, reported here is a retrospective analysis of 36 patients with N3 HNSCC

Table 1 Baseline patient, disease, and treatment characteristics

	CRT (n = 20)	RT (n = 8)	Surgery (n = 8)	All (n = 36)	p-value
Age					0.51
Median	58.5	60.5	60	59	
(range)	(43–70)	(44–78)	(48–78)	(43–78)	
Sex					0.49
Male	18 (90.0%)	6 (75.0%)	6 (75.0%)	30 (83.3%)	
Race					0.86
Black	6 (30.0%)	3 (37.5%)	2 (25.0%)	11 (30.6%)	
White	14 (70.0%)	5 (62.5%)	6 (75.0%)	25 (69.4%)	
p16					0.64
Negative	2 (10.0%)	1 (12.5%)	2 (25.0%)	5 (13.9%)	
Positive	7 (35.0%)	1 (12.5%)	2 (25.0%)	10 (27.8%)	
Unknown	11 (55.0%)	6 (75.0%)	4 (50.0%)	21 (58.3%)	
Planned neck dissection of N3 neck					0.27
Yes	11 (55.0%)	5 (62.5%)	7 (87.5%)	23 (63.9%)	
Tumor Site					0.42
Hypopharynx	1 (5.0%)	2 (25.0%)	1 (12.5%)	4 (11.1%)	
Larynx	3 (15.0%)	0 (0.0%)	0 (0.0%)	3 (8.3%)	
Oral Cavity	0 (0.0%)	0 (0.0%)	1 (12.5%)	1 (2.8%)	
Oropharynx	14 (70.0%)	5 (62.5%)	5 (62.5%)	24 (66.7%)	
Unknown	2 (10.0%)	1 (12.5%)	1 (12.5%)	4 (11.1%)	
T-Stage					0.94
T0	2 (10.0%)	1 (12.5%)	1 (12.5%)	4 (11.1%)	
T1	3 (15.0%)	2 (25.0%)	3 (37.5%)	8 (22.2%)	
T2	5 (25.0%)	2 (25.0%)	1 (12.5%)	8 (22.2%)	
T3	6 (30.0%)	1 (12.5%)	0 (0.0%)	9 (25.0%)	
T4	4 (20.0%)	2 (25.0%)	1 (12.5%)	7 (19.4%)	
RT Type					< 0.01
IMRT	13 (65.0%)	0 (0.0%)	6 (75.0%)	19 (52.8%)	
Non-IMRT	7 (35.0%)	8 (100.0%)	2 (25.0%)	17 (47.2%)	
Fraction Size					< 0.01
Median	2.11	1.67	2.0	2.0	
(range)	(1.4–2.2)	(1.2–2.0)	(1.2–2.1)	(1.2–2.2)	
RT Total Dose					0.18
Median	7000 cGy	7010 cGy	6800 cGy	7000 cGy	
(range)	(6572–7320)	(6700–7460)	(6000–7440)	(6000–7460)	
Nodal Volume					0.88
Median	40.3	37.8	48.8	42.7	
(range)	(17.3–194.8)	(15.9–81.2)	(23.1–76.0)	(15.9–194.8)	

Abbreviations: RT radiotherapy, CRT chemoradiotherapy, IMRT intensity modulated Radiotherapy

treated at a single institution. The study demonstrates overall survival and regional control of 60% and 77% at 2 years and 30% and 66% at 5 years. Distant metastases were the predominant failure pattern occurring in 53% percent of patients at 5 years. These findings are congruous with those reported in other series.

Management of patients with N3 disease often reflects institutional patterns of care and disease characteristics. In that context, identifying treatment regimens that yield the highest therapeutic ratio of cure against morbidity is difficult. Despite these challenges, a recent study compared primary surgery to chemoradiotherapy and

Table 2 Factors associated with surgery of the primary tumor (Odds ratio > 1 indicates more likelihood of undergoing surgery)

	Odds Ratio (95% CI) Radiotherapy	Odds Ratio (95% CI) Chemoradiotherapy
Age	1.01 (0.91–1.13)	0.95 (0.86–1.04)
T1	0.38 (0.02–6.35)	0.31 (0.02–4.02)
T2	1.00 (0.03–29.81)	1.25 (0.06–26.87)
T3	0.25 (0.01–7.45)	0.75 (0.05–11.31)
P16-negative	1.00 (0.03–29.81)	0.29 (0.02–3.52)
Nodal volume (cm^3)	1.00 (0.96–1.03)	1.01 (0.98–1.03)

demonstrated improved outcomes in the surgical cohort with 5-year overall survival of 80% and 46% ($p < 0.05$) for surgery and radiotherapy, respectively [11]. In this study, we were unable to define a difference in any clinical outcomes when comparing patients undergoing primary surgery, RT, or CRT. The difference in conclusions may represent a lack of numerical power to detect a difference given the small sample size and/or patient selection differences. In the aforementioned study, 76% of patients in the primary surgery group were T0, T1, or T2 classified tumors while primary chemoradiotherapy was used for only 46% of similarly classified tumors. Further, all patients with nodal disease encasing the carotid or invading deep musculature underwent primary chemoradiotherapy. When this population of patients with more advanced regional disease was excluded from the primary radiotherapy group, the significant association between treatment modalities was lost ($p = 0.07$). In contrast, neither T-stage, p16-status, or nodal volume predicted for treatment assignment in the current study, which may have contributed to the non-significant result. Thus, larger studies with greater statistical power would be valuable, however in the

absence of randomized controlled trials, the inherent selection bias that allocates patients to receive surgery vs non-surgical intervention as initial therapy will confound direct comparison of these treatment approaches on ultimate outcome.

Thirty to 80% of patients in N3 HNSCC series are comprised of oropharyngeal primaries [7–11, 13]. With data being collected from 1975 to 2010 there is likely considerable variability in the contribution of HPV-positive and HPV-negative tumors in these series. The prognostic implications of HPV status in patients with N3 disease has not been examined in N3 series. However, two recent studies evaluated the impact of tumor (T) and nodal (N) classification of HPV-positive oropharyngeal tumors. Interestingly, there was discordance between the studies regarding the impact of N3 disease. In the Princess Margaret study N3 status was considered a high-risk factor whereas in the MD Anderson analysis T4 but not N3 indicated high risk disease [14, 15]. Here, despite the small sample size, this study suggests that HPV likely confers a significant survival advantage for patients with oropharyngeal squamous cell carcinomas and N3 nodal disease as patients with p16-positive disease exhibited improved survival outcomes compared to those with p16-negative disease ($p = 0.05$). Interesting, local and regional control were similar between p16-postive and p16-negative patients whereas the incidence of distant metastases was significantly higher in the p16-negative cohort ($p < 0.05$). Given the small sample size it was not possible to evaluate the impact of treatment on p16-positive tumors.

Historically poor complete response rates to N3 nodes treated with primary RT lead to the practice of planned neck dissection. However, in the current era of CRT, clinical response of bulky adenopathy has improved [16, 17]. Analysis of Trans Tasman Radiation Oncology Group Study 98.02 demonstrated a zero incidence of isolated neck failures in patients that had a complete clinical and radiographic response [18]. More recently, Mehanna et al. demonstrated that post-CRT PET-CT-guided surveillance showed similar survival outcomes compared to planned neck dissection in those patients with N2 and N3 disease [19]. In our analysis, we found similar regional control rates in patients that underwent CRT alone with those that went on to receive planned neck dissection. Similar to the TROG data, we identified a single patient that had an isolated neck recurrence. Taken together, these data support observation in patients with complete clinical responses to CRT and suggest caution against planned neck dissections.

Chemotherapy given concurrently with radiotherapy improves outcomes in the primary and adjuvant setting [20]. Given the predominant distant metastatic pattern

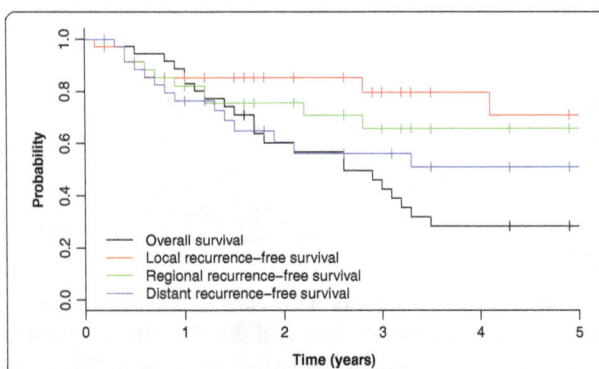

Fig. 1 Clinical outcomes of patients with N3 NHSCC treated with either primary surgery (*n* = 8), radiotherapy (*n* = 8), or chemoradiotherapy (*n* = 20)

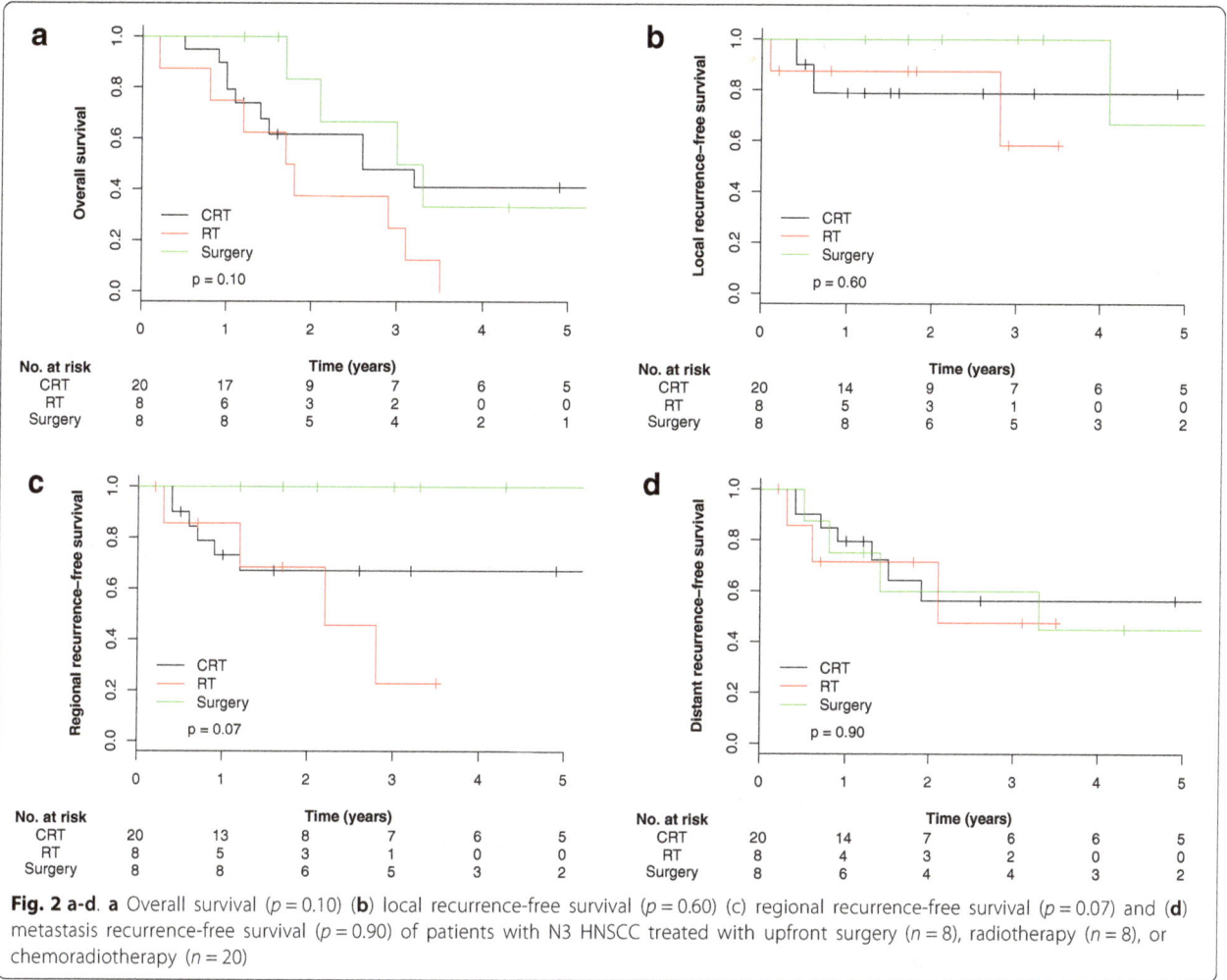

Fig. 2 a-d. **a** Overall survival (p = 0.10) (**b**) local recurrence-free survival (p = 0.60) (c) regional recurrence-free survival (p = 0.07) and (**d**) metastasis recurrence-free survival (p = 0.90) of patients with N3 HNSCC treated with upfront surgery (n = 8), radiotherapy (n = 8), or chemoradiotherapy (n = 20)

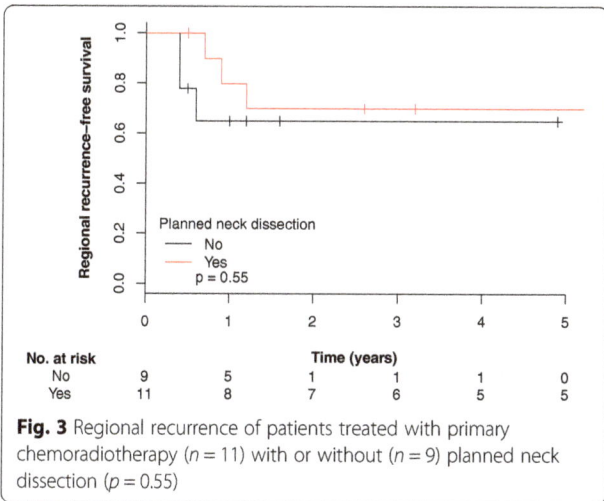

Fig. 3 Regional recurrence of patients treated with primary chemoradiotherapy (n = 11) with or without (n = 9) planned neck dissection (p = 0.55)

of failure in patients with N3 disease, a recent large randomized controlled trial evaluated the impact of induction chemotherapy followed by concurrent chemoradiotherapy in patients with advanced nodal disease. Despite the additional induction chemotherapy, there was no difference in distant failure-free or overall survival [3]. In our analysis, we did not identify a benefit in distant metastasis-free survival with the addition of chemotherapy. Given these data, newer approaches need to be explored to decrease or treat the development of metastatic disease.

This series contains several limitations inherent with retrospective analyses of an uncommon disease. First, the number of patients is small and treatment modalities varied considerably. Secondly, oropharyngeal cancers comprised a majority of the patients. Thus, it is not clear if the deduced outcomes for the overrepresented oropharyngeal tumors holds true for non-oropharyngeal cancers. Lastly, p16 data was available for a considerable portion, but not all, of our patient cohort. The majority

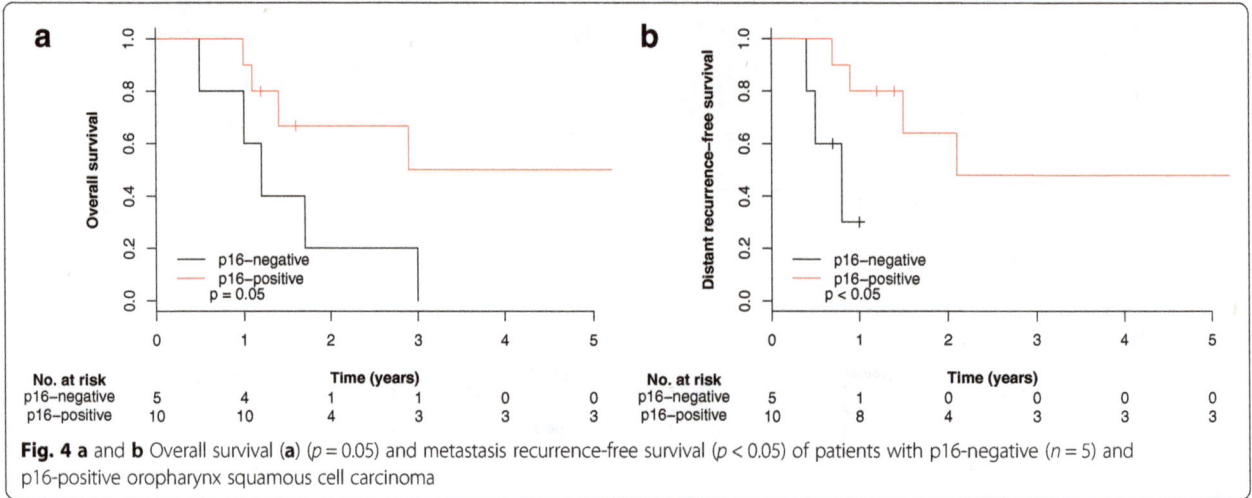

Fig. 4 a and **b** Overall survival (**a**) ($p = 0.05$) and metastasis recurrence-free survival ($p < 0.05$) of patients with p16-negative ($n = 5$) and p16-positive oropharynx squamous cell carcinoma

were p16-positive, which could imply that the p16-negative cohort is not representative of the typical p16-negative patient.

Conclusions

Several retrospective series have evaluated clinical outcomes for patient with N3 HNSCC disease. In each series, institutional practices have varied from primary radiotherapy with or without planned neck dissection to upfront surgical approaches. Despite such heterogeneous practice patterns and patient populations, reports have yielded consistent results supporting favorable locoregional control and unacceptable rates of distant failure. Although limited, existing studies suggest treatment recommendations and outcomes are heavily influence by disease presentation such as resectability [11] and patient characteristics [9]. As such, standards of care for such a rare disease will be difficult to establish given the difficulty in conducting randomized studies. Thus, larger database studies will help assess the most appropriate treatment modalities for N3 disease within particular primary tumor subsites and whether or not HPV positive patients with N3 nodes maintain a favorable prognosis. Currently, given long term survival of 30%, definitive treatment approaches should be pursed

Table 3 Patient mortality

Cause of Death	Number (%)
Locoregional disease	6 (27)
Distant metastatic disease	9 (41)
Locoregional and distant metastatic disease	4 (18)
Intercurrent disease	2 (9)
Unknown	1 (5)

barred the presence of metastatic disease at diagnosis, while newer approaches at controlling systemic disease should be investigated.

Abbreviations
BID: Twice per day; CN: Cranial nerve; CRT: Chemoradiotherapy; HNSCC: Head and neck squamous cell carcinoma; HPV: Human papillomavirus; IMRT: Intensity modulated radiotherapy; RT: Radiotherapy

Acknowledgements
Heather Geye for maintaining the University of Wisconsin Head and Neck cancer database.

Funding
This work was supported in part by NIH P50 DE026787- UW Head and Neck SPORE Grant.

Authors' contributions
MEW: Contributed to study design, data analysis, and drafting of manuscript. AMW: Contributed to study conception and manuscript editing. SC: Performed statistical analyses. TAK: Performed all radiographic analyses. CRH: Performed statistical analyses. EL: Contributed to acquisition of data. GKH: Contributed to study design. RJK: Contributed to manuscript editing. PMH: Contributed to data analysis and drafting of manuscript. All authors read and approved the final manuscript.

Author details
[1]Department of Human Oncology, University of Wisconsin, 600 Highland Avenue, K4/B100-0600, Madison, WI, Madison, WI 53792, USA. [2]Department of Surgery, Division of Otolaryngology and Head and Neck Surgery, University of Wisconsin, Madison, WI, USA. [3]Department of Biostatistics and Medical Informatics, University of Wisconsin, Madison, WI, USA. [4]Department of Radiology, University of Wisconsin, Madison, WI, USA. [5]University of Wisconsin School of Medicine and Public Health University of Wisconsin, Madison, WI, USA.

References

1. Ang KK, Harris J, Wheeler R, et al. Human papillomavirus and survival of patients with oropharyngeal cancer. N Engl J Med. 2010;363(1):24–35.
2. Bernier J, Domenge C, Ozsahin M, et al. Postoperative irradiation with or without concomitant chemotherapy for locally advanced head and neck cancer. N Engl J Med. 2004;350(19):1945–52.
3. Cohen EE, Karrison TG, Kocherginsky M, et al. Phase III randomized trial of induction chemotherapy in patients with N2 or N3 locally advanced head and neck cancer. J Clin Oncol. 2014;32(25):2735–43.
4. Cooper JS, Pajak TF, Forastiere AA, et al. Postoperative concurrent radiotherapy and chemotherapy for high-risk squamous-cell carcinoma of the head and neck. N Engl J Med. 2004;350(19):1937–44.
5. KK F, Pajak TF, Trotti A, et al. A radiation therapy oncology group (RTOG) phase III randomized study to compare hyperfractionation and two variants of accelerated fractionation to standard fractionation radiotherapy for head and neck squamous cell carcinomas: first report of RTOG 9003. Int J Radiat Oncol Biol Phys. 2000;48(1):7–16.
6. Haddad R, O'Neill A, Rabinowits G, et al. Induction chemotherapy followed by concurrent chemoradiotherapy (sequential chemoradiotherapy) versus concurrent chemoradiotherapy alone in locally advanced head and neck cancer (PARADIGM): a randomised phase 3 trial. Lancet Oncol. 2013;14(3): 257–64.
7. Igidbashian L, Fortin B, Guertin L, et al. Outcome with neck dissection after chemoradiation for N3 head-and-neck squamous cell carcinoma. Int J Radiat Oncol Biol Phys. 2010;77(2):414–20.
8. Jones AS, Goodyear PW, Ghosh S, Husband D, Helliwell TR, Jones TM. Extensive neck node metastases (N3) in head and neck squamous carcinoma: is radical treatment warranted? Otolaryngol Head Neck Surg. 2011;144(1):29–35.
9. Jung JH, Roh JL, Lee JH, et al. Prognostic factors in patients with head and neck squamous cell carcinoma with cN3 neck disease: a retrospective case-control study. Oral Surg Oral Med Oral Pathol Oral Radiol. 2014;117(2):178–85.
10. Karakaya E, Yetmen O, Oksuz DC, et al. Outcomes following chemoradiotherapy for N3 head and neck squamous cell carcinoma without a planned neck dissection. Oral Oncol. 2013;49(1):55–9.
11. Smyth JK, Deal AM, Huang B, Weissler M, Zanation A, Shores C. Outcomes of head and neck squamous cell carcinoma patients with N3 neck disease treated primarily with chemoradiation versus surgical resection. Laryngoscope. 2011;121(9):1881–7.
12. Calais G, Alfonsi M, Bardet E, et al. Randomized trial of radiation therapy versus concomitant chemotherapy and radiation therapy for advanced-stage Oropharynx carcinoma. J Natl Cancer Inst. 1999;91(24):2081–6.
13. Adelstein DJ, Li Y, Adams GL, et al. An intergroup phase III comparison of standard radiation therapy and two schedules of concurrent chemoradiotherapy in patients with unresectable squamous cell head and neck cancer. J Clin Oncol. 2003;21(1):92–8.
14. Dahlstrom KR, Garden AS, William WN Jr, Lim MY, Sturgis EM. Proposed staging system for patients with HPV-related Oropharyngeal cancer based on nasopharyngeal cancer N categories. J Clin Oncol. 2016;34(16):1848–54.
15. Huang SH, Xu W, Waldron J, et al. Refining American joint committee on cancer/Union for International Cancer Control TNM stage and prognostic groups for human papillomavirus-related oropharyngeal carcinomas. J Clin Oncol. 2015;33(8):836–45.
16. Calais G, Alfonsi M, Bardet E, et al. Randomized trial of radiation therapy versus concomitant chemotherapy and radiation therapy for advanced-stage oropharynx carcinoma. J Natl Cancer Inst. 1999;91(24):2081–6.
17. Wendt TG, Grabenbauer GG, Rodel CM, et al. Simultaneous radiochemotherapy versus radiotherapy alone in advanced head and neck cancer: a randomized multicenter study. J Clin Oncol. 1998;16(4):1318–24.
18. Corry J, Peters L, Fisher R, et al. N2-N3 neck nodal control without planned neck dissection for clinical/radiologic complete responders-results of trans Tasman radiation oncology group study 98.02. Head Neck. 2008;30(6):737–42.
19. Mehanna H, McConkey CC, Rahman JK, et al. PET-NECK: a multicentre randomised phase III non-inferiority trial comparing a positron emission tomography-computerised tomography-guided watch-and-wait policy with planned neck dissection in the management of locally advanced (N2/N3) nodal metastases in patients with squamous cell head and neck cancer. Health Technol Assess. 2017;21(17):1–122.
20. Blanchard P, Baujat B, Holostenco V, et al. Meta-analysis of chemotherapy in head and neck cancer (MACH-NC): a comprehensive analysis by tumour site. Radiother Oncol. 2011;100(1):33–40.

8

Informational and support needs of patients with head and neck cancer: current status and emerging issues

Carolyn Y. Fang* and Carolyn J. Heckman

Abstract

The objective of this article is to review and summarize the extant literature on head and neck cancer (HNC) patients' informational needs and to characterize emerging issues in this patient population in order to define priorities for future research. HNC patients may undergo challenging treatment regimens and experience treatment-related alterations in primary daily functions such as speech and eating. These changes often persist following treatment and may lead to significant deficits in quality of life and interpersonal relations. Despite empirical evidence demonstrating that receipt of adequate information and support is predictive of improved outcomes post-treatment, relatively limited attention has been paid to the informational and support needs of HNC patients. This review focuses primarily on three topic domains: (1) managing treatment-related side effects; (2) addressing alcohol and tobacco dependence; and (3) informational needs in the areas of human papillomavirus (HPV) and clinical trials. While there is increasing awareness of the rehabilitation and survivorship needs in this patient population, patients note that the impact of treatment on social activities and interactions is under-discussed and of key concern. In addition, there is a significant gap in addressing communication and informational needs of caregivers and family members who are integral for promoting healthy behaviors and self-care post-treatment. Greater integration of programs that address tobacco or alcohol dependency within a comprehensive treatment and support plan may increase patient motivation to seek help and enhance patient success in maintaining long-term abstinence. Finally, emerging patient-provider communication needs, particularly in the context of decision making about clinical trials or surrounding an HPV-related diagnosis, have been noted among both patients and healthcare providers. Future research on the development of novel programs that offer feasible and acceptable methods for addressing unmet informational and support needs is warranted and may yield benefit for improving patient-reported outcomes.

Keywords: Informational needs, Treatment side effects, Communication, Caregivers, Health behaviors, HPV

Background

Despite advances in diagnostic tools and treatment modalities, treatment for head and neck squamous cell carcinoma (HNC) can lead to considerable long-term functional impairment. Patients may experience difficulty swallowing, dry mouth, nutritional deficits, pain, and declines in social functioning, speech, and sexuality [1]. Physical and psychosocial complaints can persist even following successful therapy [2], and patients often report significant decrements in quality of life (QOL), poorer interpersonal relations, and increased social isolation [3].

Notably, empirical data indicate that patients' perceptions of having obtained adequate information and support are predictive of positive rehabilitation outcomes in the 2- to 6-year post-treatment period [4]. However, despite the complexity of treatment regimens and challenging recovery process, relatively limited attention has been paid to the informational and support needs of HNC patients. Therefore, the objective of this article is to briefly review and summarize the extant literature on informational and support needs and to characterize emerging issues in this patient population to help define priorities for future research.

* Correspondence: carolyn.fang@fccc.edu
Cancer Prevention and Control Program, Fox Chase Cancer Center, 333 Cottman Ave, Philadelphia, PA 19111, USA

Main text

Symptom management and treatment side effects

HNC patients undergoing surgical treatment may experience physical alterations on a part of their body that is highly visible (i.e. face) and with significant implications for social interactions. As a result, several studies focused on issues of postoperative changes in appearance or speech [5–7]. In a cross-sectional study of 280 surgical patients who were surveyed regarding body image [5], 75 % reported feeling concerned or embarrassed by bodily changes related to the cancer and/or its treatment at some point following diagnosis. The concerns most commonly expressed by patients involved scarring and disfigurement (42.3 %), speaking-related issues (35.8 %), loss of teeth (30.1 %), and social eating (25.1 %) [5]. Other concerns included swelling, drooling, hair loss, and weight loss. And despite patients' overall levels of satisfaction with their healthcare team, a subgroup of patients had unmet informational needs. Specifically, 25 % of patients reported dissatisfaction with the information received about the degree of scarring/disfigurement to be expected following surgery; 32 % were dissatisfied with information received about the potential effects of radiation treatment on physical appearance, and 44 % reported dissatisfaction with information about potential effects of chemotherapy on physical appearance. Factors associated with dissatisfaction included age and time since diagnosis, with younger patients reporting higher levels of dissatisfaction and body image concerns. Levels of dissatisfaction were also found to increase after surgery and remain elevated one-year post-surgery. Overall, more than one-third of patients reported that greater informational resources to help manage multiple concerns would have been helpful [5].

Among surgical patients, a desire for greater preoperative education and preparation for post-operative changes has been reported [8], particularly in the domains of speech [9] and eating [8, 10]. In an early study, questionnaires assessing informational needs and support services were completed by 125 patients who had undergone laryngectomy for treatment of their cancer and 28 spouses. Among patients, 21 % were not satisfied with the information received prior to surgery and were unaware preoperatively of the inability to speak after surgery [9]. Importantly, 61 % of patients and 81 % of spouses reported that the information provided was insufficient [9]. A smaller study evaluated informational needs and eating-related experiences among 34 patients who were recruited from an Internet-based laryngectomy support group. Similar to prior findings, most patients reported dissatisfaction with the information received, particularly with regard to the effects of laryngectomy on loss of taste and changes in eating [10]. Importantly, the majority of patients and spouses desired to have a conversation about how treatment may impact social activities and interactions with friends, family members, and other individuals in a public setting [8].

Of note, studies have revealed a potential disconnect between what doctors believe their patients are worried about and what patients say they are worried about. Healthcare professionals perceived that speech impairment and self-image were patients' primary concerns after surgery; however, patients rated concerns about the physical consequences of treatment and its interference with social activities as key concerns post-surgery [11]. Alterations in the social nature of eating are frequently reported by patients as topics that deserve more attention [8, 10]. In addition, patients desire more information on nutrition and strategies for coping with loss of smell or taste [10]. In the absence of receiving appropriate referrals to nutritionists or other support professionals, patients often turn to internet Web sites or support groups to seek the information they desire [10, 12], although the information obtained from these sources may not be reliable or accurate. While healthcare professionals may wish to avoid burdening the patient with detailed nutrition and dietary recommendations during the early stage of rehabilitation, patients do not perceive advice to "just eat something" to be particularly helpful [10], further underscoring the disconnect between patients and their providers.

In addition to swallowing and speech issues, there is growing awareness that HNC patients experience sleep disturbance. Among 58 HNC patients who completed a cross-sectional survey on sleep and fatigue, greater sleep dysfunction was associated with younger age and higher symptom burden [13]. Multiple factors may contribute to sleep dysfunction and poor sleep quality, as observed in a longitudinal, prospective study of 457 HNC patients in which pain, xerostomia, depression, presence of a tracheotomy tube, and younger age were significant predictors of poor sleep quality one-year post-diagnosis [14]. However, treatment type (surgery, radiation, or chemotherapy), primary tumor site, and cancer stage were not significantly associated with sleep quality over time.

Sleep disruption may be due to not only pain or symptom burden, but also the physiologic alterations resulting from the tumor or cancer treatment. Both radiation and surgical treatments lead to changes in the upper airway that can contribute to the development of obstructive sleep apnea (OSA) [15]. Although there have been few studies of OSA in HNC patients, the limited data available suggest that HNC patients are at increased risk of OSA [16–19]. One study of 17 HNC patients who were assessed prior to surgical treatment revealed the presence of OSA in 13 patients (76 %) [18]. A retrospective review of 56 HNC patients who had also undergone formal sleep evaluation found that patients with active disease or who had received radiation therapy were more likely to have OSA [20]. And in contrast to the general population, where obesity is a risk factor for the development of OSA, HNC patients with OSA are not more likely to be obese or overweight [15, 20, 21], suggesting that anatomic changes resulting from the tumor or cancer treatment may predispose patients to the development of OSA. Because many symptoms of OSA are nonspecific (daytime sleepiness, insomnia, dry mouth upon awakening) and could be attributed to other factors, patients may be unaware that they are suffering from a potentially treatable sleep disorder [22]. Clinicians and healthcare providers can help patients identify symptoms of OSA and provide referrals to sleep specialists if warranted.

Other unmet informational and support needs that have been identified pertain to financial and psychosocial domains. In a prospective study of 82 newly diagnosed HNC patients, informational needs commonly reported at pre-treatment included issues involving financial support (78 %), access to support groups for patient or partner (52 %), treatment side effects (50 %), and how treatment may impact QOL and functioning over the next year (43 %) [23]. Patients were hetereogenous with respect to treatments received (surgery only, radiation only, or a combination of surgery, radiation, and chemotherapy) and were re-assessed 1 month post-treatment, at which time 60 % of patients continued to report that they had not received any information regarding financial support, 34 % had not received information about support groups, and 28 % had not received information about treatment side effects or how treatment may impact functioning over time [23]. In light of the fact that study respondents had access to healthcare and were recruited from research hospital settings (which may have more resources to offer patients), it is possible that these data are underestimates of financial and other concerns than what might be found in the broader HNC patient population. To date, the informational and support needs of HNC patients who are uninsured, lack access to healthcare, or are being managed in community practices or other settings is not well-characterized.

Family caregivers often play an important role in supporting HNC patients and providing assistance during and after treatment [24, 25]. Similar to patients, caregivers of HNC patients report many unmet informational needs [24, 26]. Among 59 family caregivers of HNC patients who had completed radiation therapy, nearly 75 % reported high informational needs at diagnosis [24]. Although caregivers' needs decreased over time, over half of caregivers still had high informational needs at the end of treatment. Predominant concerns included reducing patient pain and distress across the treatment trajectory. Similarly, in a qualitative study of oral cancer patients and their family caregivers, caregivers requested more information on pain management and self-care [26]. Finally, both patients and caregivers desired more information regarding managing side effects and nutrition issues [26].

The extant literature has characterized patients' unmet informational and support needs across multiple domains, but limitations of the existing research include small sample sizes in many studies, wide variability in the timing of study assessments relative to treatment and across studies, and a reliance on predominantly cross-sectional study designs. Most studies utilized a convenience sample comprised of predominantly non-Hispanic whites, and therefore informational and support needs of HNC patients from other racial/ethnic subgroups are not well-described. In addition, the studies conducted have tended to use varied measures to assess informational needs and satisfaction with information received, thereby making it difficult to compare across studies. However, a standardized measure of satisfaction with information has been developed and evaluated specifically among HNC patients [27]. This measure, the Satisfaction with Cancer Information Profile (SCIP), assesses patient satisfaction with the amount and content of information, as well as the form and timing of the information received [27]. The use of standardized and validated measures will help promote greater consistency in the assessment and identification of informational needs over time across diverse HNC patient subgroups.

Multimedia interventions can offer a promising approach to addressing communication and information needs. In one study, partners of HNC patients received a multimedia-based program including a patient booklet, interactive computer booth and take-home DVD, which was delivered by a nurse practitioner [28]. Partners of HNC patients who received the intervention reported higher levels of satisfaction with the information provided compared to control group participants; importantly, intervention participants had lower levels of anxiety and depression at 3–6 months [28]. Other Internet-based programs that deliver content and features tailored to one's role (cancer survivor or caregiver) have been found to be well-received by oral cancer survivors and their family caregivers; and they offer the potential added ability to use online tools for communicating with other survivors and caregivers [26].

Due to the diversity of individual needs and preferences, tailored communication materials may represent the best strategy for addressing informational gaps [29, 30]. As might be expected, younger HNC patients (29–49 years of age) were more likely to report having Internet access compared to older patients (65+ years), and data suggest varied preferences regarding the format in which information is delivered [12], with some patients preferring to receive information delivered in-person by a healthcare specialist [30], whereas others are receptive to Internet-based programs [26]. Higher education level and female gender were also associated with greater preference for Internet-based programs [12]. Finally, patient financial concerns and access to healthcare services remain a significant area of informational need that is not well-addressed and one that warrants greater attention. In view of the complexity of treatment-related side effects and the extensive rehabilitation that may need to occur both during and post-treatment, strategies to address patients' informational and support needs across the continuum of care (from pre-treatment through post-treatment) are critically needed.

Alcohol and tobacco dependence

Following a cancer diagnosis and/or treatment, patients may seek to maintain or improve their health via alterations in lifestyle behaviors such as physical activity, diet, smoking, or alcohol use. Given that cancer treatment and subsequent side effects can adversely affect physical functioning and nutritional status, numerous studies have focused on the effects of physical activity or nutritional support interventions on patient outcomes (please see comprehensive reviews on physical activity [31–33] and nutrition [34–36] in HNC patients). In contrast, there have been relatively fewer studies designed to address alcohol or tobacco dependency for those patients with addiction disorders. Empirical data suggest that alcohol abuse and untreated alcohol withdrawal syndrome can lead to treatment complications and poorer outcomes, including failure of extubation or ventilator weaning and higher rates of mortality [37, 38]; however, there has been limited research focused on delivering specialized services to treat comorbid alcoholism among HNC patients [39, 40]. One US study published in 2010 found that 44.5 % of HNC survivors reported current alcohol use 1 year after diagnosis [41]. Several studies have reported various factors to be associated with ongoing alcohol use after diagnosis including: male gender, early-stage disease, longer time since treatment, receiving chemotherapy and/or radiation therapy compared to surgery, and superior oral functioning [41–43]. A 2016 Spanish study reported that alcohol use decreased by 16.7 % after diagnosis, and that receiving a surgeon's recommendation about alcohol was strongly associated with alcohol reduction or cessation [44]. Only one randomized controlled trial published in 2006 by Duffy and colleagues tested an alcohol intervention for HNC patients. Patients with HNC and tobacco, alcohol, or depression disorders, about half of whom were veterans, were randomized to a nurse-administered cognitive-behavioral and pharmacotherapy intervention for treatment of tobacco, alcohol, and depression [39]. No significant differences in 6-month alcohol consumption were observed between the intervention condition and usual care [39], attesting to the challenges of addressing alcohol disorders in this patient population.

There is a relatively larger body of research on tobacco-related complications. Continued smoking after the diagnosis of HNC impacts treatment and risk for complications, increases the likelihood of recurrence and second primary cancers, and adversely affects QOL and survival [45–48]. According to a 2015 systematic review of six studies, the survival rate for HNC patients who continued smoking after diagnosis was 21–35 % lower than patients who quit, and the recurrence rate for active smokers was 23–30 % higher than for quitters [47]. In a matched-pair study of HNC and nicotine-dependent patients published in 2007, HNC patients who stopped using tobacco also had lower rates of tobacco-related second primary tumors [46].

HNC patients, like other smokers, demonstrate ambivalence about quitting, and smoking rates among HNC patients have remained relatively constant over the last two decades despite the availability of an increased number of empirically-based pharmacotherapy and behavioral interventions to treat tobacco dependence [49]. Many HNC patients who are smokers are interested in quitting, and may even succeed in quitting unassisted, at least initially. However, a significant minority of smokers are unable to quit even after diagnosis of a smoking-related cancer, and initial quitters are at high risk for relapse. Only Duffy and colleagues' randomized controlled trial published in 2006 found a significant treatment effect of a nurse-delivered cognitive-behavioral and pharmacotherapy tobacco cessation intervention compared to usual care for HNC patients [39].

Despite the fact that evidence-based tobacco cessation interventions are available, they are woefully underutilized and have been minimally evaluated among HNC patients. Providers have not fully implemented the Public Health Service 5A guidelines for tobacco cessation (ask, advise, assess, assist, arrange) [50] among patients with tobacco-related cancers – this is likely due to a multitude of barriers that include patient factors (e.g., low motivation, self-efficacy, knowledge), provider factors (e.g., limited training, self-efficacy, time), and system factors (e.g., high cost, minimal insurance coverage). Two studies of lung and HNC patients combined demonstrated partial implementation of the 5A's, as assessed by self report and medical chart review, with 93 % of patients reporting that they were asked about tobacco use, 76–86 % advised about tobacco use, 46 % assessed for their interest in quitting, 40–65 % assisted, but only 4 % arranged with follow-up [49, 51]. A study published in 2011 found that individualized cessation programs were preferred by patients, and younger patients with early stage disease and those with partners who smoked were more interested in cessation programs [25]. A 2012 study found that delivery of 5A's was most likely to occur when patients requested cessation advice from their providers. However, according to a small qualitative study conducted at a large NCI-designated comprehensive cancer center in the Southeast published in 2009, patients do not ask providers for help quitting or maintaining abstinence, and relapsed patients are hesitant to disclose smoking due to feelings of stigma and guilt [28]. In addition, clinicians vary in the types of assistance they provide and their awareness and sensitivity to relapsed patients' concerns [28]. The advice and type of assistance offered by providers may not resonate with patients—specifically, providers reported emphasizing the long-term risks of continued smoking in their interactions with patients, but lung and HNC patients expressed a preference for a balance between risks of smoking and benefits of quitting/abstinence [52].

Few empirically-supported programs targeted for or tested specifically with HNC patients exist. The results of three randomized trials for HNC patients have been published. In the first study published in 1993, the intervention consisted of surgeon- or dentist-delivered advice to stop smoking, a contracted quit date, tailored written materials, and booster advice sessions compared to a usual care advice control condition [53]. At randomization, 88 % were current smokers. At 12-month follow-up, 70 % of participants completing the trial were continuous abstainers; among baseline smokers alone, the continuous abstinence rate was 65 %. However, the intervention effect was not statistically significant. Predictors of continuous abstinence were surgery rather than radiation only, greater stage of change, younger age, lower nicotine dependence, and race/ethnicity other than white, non-Hispanic. Based on these findings, the authors recommended systematic brief advice to stop smoking for HNC patients, with a stepped-care approach for patients less able to quit [53].

In Duffy and colleagues' study published in 2006, Veterans Affairs Medical Center (VAMC) patients with HNC and tobacco, alcohol, or depression disorders were randomized to a nurse-administered cognitive-behavioral and pharmacotherapy intervention for treatment of tobacco, alcohol, and depression [39]. Significant differences in 6-month smoking cessation rates were found with 47 % quitting in the intervention condition compared to 31 % in the usual care condition [39]. However, a recent randomized study of VAMC HNC patients published in 2016 found that receiving a $150 monetary incentive at each test visit (1, 3, and 6 months) for being biochemically-confirmed abstinent based on urine cotinine testing – in addition to being paid $50 to attend each of three cessation classes provided by the VAMC – did not result in improved cessation rates [54].

Despite the mixed results that have been reported to date, it is imperative that providers take advantage of the "teachable moment" of a diagnosis of HNC to advise smokers to quit, which can be quite effective [50]. Tobacco use and cessation should be addressed on an ongoing basis with patients throughout treatment and survivorship, including among recent quitters in order to prevent relapse. Too often, a sporadic "Band-Aid" approach is used for tobacco cessation, even among cancer patients, despite calls for nicotine dependence to be managed as a chronic disease [55, 56]. In 2015, the National Comprehensive Cancer Network published guidelines for tobacco cessation intervention among cancer patients [57], but the successful implementation of these guidelines remains to be evaluated.

Emerging issues
Human papillomavirus

A topic not commonly addressed is the impact of cancer and its treatment on sexual functioning [1, 58, 59]. In an early study, HNC patients who had extensive facial disfigurement following surgical treatment reported worse relations with their partners, increased social isolation, and reduced sexuality compared to patients with minor disfigurement [6]. Due to significant improvements in facial reconstruction techniques, extensive disfigurement is now less common; but sexual functioning may still be impacted due to treatment-related effects on breathing, swallowing, and speaking. Alterations in any of these functions can have a negative impact upon intimacy, communication, or other sexual activities. Indeed, although 85 % of HNC patients reported moderate-to-high interest in sexual relations, a majority (58 %) reported arousal problems, and 58 % did not engage in sexual intercourse [59]. Further, 51 % considered the quality of their current sexual functioning to be poor, with younger patients (<65 years) reporting significantly poorer sexual functioning than patients aged 65 or older [59].

In addition, data suggest that the incidence of human papillomavirus (HPV)-associated head and neck cancers is increasing [60–62]. Accumulating evidence point to HPV as a causal factor in the etiology of head and neck cancers that arise among non-smokers and non-drinkers [63, 64]. This emerging subgroup of HNC patients has specific informational needs, and many clinicians find themselves ill-prepared for these discussions. Patients may have questions about HPV-related disease that are difficult to answer due to limited data or physician discomfort with discussing matters related to sexual health [65].

Among HNC patients receiving an HPV-related diagnosis, informational and psychosocial needs are particularly apparent. In a qualitative study of 10 men with HPV-related HNC, the majority (8/10) sought additional HPV-specific information, mostly from the Internet [66].

Patient knowledge about HPV varied significantly, and many had questions regarding transmission of HPV infection and potential consequences for current or future partners [66]. Among 62 HNC patients who had a long-term partner, only two-thirds of patients correctly reported that they had an HPV+ tumor [67]; the remainder of patients were unsure or reported that they did not have an HPV+ tumor. Only a minority of patients (35 %) reported that their cancer was caused by HPV [67]. The majority of patients reported being uninformed about what precautions (if any) needed to be taken to prevent HPV transmission to their partner, and 39 % reported that their oncologist did not discuss issues related to HPV with them. Over half (58 %) reported seeking additional information from sources other than their oncologist [67].

The sexually-transmitted nature of HPV may create challenges for healthcare professionals who have limited experience discussing sexual health with their patients. In a qualitative study of 15 healthcare professionals who treat patients with oropharyngeal cancers, providers described two primary challenges: (1) discomfort or lack of familiarity with talking about sexual health and behaviors; and (2) limitations of scientific knowledge about the virus [68]. Patients may desire answers to specific questions about how they became infected with HPV, when they became infected, who the infection was transmitted from, and the likelihood of re-infection after cancer treatment – questions that are difficult to answer [68]. These data highlight significant challenges and gaps in patient-provider communication with respect to HPV-related issues and point to the need for additional research in this area. At present, existing data on the informational needs of patients with HPV-related cancers are quite limited as the few studies that have been conducted are based on relatively small samples of patients and physicians recruited from large academic research institutions, which may not be representative of the broader patient and healthcare provider population. As a result, little is known about the informational and support needs of patients being managed in community practices and their community providers. Studies designed to foster the development of valid and comprehensive educational and support programs to address HPV-related issues would be extremely beneficial for both patients and their providers.

Decision making about clinical trials

Another area of emerging need is the provision of informational support for clinical trials. While clinical trials are essential to the evaluation of new therapeutic regimens, a relatively small proportion of cancer patients participate in these trials [69]. This is likewise true for clinical trials specifically recruiting HNC patients, where it was reported that over 25 % of HNC trials that had been terminated, suspended, or withdrawn was due to insufficient accrual of patients [70]. Two studies investigating barriers to recruitment of HNC patients were identified. In one study, 85 healthcare professionals involved in clinical trial research (investigators, research nurses) completed a web-based survey on barriers to clinical trial recruitment. The most commonly reported barriers to recruitment (identified by more than 50 % of respondents) included patient refusal to consent due to treatment preference or aversion to randomization, the complexity and amount of information that needs to be provided to patients, and lack of time to support research [71], which is consistent with studies in other cancer patient populations [72]. Further exacerbating this situation is the complexity of the information that needs to be accurately conveyed, which can be particularly challenging for patients with limited health literacy [73].

Hence, the utilization of decision aids to assist with informed decision making about clinical trial participation has been explored as a potentially useful tool to help patients identify their values and goals, consistent with making an informed choice. To date, there have been no decision aids developed to specifically support HNC patients' informational needs and decision making about clinical trials. But prospective, randomized studies involving mixed cancer patient populations have yielded promising results. For example, among 1255 cancer patients who were randomly assigned to receive either a web-based program that provided tailored, interactive educational content about clinical trials (intervention condition) or general written information about clinical trials (control condition), intervention participants reported significantly greater increases in knowledge and greater decreases in attitudinal barriers compared to control participants [74]. Thus, tailored educational programs can effectively deliver key information about clinical trials and may help enhance communication about and preparation for decision making about clinical trials. Future research is needed to evaluate whether similar programs yield comparable benefits in addressing HNC patients' informational needs and reducing barriers to clinical trials.

Conclusion

Across studies, many patients desire additional information and support, particularly with respect to managing treatment-related side effects, maintaining one's health and healthy lifestyle behaviors after treatment, and understanding an HPV-related diagnosis. Despite the growing body of research on rehabilitation and survivorship needs in this patient population, patients note that the impact of treatment on social activities and interactions is under-discussed and of key concern. Interventions focused on swallowing and improving jaw mobility (for a review see [75]) often neglect to address the psychological and/or social aspects of eating and drinking, issues reported to be of high importance among survivors and which can contribute to decrements in emotional and social well-being. In addition, there is a significant gap in addressing communication and informational needs of caregivers and family members who provide considerable levels of support to the patient and are integral for promoting healthy behaviors and self-care during and after treatment. As caregivers often express different concerns than patients do, future studies that address caregivers' specific needs are warranted.

In addition, there is a need for more fully integrated programs to provide support for managing substance dependency issues. For example, many HNC patients express interest in quitting smoking and attempt to quit, but fewer follow through with enrolling in evidence-based smoking cessation programs or are successful in maintaining long-term abstinence. Motivational interventions to facilitate enrollment into formal programs that address alcohol or tobacco dependence among cancer patients may be beneficial [76]. Studies suggest that a cancer diagnosis and subsequent treatment window offers a "teachable moment" during which patients may be motivated to initiate and maintain healthy behaviors, including smoking cessation and decreased alcohol use [77]. Ultimately, programs addressing tobacco or alcohol dependency that are incorporated into a comprehensive treatment plan may decrease the stigma associated with substance abuse and increase patient motivation to seek help and support for staying healthy after treatment.

Finally, two emerging areas of informational needs that warrant greater attention include: (1) communication about an HPV-related diagnosis and its impact on intimacy; and (2) support for decision making about clinical trials. Although patients with HPV-related disease desire more information regarding HPV and head and neck cancer, communication and practical barriers (such as physician time constraints, limited knowledge, and patient or physician discomfort in discussing sexual health) reduce patient satisfaction with the information provided. With the increasing prevalence of HPV-related HNCs, corresponding programs that address patient and partner concerns regarding HPV-related issues are greatly needed. Similarly, multiple challenges exist in the enrollment of HNC patients to clinical trials, including limited time for conveying large amounts of complex information, addressing informational needs of patients and family members, and discussing patient preferences and values. Findings derived from other cancer patient populations suggest that novel web-based programs may not only be an effective and cost-efficient approach for delivering such information, but may also represent an acceptable and feasible format for communicating information about multiple topics that can be tailored to meet the unique needs of patients and family members.

Abbreviations

HNC: Head and neck cancer; HPV: Human papillomavirus; VAMC: Veterans Affairs Medical Center

Acknowledgements

Not applicable.

Funding

Funding from NCI Cancer Center Support Grant P30CA006927 to Fox Chase Cancer Center supported the writing of this manuscript.

Authors' contributions

CYF and CJH each reviewed the literature and contributed to writing the manuscript. Both authors read and approved the final manuscript.

Competing interests

The authors declare that they have no competing interests.

References

1. Bjordal K, Ahlner-Elmqvist M, Hammerlid E, Boysen M, Evensen JF, Biorklund A, Jannert M, Westin T, Kaasa S. A prospective study of quality of life in head and neck cancer patients. Part II: Longitudinal data. Laryngoscope. 2001;111(8):1440–52.
2. Perry AR, Shaw MA, Cotton S. An evaluation of functional outcomes (speech, swallowing) in patients attending speech pathology after head and neck cancer treatment(s): results and analysis at 12 months post-intervention. J Laryngol Otol. 2003;117(5):368–81.
3. Gritz ER, Carmack CL, de Moor C, Coscarelli A, Schacherer CW, Meyers EG, Abemayor E. First year after head and neck cancer: quality of life. J Clin Oncol. 1999;17(1):352–60.
4. de Boer MF, Pruyn JF, van den Borne B, Knegt PP, Ryckman RM, Verwoerd CD. Rehabilitation outcomes of long-term survivors treated for head and neck cancer. Head Neck. 1995;17(6):503–15.
5. Fingeret MC, Yuan Y, Urbauer D, Weston J, Nipomnick S, Weber R. The nature and extent of body image concerns among surgically treated patients with head and neck cancer. Psycho-Oncology. 2012;21(8):836–44.
6. Gamba A, Romano M, Grosso IM, Tamburini M, Cantu G, Molinari R, Ventafridda V. Psychosocial adjustment of patients surgically treated for head and neck cancer. Head Neck. 1992;14(3):218–23.
7. Penner JL. Psychosocial care of patients with head and neck cancer. Semin Oncol Nurs. 2009;25(3):231–41.
8. Happ MB, Roesch T, Kagan SH. Communication needs, methods, and perceived voice quality following head and neck surgery: A literature review. Cancer Nurs. 2004;27(1):1–9.
9. Zeine L, Larson M. Pre- and post-operative counseling for laryngectomees and their spouses: an update. J Commun Disord. 1999;32(1):51–61.
10. Lennie TA, Christman SK, Jadack RA. Educational needs and altered eating habits following a total laryngectomy. Oncol Nurs Forum. 2001; 28(4):667–74.
11. Mohide EA, Archibald SD, Tew M, Young JE, Haines T. Postlaryngectomy quality-of-life dimensions identified by patients and health care professionals. Am J Surg. 1992;164(6):619–22.

12. Fang CY, Longacre ML, Manne SL, Ridge JA, Lango MN, Burtness BA. Informational Needs of Head and Neck Cancer Patients. Heal Technol. 2012;2(1):57–62.

13. Rogers LQ, Courneya KS, Robbins KT, Rao K, Malone J, Seiz A, Reminger S, Markwell SJ, Burra V. Factors associated with fatigue, sleep, and cognitive function among patients with head and neck cancer. Head Neck. 2008;30(10):1310–7.

14. Shuman AG, Duffy SA, Ronis DL, Garetz SL, McLean SA, Fowler KE, Terrell JE. Predictors of poor sleep quality among head and neck cancer patients. Laryngoscope. 2010;120(6):1166–72.

15. Zhou J, Jolly S. Obstructive sleep apnea and fatigue in head and neck cancer patients. Am J Clin Oncol. 2015;38(4):411–4.

16. Friedman M, Landsberg R, Pryor S, Syed Z, Ibrahim H, Caldarelli DD. The occurrence of sleep-disordered breathing among patients with head and neck cancer. Laryngoscope. 2001;111(11 Pt 1):1917–9.

17. Nesse W, Hoekema A, Stegenga B, van der Hoeven JH, de Bont LG, Roodenburg JL. Prevalence of obstructive sleep apnoea following head and neck cancer treatment: a cross-sectional study. Oral Oncol. 2006;42(1):108–14.

18. Payne RJ, Hier MP, Kost KM, Black MJ, Zeitouni AG, Frenkiel S, Naor N, Kimoff RJ. High prevalence of obstructive sleep apnea among patients with head and neck cancer. J Otolaryngol. 2005;34(5):304–11.

19. Steffen A, Graefe H, Gehrking E, Konig IR, Wollenberg B. Sleep apnoea in patients after treatment of head neck cancer. Acta Otolaryngol. 2009;129(11):1300–5.

20. Faiz SA, Balachandran D, Hessel AC, Lei X, Beadle BM, William Jr WN, Bashoura L. Sleep-related breathing disorders in patients with tumors in the head and neck region. Oncologist. 2014;19(11):1200–6.

21. Qian W, Haight J, Poon I, Enepekides D, Higgins KM. Sleep apnea in patients with oral cavity and oropharyngeal cancer after surgery and chemoradiation therapy. Otolaryngol Head Neck Surg. 2010;143(2):248–52.

22. Stern TP, Auckley D. Obstructive sleep apnea following treatment of head and neck cancer. Ear Nose Throat J. 2007;86(2):101–3.

23. Llewellyn CD, McGurk M, Weinman J. How satisfied are head and neck cancer (HNC) patients with the information they receive pre-treatment? Results from the satisfaction with cancer information profile (SCIP). Oral Oncol. 2006;42(7):726–34.

24. Longacre ML, Galloway TJ, Parvanta CF, Fang CY. Medical Communication-related Informational Need and Resource Preferences Among Family Caregivers for Head and Neck Cancer Patients. J Cancer Educ. 2015;30(4):786–91.

25. Longacre ML, Ridge JA, Burtness BA, Galloway TJ, Fang CY. Psychological functioning of caregivers for head and neck cancer patients. Oral Oncol. 2012;48(1):18–25.

26. Badr H, Lipnick D, Diefenbach MA, Posner M, Kotz T, Miles B, Genden E. Development and usability testing of a web-based self-management intervention for oral cancer survivors and their family caregivers. Eur J Cancer Care. 2016;25(5):806–21.

27. Llewellyn CD, Horne R, McGurk M, Weinman J. Development and preliminary validation of a new measure to assess satisfaction with information among head and neck cancer patients: the satisfaction with cancer information profile (SCIP). Head Neck. 2006;28(6):540–8.

28. D'Souza V, Blouin E, Zeitouni A, Muller K, Allison PJ. Multimedia information intervention and its benefits in partners of the head and neck cancer patients. Eur J Cancer Care. 2016.

29. Newell R, Ziegler L, Stafford N, Lewin RJ. The information needs of head and neck cancer patients prior to surgery. Ann R Coll Surg Engl. 2004;86(6):407–10.

30. Ziegler L, Newell R, Stafford N, Lewin R. A literature review of head and neck cancer patients information needs, experiences and views regarding decision-making. Eur J Cancer Care. 2004;13:119–26.

31. Capozzi LC, Nishimura KC, McNeely ML, Lau H, Culos-Reed SN. The impact of physical activity on health-related fitness and quality of life for patients with head and neck cancer: a systematic review. Br J Sports Med. 2016;50(6):325–38.

32. Hunter KU, Jolly S. Clinical review of physical activity and functional considerations in head and neck cancer patients. Support Care Cancer. 2013;21(5):1475–9.

33. Sammut L, Ward M, Patel N. Physical activity and quality of life in head and neck cancer survivors: a literature review. Int J Sports Med. 2014;35(9):794–9.

34. Bossola M. Nutritional Interventions in Head and Neck Cancer Patients Undergoing Chemoradiotherapy: A Narrative Review. Nutrients. 2015;7(1):265.

35. Langius JAE, Zandbergen MC, Eerenstein SEJ, van Tulder MW, Leemans CR, Kramer MHH, Weijs PJM. Effect of nutritional interventions on nutritional status, quality of life and mortality in patients with head and neck cancer receiving (chemo)radiotherapy: a systematic review. Clin Nutr. 2013;32(5):671–8.

36. Nugent B, Lewis S, O'Sullivan JM. Enteral feeding methods for nutritional management in patients with head and neck cancers being treated with radiotherapy and/or chemotherapy. Cochrane Database Syst Rev. 2013;1:CD007904.

37. Chang CC, Kao HK, Huang JJ, Tsao CK, Cheng MH, Wei FC. Postoperative alcohol withdrawal syndrome and neuropsychological disorder in patients after head and neck cancer ablation followed by microsurgical free tissue transfer. J Reconstr Microsurg. 2013;29(2):131–6.

38. Deleyiannis FW, Thomas DB, Vaughan TL, Davis S. Alcoholism: independent predictor of survival in patients with head and neck cancer. J Natl Cancer Inst. 1996;88(8):542–9.

39. Duffy SA, Ronis DL, Valenstein M, Lambert MT, Fowler KE, Gregory L, Bishop C, Myers LL, Blow FC, Terrell JE. A tailored smoking, alcohol, and depression intervention for head and neck cancer patients. Cancer Epidemiol Biomark Prev. 2006;15(11):2203–8.

40. Lambert MT, Terrell JE, Copeland LA, Ronis DL, Duffy SA. Cigarettes, alcohol, and depression: characterizing head and neck cancer survivors in two systems of care. Nicotine Tob Res. 2005;7(2):233–41.

41. Potash AE, Karnell LH, Christensen AJ, Vander Weg MW, Funk GF. Continued alcohol use in patients with head and neck cancer. Head Neck. 2010;32(7):905–12.

42. Allison PJ. Factors associated with smoking and alcohol consumption following treatment for head and neck cancer. Oral Oncol. 2001;37(6):513–20.

43. Pinto FR, Matos LL, Gumz Segundo W, Vanni CM, Rosa DS, Kanda JL. Tobacco and alcohol use after head and neck cancer treatment: influence of the type of oncological treatment employed. Revista da Associacao Medica Brasileira (1992). 2011;57(2):171–6.

44. Lopez-Pelayo H, Miquel L, Altamirano J, Blanch JL, Gual A, Lligona A. Alcohol consumption in upper aerodigestive tract cancer: Role of head and neck surgeons' recommendations. Alcohol (Fayetteville, NY). 2016;51:51–6.

45. Al-Mamgani A, van Rooij PH, Mehilal R, Verduijn GM, Tans L, Kwa SL. Radiotherapy for T1a glottic cancer: the influence of smoking cessation and fractionation schedule of radiotherapy. Eur Arch Otorhinolaryngol. 2014;271(1):125–32.

46. Garces YI, Schroeder DR, Nirelli LM, Croghan GA, Croghan IT, Foote RL, Hurt RD. Second primary tumors following tobacco dependence treatments among head and neck cancer patients. Am J Clin Oncol. 2007;30(5):531–9.

47. van Imhoff LC, Kranenburg GG, Macco S, Nijman NL, van Overbeeke EJ, Wegner I, Grolman W, Pothen AJ. Prognostic value of continued smoking on survival and recurrence rates in patients with head and neck cancer: A systematic review. Head Neck. 2016;38(1 Suppl):E2214–20.

48. Zevallos JP, Mallen MJ, Lam CY, Karam-Hage M, Blalock J, Wetter DW, Garden AS, Sturgis EM, Cinciripini PM. Complications of radiotherapy in laryngopharyngeal cancer: effects of a prospective smoking cessation program. Cancer. 2009;115(19):4636–44.

49. Cooley ME, Emmons KM, Haddad R, Wang Q, Posner M, Bueno R, Cohen TJ, Johnson BE. Patient-reported receipt of and interest in smoking-cessation interventions after a diagnosis of cancer. Cancer. 2011;117(13):2961–9.

50. Fiore MC, Jaen CR. A clinical blueprint to accelerate the elimination of tobacco use. JAMA. 2008;299(17):2083–5.

51. Simmons VN, Litvin EB, Unrod M, Brandon TH. Oncology healthcare providers' implementation of the 5A's model of brief intervention for smoking cessation: patients' perceptions. Patient Educ Couns. 2012;86(3):414–9.

52. Simmons VN, Litvin EB, Patel RD, Jacobsen PB, McCaffrey JC, Bepler G, Quinn GP, Brandon TH. Patient-provider communication and perspectives on smoking cessation and relapse in the oncology setting. Patient Educ Couns. 2009;77(3):398–403.

53. Gritz ER, Carr CR, Rapkin D, Abemayor E, Chang LJ, Wong WK, Belin TR, Calcaterra T, Robbins KT, Chonkich G, et al. Predictors of long-term smoking

cessation in head and neck cancer patients. Cancer Epidemiol Biomark Prev. 1993;2(3):261–70.

54. Ghosh A, Philiponis G, Bewley A, Ransom ER, Mirza N. You can't pay me to quit: the failure of financial incentives for smoking cessation in head and neck cancer patients. J Laryngol Otol. 2016;130(3):278–83.

55. Foulds J, Schmelzer AC, Steinberg MB. Treating tobacco dependence as a chronic illness and a key modifiable predictor of disease. Int J Clin Pract. 2010;64(2):142–6.

56. Steinberg MB, Schmelzer AC, Richardson DL, Foulds J. The case for treating tobacco dependence as a chronic disease. Ann Intern Med. 2008;148(7):554–6.

57. Shields PG. New NCCN Guidelines: Smoking Cessation for Patients With Cancer. J Natl Compr Canc Netw. 2015;13(5 Suppl):643–5.

58. Metcalfe MC, Fischman SH. Factors affecting the sexuality of patients with head and neck cancer. Oncol Nurs Forum. 1985;12(2):21–5.

59. Monga U, Tan G, Ostermann HJ, Monga TN. Sexuality in head and neck cancer patients. Arch Phys Med Rehabil. 1997;78(3):298–304.

60. Auluck A, Hislop G, Bajdik C, Poh C, Zhang L, Rosin M. Trends in oropharyngeal and oral cavity cancer incidence of human papillomavirus (HPV)-related and HPV-unrelated sites in a multicultural population: the British Columbia experience. Cancer. 2010;116(11):2635–44.

61. Chaturvedi AK, Engels EA, Pfeiffer RM, Hernandez BY, Xiao W, Kim E, Jiang B, Goodman MT, Sibug-Saber M, Cozen W, et al. Human Papillomavirus and Rising Oropharyngeal Cancer Incidence in the United States. J Clin Oncol. 2011;29(32):4294–301.

62. Ryerson AB, Peters ES, Coughlin SS, Chen VW, Gillison ML, Reichman ME, Wu X, Chaturvedi AK, Kawaoka K. Burden of potentially human papillomavirus-associated cancers of the oropharynx and oral cavity in the US, 1998–2003. Cancer. 2008;113(10 Suppl):2901–9.

63. D'Souza G, Dempsey A. The role of HPV in head and neck cancer and review of the HPV vaccine. Prev Med. 2011;53 Suppl 1:S5–S11.

64. Marur S, D'Souza G, Westra WH, Forastiere AA. HPV-associated head and neck cancer: a virus-related cancer epidemic. Lancet Oncol. 2010;11(8):781–9.

65. Evans M, Powell NG. Sexual health in oral oncology: Breaking the news to patients with human papillomavirus–positive oropharyngeal cancer. Head Neck. 2014;36(11):1529–33.

66. Baxi SS, Shuman AG, Corner GW, Shuk E, Sherman EJ, Elkin EB, Hay JL, Pfister DG. Sharing a diagnosis of HPV-related head and neck cancer: The emotions, the confusion, and what patients want to know. Head Neck. 2013;35(11):1534–41.

67. Milbury K, Rosenthal DI, El-Naggar A, Badr H. An exploratory study of the informational and psychosocial needs of patients with human papillomavirus-associated oropharyngeal cancer. Oral Oncol. 2013;49(11):1067–71.

68. Dodd RH, Marlow LAV, Waller J. Discussing a diagnosis of human papillomavirus oropharyngeal cancer with patients: An exploratory qualitative study of health professionals. Head Neck. 2016;38(3):394–401.

69. Murthy VH, Krumholz HM, Gross CP. Participation in cancer clinical trials: Race-, sex-, and age-based disparities. JAMA. 2004;291(22):2720–6.

70. Haddad RI, Chan AT, Vermorken JB. Barriers to clinical trial recruitment in head and neck cancer. Oral Oncol. 2015;51(3):203–11.

71. Kaur G, Hutchison I, Mehanna H, Williamson P, Shaw R, Tudur Smith C. Barriers to recruitment for surgical trials in head and neck oncology: a survey of trial investigators. BMJ Open. 2013;3:e002625. doi:10.1136/bmjopen-2013-002625.

72. Jenkins V, Farewell D, Batt L, Maughan T, Branston L, Langridge C, Parlour L, Farewell V, Fallowfield L. The attitudes of 1066 patients with cancer towards participation in randomised clinical trials. Br J Cancer. 2010;103(12):1801–7.

73. Evans KR, Lewis MJ, Hudson SV. The role of health literacy on African American and Hispanic/Latino perspectives on cancer clinical trials. J Cancer Educ. 2012;27(2):299–305.

74. Meropol NJ, Wong YN, Albrecht T, Manne S, Miller SM, Flamm AL, Benson 3rd AB, Buzaglo J, Collins M, Egleston B, et al. Randomized Trial of a Web-Based Intervention to Address Barriers to Clinical Trials. J Clin Oncol. 2016;34(5):469–78.

75. Cousins N, MacAulay F, Lang H, MacGillivray S, Wells M. A systematic review of interventions for eating and drinking problems following treatment for head and neck cancer suggests a need to look beyond swallowing and trismus. Oral Oncol. 2013;49(5):387–400.

76. Schnoll RA, Rothman RL, Lerman C, Miller SM, Newman H, Movsas B, Sherman E, Ridge JA, Unger M, Langer C, et al. Comparing cancer patients who enroll in a smoking cessation program at a comprehensive cancer center with those who decline enrollment. Head Neck. 2004;26(3):278–86.

77. Simmons VN, Litvin EB, Jacobsen PB, Patel RD, McCaffrey JC, Oliver JA, Sutton SK, Brandon TH. Predictors of smoking relapse in patients with thoracic cancer or head and neck cancer. Cancer. 2013;119(7):1420–7.

9

Response to R-CHOP in HPV-related squamous cell carcinoma of base of tongue

Ting Martin Ma[1], Hyunseok Kang[2], Steven P. Rowe[3] and Ana P. Kiess[1*]

Abstract

Background: Synchronous squamous cell carcinoma of the head and neck (HNSCC) and non-Hodgkin's lymphoma is a rare clinical scenario. It is unknown whether the R-CHOP chemotherapy for lymphoma would also be active against HNSCC. Herein, we present such a case and a review of the literature.

Case presentation: A 64 year-old female presented with painless jaundice. CT demonstrated a retroperitoneal mass and pathology showed follicular lymphoma. A base-of-tongue HPV[+] squamous cell carcinoma was found incidentally on staging CT. R-CHOP chemotherapy was initiated. After 3 cycles of R-CHOP the lymphoma had a complete metabolic response and, unexpectedly, the HNSCC also demonstrated excellent response. The patient received another 3 cycles followed by radiation to the HNSCC and to date is in remission for both cancers.

Conclusions: This case highlights the exquisite sensitivity of HPV-related HNSCC, which should be taken into consideration in treatment prioritization of a concurrent diagnosis of a second cancer.

Keywords: Squamous cell carcinoma, Non-Hodgkin's lymphoma, R-CHOP, Synchronous, HPV

Background

Squamous cell carcinoma (SCC) accounts for more than 90% of tumors in the head and neck [1]. For patients with head and neck squamous cell carcinoma (HNSCC), a synchronous second primary cancer (SPC) has been reported in 1–5% of cases [2, 3]. Typically SPCs are also SCCs. An SPC of lymphogenic origin is extremely rare. In one study, 3.5% of the SPCs were non-Hodgkin lymphoma (NHL) with a majority of the index primaries seen in the oropharynx (39.2%) [3]. With the emergence of human papillomavirus (HPV) as a distinct risk factor for oropharyngeal HNSCC, the risk of SPC carried by oropharyngeal cancers has decreased [2]. On the other hand, there is a growing body of evidence demonstrating that patients with NHL or chronic lymphoid leukemia are immunosuppressed, partially attributed to disease biology itself, and are more susceptible to other malignancies including cutaneous SCC [4–10]. Various mechanisms of immune escape in NHL have been described, including impaired HLA-mediated cancer cell recognition [11], deranged apoptotic mechanisms, and changes in the tumor microenvironment involving regulatory T cells and tumor-associated macrophages [12–15].

Here, we report a unique case of synchronous follicular lymphoma and HPV[+] squamous cell carcinoma at base of tongue in which the SCC demonstrated an excellent response after only 3 cycles of R-CHOP chemotherapy. We also review the literature and cite other cases of synchronous SCC of aerodigestive tract and lymphoma treated with upfront R-CHOP chemotherapy, with a discussion of possible mechanisms of how component(s) of R-CHOP chemotherapy led to the regression of SCC.

Case presentation

A 64 year-old Caucasian female former smoker (4 pack-year) originally presented to the emergency department with painless jaundice. Physical exam revealed an afebrile female with scleral icterus and jaundice. Her abdomen was soft, non-tender, and non-distended in all quadrants with normal bowel sounds and no organomegaly. CT imaging demonstrated a large (10 cm) retroperitoneal mass, necessitating biliary stenting. Fine needle aspiration of the mass

* Correspondence: akiess1@jhmi.edu

[1]Department of Radiation Oncology and Molecular Radiation Sciences, The Johns Hopkins University School of Medicine, Baltimore, MD 21231, USA

Full list of author information is available at the end of the article

revealed a CD10$^+$clonal B cell population by flow cytometry, consistent with presumptive B cell lymphoma. During the staging workup for the lymphoma, right-sided cervical level IIA and III lymphadenopathy was found incidentally during a routine dental check-up, which was initially thought to be of the same disease process. She had no supraclavicular or axillary lymphadenopathy. CT demonstrated right level II/III LN and possible right base of tongue (BOT) mass. Flexible laryngoscopy revealed an exophytic mass involving the right BOT that extended to the right glosso-tonsillar sulcus and beyond the midline measuring approximately 3 cm (Fig. 1). Excisional biopsy of two right cervical lymph nodes unexpectedly demonstrated squamous cell cancer (SCC) that was positive for p16 and HPV. Subsequently, positron emission tomography/computed tomography (PET/CT) demonstrated an FDG-avid right BOT mass (2.3 × 0.9 cm) with right-sided level IIA, IIB and III lymphadenopathy (all < 3 cm), consistent with biopsy-proven HPV-associated SCC (Fig. 2). There was also an intensely FDG-avid retroperitoneal mass (8.2 × 13.4 × 10.7 cm) along with left mesenteric, left periaortic, and left retroperitoneal lymph nodes (Fig. 3). Laparoscopic biopsy of gastroepiploic, mesenteric, and gastrocolic lymph nodes confirmed follicular lymphoma. Pathology showed relatively low number of centroblasts (fewer than 15 per high power field) compatible with low grade follicular lymphoma (WHO grade 1–2) with significantly elevated Ki-67 proliferation index (~ 80%) suggesting clinical behavior similar to WHO grade 3 follicular lymphoma. Omentum and liver were not involved. Therefore, a diagnosis of synchronous stage IV T2N2bM0 HPV$^+$ SCC of right BOT and stage IIAX follicular lymphoma was made. At the time, she was relatively asymptomatic from the BOT cancer. She denied dysphagia, odynophagia, trismus, otalgia, or speech or voice change. She also denied night sweats, fevers, significant weight loss, or infectious symptoms. Videofluoroscopic swallow study evaluation was normal. ECOG performance status was 1. After stenting, the patient's bilirubin normalized and she was asymptomatic. Her case was discussed at multidisciplinary case conferences, and the initial plan was to treat the BOT cancer first due to its likely curability and shorter treatment course.

One month later, however, the patient was admitted to the hospital because of worsening abdominal pain. Given concern for lymphoma becoming increasingly symptomatic, R-CHOP (rituximab, cyclophosphamide, doxorubicin, vincristine, and prednisone) chemotherapy was initiated. She tolerated therapy well and had resolution of abdominal pain. After completion of 3 cycles of R-CHOP, PET/CT scan demonstrated interval markedly decreased size and uptake of the retroperitoneal mass, as well as interval resolution of the FDG-avid BOT lesion, and most of the FDG-avid cervical lymph nodes (Figs. 2 and 3). She had no symptoms referable to lymphoma at this time. Nasopharyngolaryngoscopy also revealed no residual fullness in the area of the right BOT (Fig. 1). After completion of another 3 cycles of R-CHOP (in total 6 cycles), PET/CT scan demonstrated sustained metabolic resolution of the abdominal mass. However, FDG-avid right BOT lesion as well as right cervical level II and III nodes had become slightly more prominent compared to the end of cycle 3. The decision was made to start 7-week concurrent chemoradiation with weekly cisplatin 40 mg/m^2 for the SCC. Unfortunately, she was found to be neutropenic and cisplatin was switched to cetuximab. At the end of the first cetuximab infusion, she developed a Grade 3 infusion reaction with rigors and chest pain and was diagnosed with NSTEMI. An attempt to re-initiate cisplatin treatment after ANC normalized was unsuccessful as patient experienced fever and altered mental status necessitating hospital admission. She had received a total of one dose of cetuximab and two doses of cisplatin before the decision was made to proceed with radiation therapy (RT) without further chemotherapy. In total, the patient received 6996 cGy, 212 cGy per day in 33 fractions with coverage of the oropharynx and bilateral neck using tomotherapy-based image-guided intensity-modulated radiation therapy. Despite experiencing significant anterior mouth sores from cetuximab early in treatment, as well as significant oropharynx mucositis late in treatment, she was ultimately

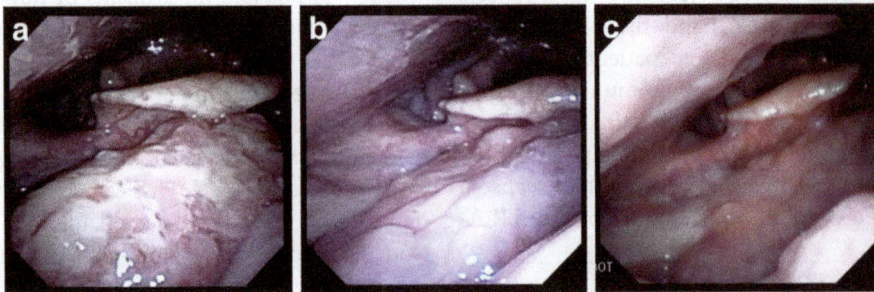

Fig. 1 Flexible nasopharyngolaryngoscopy view of the right BOT mass before treatment (**a**), after 3 cycles of R-CHOP chemotherapy (**b**) and after the completion of 6 cycles of R-CHOP chemotherapy (**c**)

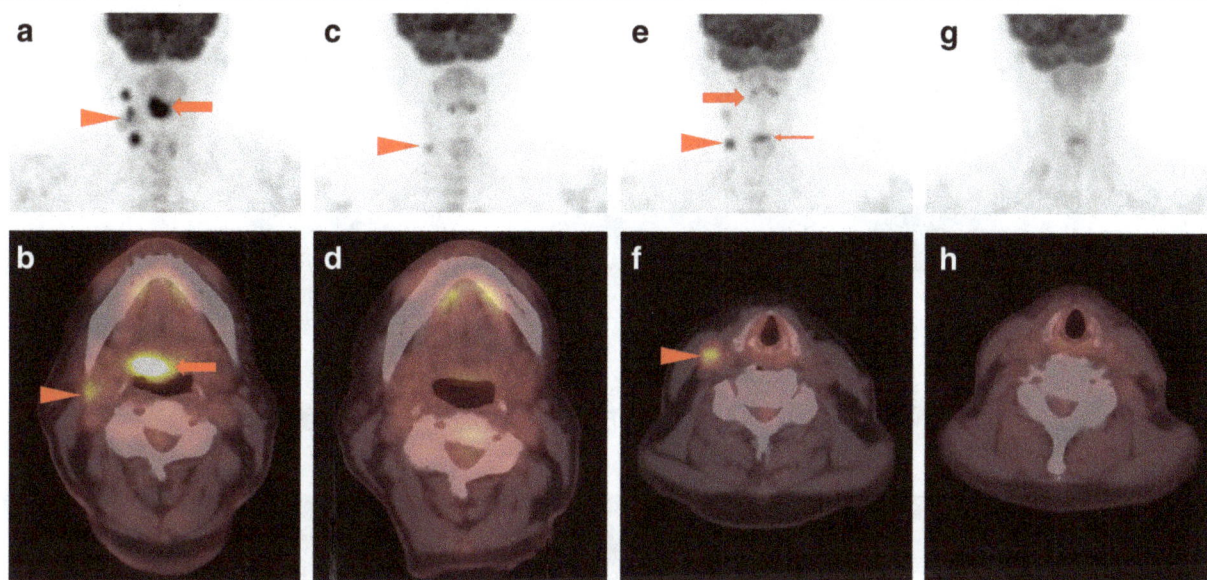

Fig. 2 a Baseline head and neck maximum intensity projection (MIP) image demonstrating focal FDG uptake in the patient's BOT HNSCC (red arrow) as well as ipsilateral cervical adenopathy (red arrowhead). **b** Representative axial PET/CT slice from the same time point as in (**a**) which delineates the BOT HNSCC (red arrow) and also highlights one of the right-sided cervical lymph nodes (red arrowhead). **c** Head and neck MIP image following 3 cycles of R-CHOP demonstrates complete metabolic response in the patient's BOT HNSCC and partial response in the ipsilateral cervical adenopathy (red arrowhead). **d** Axial PET/CT image from the same time point as (**c**) shows no abnormal uptake at the BOT (persistently FDG-avid cervical nodes are not shown on this slice). **e** Head and neck MIP image following completion of R-CHOP therapy demonstrates very subtle increased uptake in the BOT HNSCC (red arrow, barely visible) and increasing uptake in ipsilateral cervical lymph nodes (red arrowhead). Note normal physiologic activity in the vocal cords (thin red arrow). **f** Representative axial PET/CT image through the neck shows an FDG-avid right level III lymph node compatible with residual HNSCC. **g** Head and neck MIP and (**h**) axial PET/CT images following completion of chemoradiation therapy show no evidence of metabolically active primary or nodal HNSCC

able to complete RT without an enteral feeding tube. At 3-month follow-up, she had no clinical or radiographic evidence of disease on exam or PET/CT scan. At the time of this manuscript submission, 3 years after completion of the radiation therapy, she remained in remission for both cancers.

Discussion

SCC is the most common malignant tumor of the head and neck and may arise in the oral cavity, pharynx, larynx, or sinonasal cavities. Although most HNSCCs are related to alcohol and/or tobacco use, the incidence of HPV-associated HNSCC is on the rise worldwide [16]. In the United States, more than half of cancers diagnosed in the oropharynx are linked to HPV type 16 [17]. Interestingly, one Danish study demonstrated that HPV infection is associated with an increased incidence of both Hodgkin and NHL using conization as a surrogate marker [18]. Therefore it is plausible that in this case, chronic immune activation induced by persistent HPV infection and the failure of the immune system to clear HPV infection and to control lymphoma development could have contributed to lymphomagenesis in addition to its role in the pathogenesis of HNSCC.

HPV+ OPC is a distinct type of OPC and has very different biology compared to its HPV- counterparts. Patients with HPV-related OPCs have a more favorable prognosis, in part due to the natural biology of the cancer and in part because these tumors are more responsive to chemotherapy and radiotherapy than HPV- cancers [19, 20]. Definitive treatment of locoregionally advanced (III/IV) OPC often requires a multimodality approach that may include chemotherapy, RT, concurrent chemoradiation (CRT) and/or surgery. Cisplatin is considered the gold standard for CRT, with cetuximab as an alternative agent [21]. Other common chemotherapy agents including paclitaxel, docetaxel, 5-FU, hydroxyurea and carboplatin have also been used in treating OPC.

An unexpected observation in this case was the excellent response of BOT HNSCC to R-CHOP chemotherapy intended for follicular lymphoma, even after only 3 cycles. Despite slight regrowth seen at the end of cycle 6, the SCC responded very well to the initial 3 cycles of R-CHOP, judged by the interval resolution of the FDG-avid BOT lesion and most of the FDG-avid cervical lymph nodes and negative nasopharyngolaryngoscopy results. The patient was also free of symptoms from SCC. The observed effect of R-CHOP on HPV+ head and neck cancer was unexpected because components of this regimen do not overlap with any routine chemotherapy regimen for HNSCC. A literature search

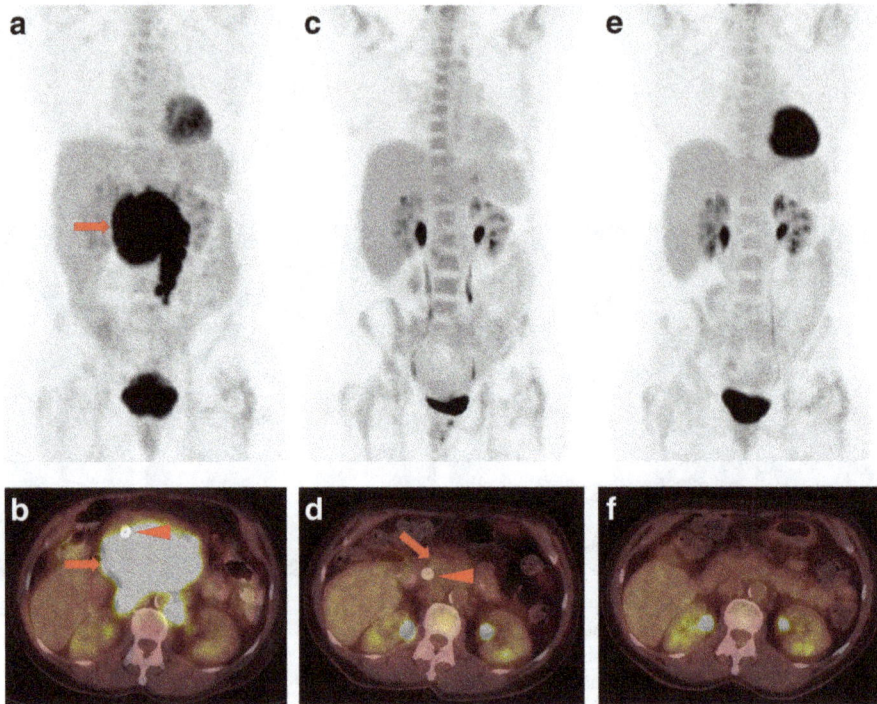

Fig. 3 a Baseline whole-body MIP image demonstrating intense FDG uptake in a large retroperitoneal mass (red arrow) compatible with patient's follicular lymphoma. **b** Representative axial PET/CT image from the same time point as in (**a**) showing the large, FDG-avid mass (red arrow). Note the common bile duct stent (red arrowhead) that is markedly anteriorly displaced by the lymphomatous mass and explains the patient's presentation with obstructive jaundice. **c** Whole-body MIP image following three cycles of R-CHOP shows no residual metabolically active lymphoma. **d** Representative axial PET/CT image from the same time point as in (**c**) is notable for the presence of minimal residual abnormal soft tissue in the retroperitoneum (red arrow, Lugano 2), with uptake equal to blood pool, compatible with a complete metabolic response. The common bile duct stent is in near-orthotopic location now that the retroperitoneal mass has dramatically reduced in size (red arrowhead). **e** Whole-body MIP image at the end of therapy, again demonstrating no metabolically active tumor. **f** Representative axial PET/CT image from the same time point as in (**e**) again depicts the complete metabolic response (Lugano 1) and also the removal of the common bile duct stent

revealed 3 case reports of synchronous SCC of aerodigestive tract and lymphoma treated with upfront R-CHOP chemotherapy (Table 1). Lymphoma achieved complete response in 2 cases [22, 23] and partial response in the other [24]. In contrast, SCC achieved partial response in 1 case [22] and stability/progression in 2 cases [23, 24]. Of note, none of these cases were HPV-related SCC.

Among the components of R-CHOP, only 2 agents have been evaluated as single chemotherapy agents in HNSCC. Cyclophosphamide had a response rate of 36% in 77 patients in one study [25] and doxorubicin had a response rate of 24% in another study [25]. Vinblastine, a closely related agent to vincristine, demonstrated a response rate of 29% [25]. However, these early studies should be interpreted with caution due to lower

Table 1 Case reports of synchronous SCC of aerodigestive tract and lymphoma treated with upfront R-CHOP chemotherapy

Study	Patient characteristics	Index primary	Synchronous secondary primary	Treatment regimen	Response	Remarks
Morita et al., 2009 [22]	75-year-old female	DLBCL (lower lip)	SCC (buccal mucosa)	6 cycles of R-THP-COP	Complete response for DLBCL, partial response for SCC	SCC was subsequently treated with tegafur, gimeracil and oteracil potassium with partial response
Oikonomou et al., 2013 [24]	72-year-old male, 20 pack-yr smoking hx	BALT Lymphoma (LLL)	low-differentiated lung SCC (RML)	3 cycles of R-CHOP	Significant reduction in size of lymphoma and stability of the lung SCC	9-month follow-up CT revealed progression of the lung cancer with distant metastatic disease
Fujii et al., 2014 [23]	68-year-old female	DLBCL (Left cervical LNs)	Lung SCC (RUL and hilar and mediastinal LNs)	3 cycles of R-CHOP	Complete response for DLBCL; pulmonary SCC and right hilar LN stable/increased	Radical surgery performed after 3 cycles of R-CHOP to resect lung SCC

DLBCL diffuse large B-cell lymphoma, *SCC* squamous cell carcinoma, *BALT* bronchial-associated lymphoid tissue, *LLL* left lower lobe, *RML* right middle lobe, *RUL* right upper lobe, *LN* lymph node, *R-THP-COP* rituximab, pirarubicin, cyclophosphamide, vincristine, and prednisolone

prevalence of HPV-related SCC during the study period [16], limited size, and a lack of information concerning prior treatment and nutritional and performance status.

Historically, these agents have also been evaluated as combination therapies with other chemotherapy agents, mostly in the 1980's and 1990's. Many cyclophosphamide combinations have been reported, as this is an agent with very broad activity in a variety of epithelial tumors. The most common combination utilized was with bleomycin, methotrexate, and 5-FU. The overall response rate was 47% (132/279) with a range of 11–69% [26].

Vincristine has been mostly reported as a combinatorial agent with cyclophosphamide, cisplatin, bleomycin, methotrexate, and 5-FU in HNSCC [26–28]. For example, the combination of vincristine, bleomycin, and methotrexate produced a response rate of the primary tumor in 61% [29]. As part of the CABO (cisplatin, methotrexate, bleomycin and vincristine) regimen, the overall response rate was 34% in a phase III trial of recurrent or metastatic HNSCC [30].

The role of B cells in solid tumors has also been under intense examination. B cells can exert their tumorigenic effects by secretion of paracrine factors that sustain chronic inflammation [31], deposition of immune complexes and Fcγ receptor-dependent activation of myeloid cells, and by enhancing T_H2-type $CD4^+$ T helper cells while repressing $CD4^+$ T_H1 cells which influence $CD8^+$ cytotoxic T cell activity [32]. As human SCCs of the vulva and head and neck exhibit hallmarks of B cell infiltration, it is postulated that rituximab, a chimeric monoclonal antibody against CD20 that leads to B cell depletion [33], could be considered in solid tumors [32]. Indeed, in a preclinical murine model of HPV16-related SCC, administration of rituximab to mice bearing preexisting SCCs improved response to platinum- and taxol-based chemotherapy, although it was ineffective as a single agent. This process was dependent on expression of an altered repertoire of chemokines expressed by macrophages, resulting in increased recruitment of cytotoxic T lymphocytes. A pilot clinical study in advanced colon cancer patients treated with rituximab reported encouraging tumor regressions [34]. Therefore it is possible that depletion of B cells with rituximab also played a role in the response of HNSCC to R-CHOP in this case. It should be noted that in addition to B cell depletion from rituximab, the treatment of lymphoma with R-CHOP possibly led to broad immunologic changes, restoring immune function in general.

The excellent response could also be attributed to the inherent treatment-sensitive biology of HPV^+ SCC. HPV^+ patients have better progression-free survival, lower locoregional failure rates, and improved 3-year overall survival in the setting of treatment with sequential chemoradiation and even after radiotherapy alone [35]. Therefore HPV

positivity may confer a more favorable prognosis in a "platform-independent" manner. In a prospective trial of low-risk HPV^+ patients (T1-3 N0-N2b), 3 cycles of induction chemotherapy with cisplatin, paclitaxel, and cetuximab achieved an excellent complete clinical response (cCR) rate of 70%, which subsequently enabled them to be treated with a substantially lower dose of radiation (54Gy vs. 69.3Gy) [36]. In fact, the benefit of chemotherapy is unclear in this selected group of low-risk patients and efforts are underway to evaluate if chemotherapy can be omitted altogether ([35] and clinical trial NCT02254278).

In the present case, we would not have been able to observe the therapeutic effect of R-CHOP on SCC had we decided to treat SCC first with concurrent CRT. The main reason we prioritized treating lymphoma was the concern that the index retroperitoneal mass represented transformed lymphoma. However, this could not be ascertained without a tissue biopsy which was contraindicated due to the large size and vascularity of the mass. In addition, the high proliferation rate of the surrounding nodal disease, bulky disease, and relatively good prognosis of SCC all conspired for an upfront aggressive chemotherapy regimen like R-CHOP.

Conclusions

We report a case of synchronous retroperitoneal follicular lymphoma and HPV^+ BOT HNSCC in a 64 year-old female patient in which HNSCC had an excellent response to R-CHOP chemotherapy before definitive chemoradiation therapy. Although there are published case reports of synchronous SCC of the aerodigestive tract and NHL [22–24, 37–48], this is the first to report a dramatic response of SCC to R-CHOP. This case highlights the exquisite sensitivity of HPV-related HNSCC, which should be taken into consideration in treatment prioritization in the setting of a concurrent diagnosis of a second cancer. The exact agent(s) responsible for the observed response is unclear but the immunomodulatory effect of rituximab and/or the cytotoxic effect of cyclophosphamide, doxorubicin and vincristine could each have played a role.

Abbreviations
5-FU: 5-fluorouracil; BOT: Base of tongue; CABO: Cisplatin, methotrexate, bleomycin and vincristine; cCR: Complete clinical response; CRT: Concurrent chemoradiation; CT: Computed tomography; EGFR: Epidermal growth factor receptor; HNSCC: Squamous cell carcinoma of the head and neck; HPV: Human papillomavirus; NSTEMI: non-ST-elevation myocardial infarction; OPC: Oropharyngeal cancer; PET/CT: Positron emission tomography/computed tomography; R-CHOP: Rituximab, cyclophosphamide, doxorubicin, vincristine, and prednisone; RT: Radiation therapy; SCC: Squamous cell carcinoma; SPC: Second primary cancer

Authors' contributions
APK and HK were directly involved in the care of the patient described in this report and were responsible for the study concept and design. Patient data were acquired and analyzed by TMM and SPR. SPR supervised analysis of the radiographic images. TMM and SPR drafted the manuscript. All authors read and approved the final manuscript.

Competing interests
The authors declare that they have no competing interests.

Author details
[1]Department of Radiation Oncology and Molecular Radiation Sciences, The Johns Hopkins University School of Medicine, Baltimore, MD 21231, USA. [2]Department of Oncology, The Johns Hopkins University School of Medicine, Baltimore, MD 21287, USA. [3]The Russell H. Morgan Department of Radiology and Radiological Science, The Johns Hopkins University School of Medicine, Baltimore, MD 21287, USA.

References
1. Sanderson RJ, Ironside JA. Squamous cell carcinomas of the head and neck. BMJ. 2002;325:822–7.
2. Jain KS, Sikora AG, Baxi SS, Morris LG. Synchronous cancers in patients with head and neck cancer: risks in the era of human papillomavirus-associated oropharyngeal cancer. Cancer. 2013;119:1832–7.
3. Krishnatreya M, Rahman T, Kataki AC, Das A, Das AK, Lahkar K. Synchronous primary cancers of the head and neck region and upper aero digestive tract: defining high-risk patients. Indian J Cancer. 2013;50:322–6.
4. Levi F, Randimbison L, Te VC, La Vecchia C. Non-Hodgkin's lymphomas, chronic lymphocytic leukaemias and skin cancers. Br J Cancer. 1996;74:1847–50.
5. Jones SE, Griffith K, Dombrowski P, Gaines JA. Immunodeficiency in patients with non-Hodgkin lymphomas. Blood. 1977;49:335–44.
6. Brewer JD, Habermann TM, Shanafelt TD. Lymphoma-associated skin cancer: incidence, natural history, and clinical management. Int J Dermatol. 2014;53:267–74.
7. Brewer JD, Shanafelt TD, Khezri F, Sosa Seda IM, Zubair AS, Baum CL, Arpey CJ, Cerhan JR, Call TG, Roenigk RK, et al. Increased incidence and recurrence rates of nonmelanoma skin cancer in patients with non-Hodgkin lymphoma: a Rochester epidemiology project population-based study in Minnesota. J Am Acad Dermatol. 2015;72:302–9.
8. Hartley BE, Searle AE, Breach NM, Rhys-Evans PH, Henk JM. Aggressive cutaneous squamous cell carcinoma of the head and neck in patients with chronic lymphocytic leukaemia. J Laryngol Otol. 1996;110:694–5.
9. Dasanu CA, Alexandrescu DT. Risk for second nonlymphoid neoplasms in chronic lymphocytic leukemia. MedGenMed. 2007;9:35.
10. Agnew KL, Ruchlemer R, Catovsky D, Matutes E, Bunker CB. Cutaneous findings in chronic lymphocytic leukaemia. Br J Dermatol. 2004;150:1129–35.
11. Drenou B, Le Friec G, Bernard M, Pangault C, Grosset JM, Lamy T, Fauchet R, Amiot L. Major histocompatibility complex abnormalities in non-Hodgkin lymphomas. Br J Haematol. 2002;119:417–24.
12. Laurent C, Charmpi K, Gravelle P, Tosolini M, Franchet C, Ysebaert L, Brousset P, Bidaut A, Ycart B, Fournie JJ. Several immune escape patterns in non-Hodgkin's lymphomas. Oncoimmunology. 2015;4:e1026530.
13. Upadhyay R, Hammerich L, Peng P, Brown B, Merad M, Brody JD. Lymphoma: immune evasion strategies. Cancers. 2015;7:736–62.
14. Menter T, Tzankov A. Mechanisms of immune evasion and immune modulation by lymphoma cells. Front Oncol. 2018;8:54.
15. Dalla-Favera R. Molecular genetics of aggressive B-cell lymphoma. Hematol Oncol. 2017;35(Suppl 1):76–9.
16. Gillison ML, Chaturvedi AK, Anderson WF, Fakhry C. Epidemiology of human papillomavirus-positive head and neck squamous cell carcinoma. J Clin Oncol. 2015;33:3235–42.
17. Chaturvedi AK, Engels EA, Pfeiffer RM, Hernandez BY, Xiao W, Kim E, Jiang B, Goodman MT, Sibug-Saber M, Cozen W, et al. Human papillomavirus and rising oropharyngeal cancer incidence in the United States. J Clin Oncol. 2011;29:4294–301.
18. Intaraphet S, Farkas DK, Johannesdottir Schmidt SA, Cronin-Fenton D, Sogaard M. Human papillomavirus infection and lymphoma incidence using cervical conization as a surrogate marker: a Danish nationwide cohort study. Hematol Oncol. 2017;35:172–6.
19. Kumar B, Cipolla MJ, Old MO, Brown NV, Kang SY, Dziegielewski PT, Durmus K, Ozer E, Agrawal A, Carrau RL, et al. Surgical management of oropharyngeal squamous cell carcinoma: survival and functional outcomes. Head Neck. 2016;38(Suppl 1):E1794–802.
20. Ang KK, Harris J, Wheeler R, Weber R, Rosenthal DI, Nguyen-Tan PF, Westra WH, Chung CH, Jordan RC, Lu C, et al. Human papillomavirus and survival of patients with oropharyngeal cancer. N Engl J Med. 2010;363:24–35.
21. Bonner JA, Harari PM, Giralt J, Azarnia N, Shin DM, Cohen RB, Jones CU, Sur R, Raben D, Jassem J, et al. Radiotherapy plus cetuximab for squamous-cell carcinoma of the head and neck. N Engl J Med. 2006;354:567–78.
22. Morita Y, Kimoto N, Ogawa H, Omata T, Morita N. Squamous cell carcinoma and malignant lymphoma as synchronous malignant Tumours in the oral cavity. Asian J Oral Maxillofac Surg. 2009;21:64–8.
23. Fujii M, Shirai T, Asada K, Saito Y, Hirose M, Suda T. Synchronous diffuse large B-cell lymphoma and squamous cell lung carcinoma. Respirol Case Rep. 2014;2:33–5.
24. Oikonomou A, Astrinakis E, Kotsianidis I, Kaloutsi V, Didilis V, Tsatalas K, Prassopoulos P. Synchronous BALT lymphoma and squamous cell carcinoma of the lung: coincidence or linkage? Case Rep Oncol Med. 2013;2013:420393.
25. Carter SK. The chemotherapy of head and neck cancer. Semin Oncol. 1977;4:413–24.
26. Al-Sarraf M. Chemotherapy strategies in squamous cell carcinoma of the head and neck. Crit Rev Oncol Hematol. 1984;1:323–55.
27. Richman SP, Livingston RB, Gutterman JU, Suen JY, Hersh EM. Chemotherapy versus chemoimmunotherapy of head and neck cancer: report of a randomized study. Cancer Treat Rep. 1976;60:535–9.
28. Clavel M, Cognetti F, Dodion P, Wildiers J, Rosso R, Rossi A, Gignoux B, Van Rymenant M, Cortes-Funes H, Dalesio O, et al. Combination chemotherapy with methotrexate, bleomycin, and vincristine with or without cisplatin in advanced squamous cell carcinoma of the head and neck. Cancer. 1987;60:1173–7.
29. Figueroa-Valles NR, Marcial VA, Velez-Garcia E, Cintron J, Vallecillo LA. Multidrug chemotherapy (vincristine-bleomycin-methotrexate) followed by radiotherapy in inoperable carcinomas of the head and neck: a pilot study of the radiation therapy oncology group. Am J Clin Oncol. 1982;5:399–404.
30. Clavel M, Vermorken JB, Cognetti F, Cappelaere P, de Mulder PH, Schornagel JH, Tueni EA, Verweij J, Wildiers J, Clerico M, et al. Randomized comparison of cisplatin, methotrexate, bleomycin and vincristine (CABO) versus cisplatin and 5-fluorouracil (CF) versus cisplatin (C) in recurrent or metastatic squamous cell carcinoma of the head and neck. A phase III study of the EORTC head and neck Cancer cooperative group. Ann Oncol. 1994;5:521–6.
31. Pillai S, Mattoo H, Cariappa A. B cells and autoimmunity. Curr Opin Immunol. 2011;23:721–31.
32. Coussens LM, Zitvogel L, Palucka AK. Neutralizing tumor-promoting chronic inflammation: a magic bullet? Science. 2013;339:286–91.
33. Kessel A, Rosner I, Toubi E. Rituximab: beyond simple B cell depletion. Clin Rev Allergy Immunol. 2008;34:74–9.
34. Tan TT, Coussens LM. Humoral immunity, inflammation and cancer. Curr Opin Immunol. 2007;19:209–16.
35. O'Sullivan B, Huang SH, Siu LL, Waldron J, Zhao H, Perez-Ordonez B, Weinreb I, Kim J, Ringash J, Bayley A, et al. Deintensification candidate subgroups in human papillomavirus-related oropharyngeal cancer according to minimal risk of distant metastasis. J Clin Oncol. 2013;31:543–50.
36. Marur S, Li S, Cmelak AJ, Gillison ML, Zhao WJ, Ferris RL, Westra WH, Gilbert J, Bauman JE, Wagner LI, et al. E1308: phase II trial of induction chemotherapy followed by reduced-dose radiation and weekly Cetuximab in patients with HPV-associated Resectable squamous cell carcinoma of the oropharynx- ECOG-ACRIN Cancer research group. J Clin Oncol.
37. Kaur P, Khurana A, Chauhan AK, Singh G, Katari SP. Non-Hodgkin's lymphoma of thyroid synchronously with squamous cell carcinoma base of tongue: a rare coincidence and treatment strategy. Intl J Head Neck Surg. 2014;5:155–7.
38. Sun Y, Shi YF, Zhou LX, Chen KN, Li XH. Synchronous pulmonary squamous cell carcinoma and mantle cell lymphoma of the lymph node. Case Rep Gen. 2011;2011:945181.
39. Hadjileontis CG, Kostopoulos IS, Kaloutsi VD, Nikolaou AC, Kotoula VA, Papadimitriou CS. An extremely rare case of synchronous occurrence in the

larynx of intravascular lymphoma and in situ squamous cell carcinoma. Leuk Lymphoma. 2003;44:1053–7.

40. Tezer MS, Tuncel U, Uzlugedik S, Uzun M, Kulacoglu S, Unal A. Coexistence of laryngeal squamous cell carcinoma and non-Hodgkin's lymphoma with nasopharyngeal involvement. J Laryngol Otol. 2006;120:e2.

41. Nigri PT, Khasgiwala CK. Unusual presentation of head and neck neoplasm. Laryngoscope. 1982;92:1245–6.

42. Shudo A, Takenobu T, Hirai Y, Yamamoto S, Taniike N, Usami Y. A case of synchronous squamous cell carcinoma of the mandibular gingiva and primary malignant lymphoma of the neck. Japanese J Oral Maxillofac Surg. 2017;63:45–50.

43. Park JH, Lee JH, Lim Y, Lee YJ, Lee DY. Synchronous occurrence of primary cutaneous anaplastic large cell lymphoma and squamous cell carcinoma. Ann Dermatol. 2016;28:491–4.

44. Kader I, Leavers B, Shashinder S, Wylie B, Chi KK, Sundaresan P. Synchronous or metachronous lymphoma and metastatic cutaneous squamous cell carcinoma in the head and neck region: a diagnostic and management dilemma. J Laryngol Otol. 2016;130(Suppl 4):S45–9.

45. Watanabe N, Inohara H, Akahani S, Yamamoto Y, Moriwaki K, Kubo T. Synchronous squamous cell carcinoma and malignant lymphoma in the head and neck region. Auris Nasus Larynx. 2007;34:273–6.

46. Fonseca D, Musthyala B, Ahmed F, Murthy SS, Raju KV. A tale of synchronous lung carcinoma and diffuse large B-cell lymphoma of ileum: a rare combination. Lung India. 2015;32:398–401.

47. Heidemann LN, Johansen J, Larsen SR, Sorensen JA. Four synchronous cancers in a patient with tongue pain as the only symptom. BMJ Case Rep. 2016;2016. https://www.ncbi.nlm.nih.gov/pubmed/2715.

48. Raldow AC, Brown JG, Chau N, Davids MS, Margalit DN, Tishler RB, Ng A, Schoenfeld JD. Synchronous squamous cell carcinoma and diffuse large B-cell lymphoma of the head and neck: the odd couple. BJR Case Rep. 2016;2:1–4.

10

Costimulatory and coinhibitory immune checkpoint receptors in head and neck cancer: unleashing immune responses through therapeutic combinations

Ruth J. Davis[1], Robert L. Ferris[2,3,4] and Nicole C. Schmitt[1,5]*

Abstract

Head and neck squamous cell carcinoma (HNSCC) represents a model of escape from anti-tumor immunity. The high frequency of p53 tumor suppressor loss in HNSCC leads to genomic instability and immune stimulation through the generation of neoantigens. However, the aggressive nature of HNSCC tumors and significant rates of resistance to conventional therapies highlights the ability of HNSCC to evade this immune response. Advances in understanding the role of co-stimulatory and immune checkpoint receptors in HNSCC-mediated immunosuppression lay the foundation for development of novel therapeutic approaches. This article provides an overview of these co-stimulatory and immune checkpoint pathways, as well as a review of preclinical and clinical evidence supporting the modulation of these pathways in HNSCC. Finally, the synergistic potential of combining these approaches is discussed, along with an update of current clinical trials evaluating combinations of immune-based therapies in HNSCC patients.

Keywords: Head and neck cancer, Immune checkpoints, Costimulatory receptors, CD137, CD40, OX40, PD-1, CTLA-4, Cetuximab, Immunotherapy

Abbreviations: APC, Antigen-presenting cell; CTLA-4, Cytotoxic T lymphocyte-associated protein 4; EGFR, Epidermal growth factor receptor; HNSCC, Head and neck squamous cell carcinoma; HPV, Human papillomavirus; IMRT, Intensity modulated radiation therapy; LAG-3, Lymphocyte-activation gene 3; mAb, Monoclonal antibody; MDSC, Myeloid-derived suppressor cell; MHC, Major histocompatibility complex; NSCLC, Non small-cell lung cancer; PBMC, Peripheral blood mononuclear cell; PD-1, Programmed death-1; PD-L1, programmed death-1 ligand; TCR, T-cell receptor; TIM-3, T-cell immunoglobulin mucin 3; TLR, Toll-like receptor; TLR, Toll-like receptor; TME, Tumor microenvironment; Treg, Regulatory T-cell

Background

Head and neck squamous cell carcinoma (HNSCC) is the sixth most common cancer in the world, affecting over 500,000 people each year [1]. While HPV-associated HNSCC responds well to standard anti-cancer therapies, five-year survival rates of carcinogen-induced HNSCC are 60 % or less [1]. This poor prognosis despite advances in chemotherapy, radiation, and surgical protocols highlights the need for treatments with greater efficacy in the HPV- population, and improved toxicity profiles for HPV+ patients. Advances in understanding the role of the immune system in preventing development and growth of HNSCC has led to renewed focus on immune-targeting therapies as a means of achieving these goals.

In a process termed immune surveillance, recognition of non-self antigens on tumor cells allows for their destruction by the host immune system [2]. The high frequency of p53 tumor suppressor loss in HNSCC

* Correspondence: nicole.schmitt@nih.gov
[1]Tumor Biology Section, Head and Neck Surgery Branch, National Institute on Deafness and Other Communication Disorders, National Institutes of Health, 10 Center Drive, Room 5B-39, Bethesda, MD 20892, USA
[5]Department of Otolaryngology-Head and Neck Surgery, Johns Hopkins School of Medicine, 6420 Rockledge Drive, Suite 4920, Bethesda, MD 20817, USA
Full list of author information is available at the end of the article

leads to significant genomic instability and the generation of neoantigens, which can activate the immune system and attract infiltrates of effector T-lymphocytes and natural killer (NK) cells into the tumor [3–5]. These adaptive anti-tumor immune responses have been correlated with improved outcomes in many cancers, including HNSCC [6, 7]. However, in order for a clinically significant cancer to develop, the tumor must escape from this anti-cancer immunity through a variety of mechanisms [8]. HNSCC represents an ideal model for understanding and targeting these mechanisms of immune escape in order to unleash the full power of the immune response that can be induced by its characteristically high genetic alteration rate. On the other hand, HPV+ HNSCC is an excellent model of viral-induced cancer, in which oncoproteins such as E6 and E7 are by definition antigenic and therefore tumor development is predicated upon evasion of antiviral immunity [9].

Once recruited to the tumor microenvironment, T-cells interact with antigen-presenting cells (APCs) at the "immune synapse," and require two simultaneous signals from APCs before they can be activated to mediate their anti-tumor effects (Fig. 1). The first, "signal one,"

occurs through interaction of the T-cell receptor (TCR) on the surface of the T-cell and a major histocompatibility complex (MHC) molecule presenting tumor antigen on the surface of an APC (Fig. 1, blue). The second, "signal two" is made up of interactions between co-stimulatory molecules on the surface of APCs and T-cells, such as B7 on the APC surface and CD28 on the T-cell (Fig. 1, green) [2]. Both of these signals must also occur in the context of a third signal made up of immune-activating cytokines such as IL-12, type I (IFNα/β) or type II (IFNγ) interferon [10, 11].

In contrast to these co-stimulatory molecules, the inhibitory "immune checkpoints" prevent T-cell activation. These checkpoints normally function to prevent exaggerated immune responses and subsequent autoimmune disease. However, HNSCC subverts this physiologic function in order to suppress tumor-directed immune activation. The two best known checkpoints include programmed death-1 (PD-1) and cytotoxic T-lymphocyte-associated protein 4 (CTLA-4), both of which are the targets of FDA-approved inhibitory antibodies [12].

Like other cancers, HNSCC tumor cells mediate immunosuppression in the tumor microenvironment (TME) through mechanisms including upregulation of PD-L1

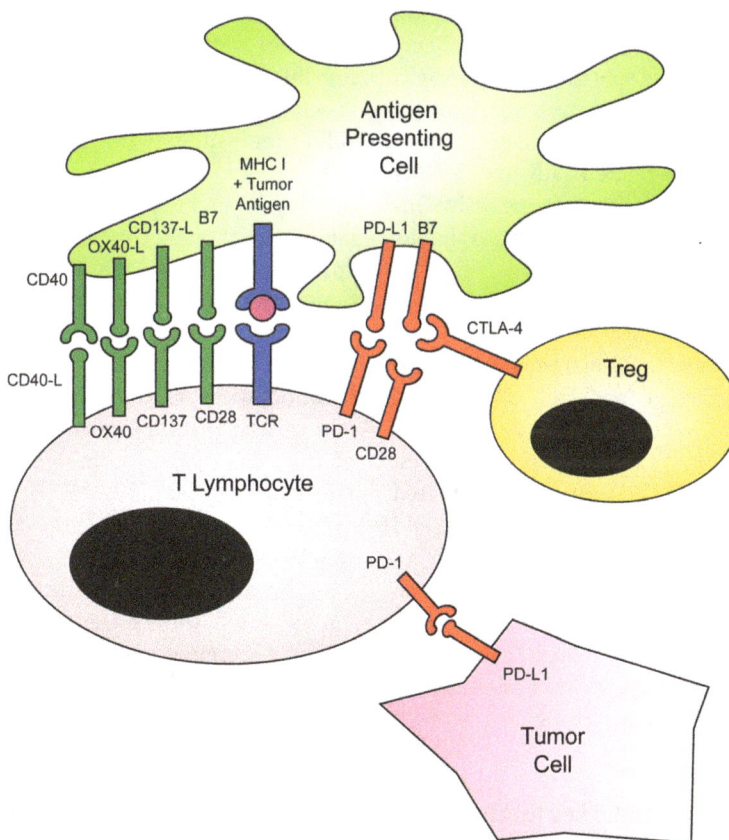

Fig. 1 The Immune Synapse. The balance between costimulatory (*green*) and coinhibitory signals (*red*) alters the net stimulating effect of TCR signaling mediated through antigen presentation on MHC (*blue*). Adapted from Ferris RL, J Clin Oncol. 2015;33(29):3293–304

expression and release of immunosuppressive factors [13]. In addition, recruitment or differentiation of immunosuppressive regulatory T cells (Tregs) and myeloid-derived suppressor cells (MDSCs) represent key mechanisms of immune escape. This review will focus on co-stimulatory receptors, inhibitory checkpoint receptors, and combination immunotherapies in HNSCC.

Review

Activating co-stimulatory receptors to enhance anti-tumor immune responses

As mentioned previously, the co-stimulatory receptors that make up "signal two" play a central role in the activation of tumor-fighting T-cells. Absence of this co-stimulatory signal can lead to induction of T-cell anergy or apoptosis and decreased strength of the immune response. In addition to the classically described CD28/B7, other key co-stimulatory interactions between T-cells and APCs, respectively, include CD137/CD137-L, OX40/ OX40-L, and CD40-L/CD40 (Fig. 1). These costimulatory receptors are members of the tumor necrosis factor receptor superfamily. Decreased expression of CD137, OX40, CD27, and CD28 have been observed on T-cells derived from HNSCC patients compared to those from healthy controls, emphasizing the potential benefits of targeting these co-stimulatory pathways in this population [14–16]. Agonists of co-stimulatory receptors are currently under investigation in multiple trials for HNSCC and other malignancies. Liver toxicity and cytokine storm symptoms have been reported with costimulatory agonists, but these immune-related adverse events (irAEs) may be dose-dependent. Though extensive information on irAEs of these agents is not yet available, they appear to be well tolerated [17].

CD137

CD137 (also known as 4-1BB) is a costimulatory receptor expressed on the surface of activated T-cells, NK cells, and dendritic cells. When bound by its ligand (CD137-L) on the surface of APCs such as macrophages, dendritic cells, and B cells, trimerization of activated CD137 enhances proliferation, cytotoxic capacity, and survival of T-cells [18]. Stimulation of CD137 with an anti-CD137 monoclonal antibody (mAb) has been shown to induce T-cell mediated eradication of established solid tumors in mice [19]. Although anti-CD137 mAb has not been effective as a monotherapy in HNSCC models, it has been shown to synergize with chemoradiation in a model of HPV+ HNSCC to inhibit tumor growth [20, 21].

Two humanized monoclonal antibodies (mAb) against CD137 have been developed including urelumab (IgG4) and PF-05082566 (IgG2) [12]. These antibodies have been evaluated in early phase trials in melanoma, non-

small cell lung cancer (NSCLC) and lymphoma, as monotherapy or in combination with rituximab [12]. Studies of CD137 mAb in combination with other immunotherapies are underway in solid cancers including HNSCC, and are discussed further below.

CD40-L

CD40-L expressed on the surface of activated CD4 T-cells binds to CD40 on APCs, playing a key role in the "helper" T-cell function to activate APCs to prime CD8 T-cells [22]. Expression of both CD40 and CD40-L decrease with increasing HNSCC stage, and surgical resection results in increased APC expression of CD40 [23]. These data implicate downregulation of this co-stimulatory pathway in HNSCC immune escape, with subsequent reversal following surgical resection of the tumor bulk. In addition to its expression on immune cells, CD40 has also been identified on HNSCC cell lines and human HNSCC tumors [24, 25]. The precise role of CD40 in this context is controversial, as ligation of CD40 has been shown to inhibit growth of HNSCC cell lines while also inhibiting cancer cell apoptosis and increasing secretion of proangiogenic cytokines [24, 25]. In vitro studies of agonistic CD40 mAb induced APC activation and maturation, and recombinant CD40L increased the ability of APCs to cross-prime naïve T-cells to tumor antigens [26, 27]. These data suggest a role for this approach in augmenting responses to tumor vaccines, which has been demonstrated in a murine solid tumor model [28].

A variety of CD40-targeting therapies have been developed, including agonistic mAbs and recombinant ligands. Although this approach has not been studied specifically in the HNSCC population, one HNSCC patient treated in a phase I trial of recombinant CD40-L experienced a durable and complete response [29]. Phase I trials of agonistic CD40 mAb alone and in combination with standard therapies have shown promise in a variety of solid tumors, encouraging further studies of this approach in combination with other immune-targeting therapies [30–32].

OX40

Like CD137, OX40 is a co-stimulatory molecule expressed on the T-cell surface that promotes T-cell proliferation, cytokine secretion and memory function when bound by its ligand (OX40-L) [12]. The relevance of OX40 to the local immune response in HNSCC has been demonstrated by the observation that close to 30% of T-cells within the tumor and tumor-draining lymph nodes of HNSCC patients expressed OX40, compared to none of the peripheral blood mononuclear cells (PBMCs) [33]. OX40 is also expressed on regulatory T-cells (Tregs), and appears to inhibit Treg-mediated immunosuppression [34].

Although not explicitly evaluated in HNSCC models, OX40 agonism has improved tumor-free survival in a number of solid tumor models through expansion of tumor-specific CD4+ T-cells [34]. An agonistic OX40 mAb was also shown to synergize with cytolytic therapy through apoptosis of Tregs and enhanced CD8 T-cell response [35]. In a sarcoma model, surgical resection followed by adjuvant anti-OX40 treatment resulted in improved survival and increased antigen-specific T-cell proliferation compared to surgical treatment alone [36].

A phase I trial of the murine agonistic anti-human OX40 mAb 9B12 in patients with refractory solid tumors demonstrated a mild toxicity profile and promising immunologic correlates (NCT01644968) [37]. Although no objective responses were observed, 12 out of the 30 patients experienced regression of at least one metastatic tumor deposit [37]. Additional therapies targeting OX40, including the anti-OX40 mAbs MEDI6469, MEDI0562, PF-04518600, and the OX40L fusion protein MEDI6383, are currently in phase I trials in patients with advanced solid tumors (NCT02205333, NCT02318394, NCT02315066, NCT02221960). In addition, based on the promising preclinical data combining anti-OX40 treatment with surgery [36], a phase Ib trial of OX40 agonistic mAb MEDI6469 prior to definitive surgical resection is currently recruiting patients with locoregionally advanced HNSCC (NCT02274155).

Inhibiting immune checkpoint receptors to enhance anti-tumor immune responses

A reciprocal approach to agonism of co-stimulatory receptors is the inhibition of the immunosuppressive checkpoint receptors. These molecules are upregulated by immune activation, and serve a physiologic role by preventing excessive inflammation and autoimmune disease. However, when overexpressed in the TME, these checkpoints contribute to tumor-promoting immunosuppression, and therefore represent a promising target for disinhibiting immune responses against tumor cells and improving HNSCC patient outcomes. Immune-related adverse events (irAEs) may occur in patients treated with these drugs, including rash, gastrointestinal symptoms, thyroid disorders or autoimmune pneumonitis; however these irAEs are now easily recognized and treated with steroids and/or cessation of the drug in most cases [38].

PD-1/PD-L1

PD-1 is expressed by activated CD8 T-cells, NK cells, B cells, monocytes, and dendritic cells, and normally serves to prevent overactivation of the immune response [12]. However, chronic antigen exposure can lead to chronic upregulation of PD-1 and subsequent T-cell fatigue [39]. Ligation by PD-L1 inhibits activation signaling through

the TCR. PD-L1 is expressed by the majority of HNSCC tumors, and blockade of PD-L1 has been shown to synergize with T-cell immunotherapy in an animal model of HNSCC [40]. CD8 T-cells derived from HPV+ HNSCC samples expressed high levels of PD-1, and HPV+ HNSCC cells were observed to express greater levels of PD-L1 compared to HPV- samples [41, 42]. In addition, infiltration of T-cells expressing PD-1 has been associated with a better prognosis in HPV+ disease, emphasizing the role of prior immune activation in patient prognosis [42].

A variety of antibodies have been developed against both PD-1 and PD-L1, including pembrolizumab (anti-PD1 mAb; FDA approved for HNSCC, melanoma and NSCLC) and nivolumab (anti-PD1; FDA approved for melanoma, NSCLC, and renal cell carcinoma). Numerous clinical trials targeting the PD-1/PD-L1 pathway have been extensively discussed in recent reviews [2, 13, 43]. Therefore we will only briefly highlight a few current late-phase trials in HNSCC, then further discuss checkpoint inhibitor combination trials below. Of note, the Keynote 40 and Keynote 48 phase III trials comparing pembrolizumab to standard of care are currently recruiting patients with recurrent or metastatic HNSCC who have failed platinum-based treatment (NCT02252042), or as first-line therapy (NCT02358031). The Keynote 55 phase II trial is evaluating pembrolizumab in HNSCC patients who have failed both platinum and cetuximab therapy (NCT02255097). Pembrolizumab was recently FDA approved based on long-term data from the KEYNOTE-012 trial including HNSCC patients with recurrent or metastatic HNSCC on or following platinum-based chemotherapy. KEYNOTE-012 showed an overall response rate of 17.7 %, median overall survival of 8.5 months, and 6-month progression-free survival (PFS) rate of 25 %; 12 % of patients had grade 3–4 adverse events [44]. The Checkmate 141 phase III trial comparing nivolumab to investigator's choice in patients with recurrent or metastatic, platinum-refractory HNSCC (NCT02105636) was stopped early due to significant survival benefit including a 30 % reduction in risk of death and doubling of one-year survival from 17 to 36 % [45]. Median overall survival in Checkmate 141 was 7.5 months with nivolumab vs. 5.1 months for investigator's choice therapy; overall response rate ranged from 18–33 %, with higher response rates noted in patients whose tumors expressed higher levels of PD-L1 [46]. Similar to KEYNOTE-012, in Checkmate 141 the rate of grade 3–4 adverse events was 13 % [45, 46].

CTLA-4

CTLA-4 is transiently expressed by activated T-cells upon binding of an antigen-bearing MHC molecule to the TCR, thereby limiting exaggerated immune responses [47]. CTLA-4 is also constitutively expressed on the surface of Tregs in the HNSCC microenvironment [48]. In animal models, CTLA-4 expression was necessary to the immunosuppressive function of Tregs, and conditional knockout of CTLA-4 in Tregs protected from tumor development [49]. CTLA-4 binds B7 ligands CD80 and CD86 with higher affinity than CD28, thereby competitively inhibiting "signal two" in the T-cell activation cascade [47]. Preclinical studies in solid tumor models demonstrated regression of established tumors and the rejection of further tumor challenge following anti-CTLA-4 mAb treatment [50].

Since that time, two humanized anti-CTLA-4 mAbs, ipilimumab (IgG1) and tremelimumab (IgG2), have been developed and evaluated in phase III trials in advanced melanoma [47]. Based on results of two phase III trials of ipilimumab demonstrating enhanced survival and improved tumor responses, ipilimumab became the first FDA-approved checkpoint inhibitor in 2011 [51, 52]. For patients with platinum-refractory, recurrent or metastatic, PD-L1-negative HNSCC, an ongoing phase II/III study includes tremelimumab and durvalumab (anti-PD-L1) as separate monotherapies or in combination (NCT02319044). Trials combining multiple checkpoint inhibitors are further discussed below.

LAG-3

LAG-3 is another inhibitory checkpoint that is expressed on the surface of Tregs in HNSCC patients [53]. LAG-3 has been identified as a key regulatory molecule involved in prevention of autoimmune disease, as well as the development of tumor tolerance [54, 55]. Knockout of LAG-3 in murine models has been shown to reduce the immunosuppressive activity of Tregs, and conversely ectopic expression of LAG-3 has been shown to confer immunosuppressive capacity upon CD4 T-cells [56]. In addition to playing a role in the immunosuppressive functions of Tregs, LAG-3 expression has also been observed on effector CD8 T-cells at the immunologic synapse [57]. Anti-LAG-3 mAb treatment in solid tumor models has shown success in inhibiting primary tumor growth through activation of antigen-specific T-cells in the TME [55]. In murine solid tumor models, LAG-3 and PD-1 co-expression has been identified on the surface of TILs, and combination anti-LAG-3 and anti-PD-1 antibody treatment cured the majority of established tumors in mice [58]. Early phase clinical trials evaluating anti-LAG-3 mAb in combination with other checkpoint inhibitors are reviewed in Table 1.

TIM-3

TIM-3 represents an additional inhibitory checkpoint that has been implicated both in the immunosuppressive function of Tregs and in the exhaustion of effector T cells in the TME. Elevated expression of TIM-3 has been observed on intratumoral Tregs derived from patients with HNSCC and non-small cell lung cancer, and has been observed to correlate with worse clinical outcomes [53, 59]. TIM-3 has also been implicated in the exhaustion of effector T cells through upregulation of TCR signaling [60]. Anti-TIM-3 mAbs have been shown to modestly inhibit solid tumor growth in murine models, and have induced more impressive control of tumor growth in combination with CTLA-4 and PD-1 targeting therapies [61, 62].

B7-H3

Initially identified as a co-stimulatory receptor of T cell function [63], B7-H3 has since been described as a co-inhibitory checkpoint expressed in a variety of tumor types [64, 65]. Although the specific immunological role of B7-H3 in cancer remains controversial, B7-H3 expression has been correlated with poor prognosis in multiple cancer types, including HNSCC [66]. Antibodies targeting the B7-H3 molecule have been shown to exhibit antitumor activity in solid tumor models with surface expression of B7-H3 [67]. Early phase trials combining these agents with other checkpoint inhibitors are currently underway (Table 1).

Combination immunotherapies for maximal enhancement of anti-tumor immune responses

Although many of the above mentioned immunotherapy approaches have shown significant efficacy in certain patients, there is room for improvement with regards to expanding response rates. Current efforts focus on the rational combination of immunotherapy approaches in order to increase the breadth and depth of patient responses (Table 1). It is important to note, however, that combination immunotherapies may increase the frequency and/or severity of immune-related adverse events [38].

Cetuximab

Cetuximab is a human-mouse chimeric IgG1 antibody against epidermal growth factor receptor (EGFR) that is FDA approved as a monotherapy for recurrent/metastatic HNSCC, in combination with radiation therapy for advanced HNSCC, and in combination with chemoradiation for recurrent/metastatic HNSCC [13]. Although more than 80 % of HNSCC tumors overexpress EGFR, only 10-20 % of patients respond to cetuximab treatment [68]. In patients who respond, cetuximab is thought to mediate part of its effect through inhibition of EGFR signaling and downstream proliferation signals. However, evidence suggests that much of the therapeutic effect of cetuximab is derived from activation of NK cells and antibody-dependent cell-mediated cytotoxicity (ADCC) [43]. Extracellular binding of cetuximab to EGFR exposes the constant region (Fc) of cetuximab to binding by the

Table 1 Current Combination Immunotherapy Trials Including HNSCC Patients

Targets	Treatments	Phase	Clinical Trial ID	Patient Eligibility	Status
Costimulatory/Checkpoint Combinations					
CD137 (4-1BB) PD-L1	PF-05082566 + Avelumab	Ib/II	NCT02554812	Advanced/metastatic solid tumors	Recruiting
CD137 (4-1BB) PD-1	PF-05082566 + Pembrolizumab	I	NCT02179918	Advanced/metastatic solid tumors	Recruiting
OX40 PD-L1	MEDI6383 +/−Durvalumab	I	NCT02221960	Recurrent or metastatic solid tumors	Recruiting
OX40 CTLA-4 PD-L1	MEDI6469 Alone, + Tremelimumab, or + Durvalumab	Ib/II	NCT02205333	Advanced solid tumors	Ongoing, not recruiting
CD27 PD-L1	Varlilumab + Atezolizumab	I/II	NCT02543645	Advanced cancers including HNSCC	Recruiting
CD27 PD-1	Varlilumab + Nivolumab	I/II	NCT02335918	Advanced solid tumors	Recruiting
Checkpoint/Checkpoint Combinations					
CTLA-4 B7-H3	Ipilimumab + MGA271	I	NCT02381314	Advanced/metastatic B7-H3+ HNSCC, melanoma, or NSCLC	Recruiting
CTLA-4 PD-L1	Tremelimumab + Durvalumab	III	NCT02551159	HNSCC with no prior chemotherapy	Recruiting
CTLA-4 PD-L1	Tremelimumab + Durvalumab	I	NCT02262741	Recurrent or metastatic HNSCC	Recruiting
CTLA-4 PD-L1	Tremelimumab + Durvalumab (monotherapy or combination)	II	NCT02319044	Recurrent or metastatic HNSCC	Ongoing, not recruiting
CTLA-4 PD-L1 Vaccine	Tremelimumab + Durvalumab + PolyICLC	I/II	NCT02643303	Advanced solid tumors including HPV- HNSCC or HPV+ HNSCC after prior treatment failure	Not yet recruiting
PD-L1 CTLA-4	Durvalumab +/−Tremelimumab	III	NCT02369874	Recurrent or metastatic HNSCC	Recruiting
PD-1 B7-H3	Pembrolizumab + MGA271	I	NCT02475213	B7-H3+ advanced HNSCC	Recruiting
PD-L1 HPV E7	Durvalumab + ADXS 11–001	I/II	NCT02291055	Recurrent or metastatic HPV-associated HNSCC	Ongoing, not recruiting
LAG-3 PD-1	BMS-986016 +/− Nivolumab	I	NCT01968109	Advanced solid tumors	Recruiting
LAG-3 PD-1	LAG525 +/− PDR001	I/II	NCT02460224	Advanced solid tumors	Recruiting
TIM-3 PD-1	MBG453 +/−PDR001	I/II	NCT02608268	Advanced solid malignancies	Recruiting
Cetuximab Combinations					
CD137 (4-1BB)	Urelumab + Cetuximab	Ib	NCT02110082	Advanced/metastatic HNSCC or CRC	Ongoing, not recruiting
CTLA-4	Iplimumab + Cetuximab + IMRT	Ib	NCT01860430, NCT01935921	Stage III-IVB HNSCC p16- or intermediate-risk p16+	Recruiting
TLR8	Cetuximab + SOC Chemo (CDDP + 5-FU) +/− VTX-2337	II	NCT01836029	Recurrent or metastatic HNSCC	Ongoing, not recruiting
TLR8	Cetuximab + VTX-2337 window of opportunity before surgery	Ib	NCT02124850	Stage II-IVA resectable HNSCC	Recruiting

activating Fc receptor (CD16/FcγRIII) expressed on NK cells. This activation signal induces ADCC mediated by NK cells resulting in tumor cell lysis (Fig. 2). The variability of patient response to cetuximab is thought to be in part due to polymorphisms in NK cell FcγRIII, which lead to variation in its affinity for the Fc region of cetuximab [69].

In addition to mediating ADCC, cetuximab-activated NK cells have been shown to promote maturation of

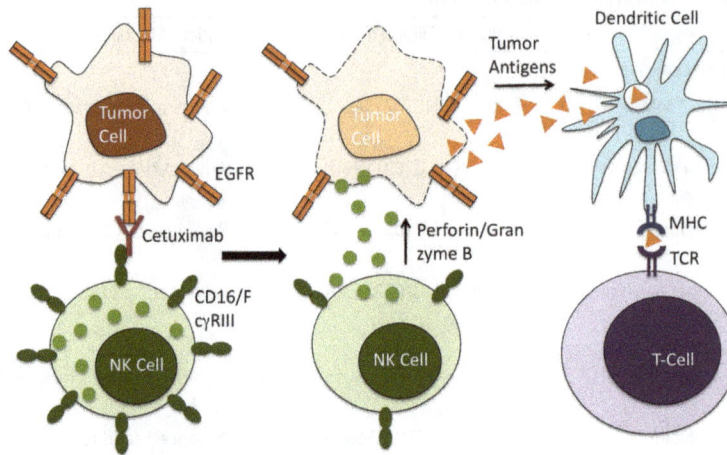

Fig. 2 Cetuximab-Mediated ADCC. The Fab portion of Cetuximab binds to EGFR on the surface of tumor cells, while its Fc region binds to the Fc receptor CD16/FcγRIII on the NK cell surface. This leads to NK cell activation and release of cytolytic granules containing perforin and granzyme B that result in tumor cell lysis and release of tumor antigen. This tumor antigen is subsequently presented on APCs to activate antigen-specific T-cells

APCs and the development of an adaptive immune response [68]. Recent evidence also suggests that cetuximab treatment decreases the function of immunosuppressive myeloid cells [70]. Increased numbers of monocytic MDSCs were observed in patients who did not respond to cetuximab therapy, suggesting potential for improving responses through combining cetuximab with MDSC-targeting treatments [70]. Given the low response rate to cetuximab as a monotherapy or in combination with standard therapies, recent efforts have focused on combining cetuximab with additional immunotherapies to enhance ADCC.

Human NK cells have been shown to upregulate surface expression of CD137 following exposure to cetuximab and EGFR-expressing cell lines [71]. In preclinical studies, sequential treatment with cetuximab followed by anti-CD137 mAb eradicated established tumors in an NK-cell dependent manner [71]. In addition to this enhancement of ADCC, preclinical evidence also supports a mechanistic role for the adaptive immune "vaccinal effect." Mice previously cured with this combination therapy rejected rechallenge with both EGFR-positive and negative cell lines, which supports immunologic memory and epitope spreading [72]. Based on this promising preclinical data, a phase Ib trial combining cetuximab with the anti-CD137 mAb urelumab is currently underway (NCT02110082).

In addition to FcγRIII polymorphisms, proposed mechanisms of resistance to cetuximab-mediated ADCC include an increase in the number of Tregs within the HNSCC TME following cetuximab treatment [73]. These CTLA-4+ Tregs were shown to suppress cetuximab-mediated ADCC, and their increased numbers correlated with poor patient prognosis [73]. *Ex*

vivo treatment of HNSCC tumor-infiltrating lymphocytes with the anti-CTLA-4 mAb ipilimumab depleted Tregs and restored NK cell-mediated ADCC [73]. Based on this promising preclinical data, two phase Ib studies combining ipilimumab with intensity modulated radiation therapy (IMRT) and cetuximab are currently recruiting patients with untreated advanced HNSCC (NCT01860430, NCT01935921).

Toll like receptor agonists

Toll-like receptors (TLRs) are transmembrane receptors that recognize microbial invasion and respond through activation of the innate immune system [74]. TLR7 and TLR8 have been particular targets for improving anticancer immunity. An early topical TLR7/8 agonist, imiquimod, is FDA approved for actinic keratosis and basal cell carcinoma. In addition, novel stabilized immunemodulatory RNA (SIMRA) compounds are also under study for their dual TLR7/8 agonism [75]. However, recent development of a potent and selective TLR8 agonist has focused attention on this endosomal TLR that is naturally activated by viral single-stranded RNA. Stimulation of TLR8 results in activation of dendritic cells and macrophages and subsequent secretion of immune-activating cytokines. TLR8 signaling has also been implicated in reversal of Treg function [76]. VTX-2337, a TLR8 agonist, has been shown to induce TNFα and IL-12 secretion by monocytes and myeloid dendritic cells, in addition to increasing NK cell cytotoxicity and secretion of IFNγ [77]. VTX-2337 has also been reported to enhance rituximab and trastuzumab-induced ADCC in lymphoma and breast cancer cells lines, respectively [77]. Subsequent preclinical studies using PBMCs from healthy individuals and HNSCC patients demonstrated the ability of VTX-2337 to enhance cetuximab-mediated ADCC against HNSCC cells [78].

Based on these promising preclinical data regarding selective TLR8 agonism, VTX-2337 was studied in a phase I trial in advanced solid tumors [79]. This trial demonstrated clinical tolerability in addition to increases in plasma levels of immune-activating cytokines G-CSF, monocyte chemoattractant protein-1, macrophage inflammatory protein-1β, and TNFα when administered at higher doses. Based on this information, phase II placebo-controlled trials of combination therapy with VTX-2337 have been initiated, including a comparison of chemotherapy + cetuximab + VTX-2337 to chemotherapy + cetuximab alone in recurrent or metastatic HNSCC (NCT01836029). In addition, a phase Ib study of neoadjuvant cetuximab + VTX-2337 vs. cetuximab + VTX-2337 + nivolumab is currently recruiting patients with stage II-IVA surgically resectable HNSCC (NCT02124850).

Checkpoint inhibitors

Although the degree and durability of response to checkpoint inhibitor monotherapy has been impressive, objective response rates remain low. For example, preliminary data from the KEYNOTE-012 expansion cohort showed an objective response in 18.2 % of recurrent/metastatic HNSCC patients treated with pembrolizumab monotherapy [80]. For this reason, much attention is currently directed towards combining checkpoint inhibitors with a variety of immune-based therapies to achieve higher response rates in both preclinical and clinical studies (Table 1).

Signaling through various immune checkpoints and downregulation of costimulatory receptors each represent a distinct mechanism of tumor-mediated immunosuppression. Combining inhibitors that target different checkpoints is a logical strategy to generate synergy and target potential mechanisms of resistance to therapy. For example, melanoma patients with high PD-L1 expression did not respond to anti-CTLA4 mAb and radiation, implicating PD-1/PD-L1 signaling in this resistance (NCT01497808) [81]. However, in preclinical studies of melanoma, combined targeting of CTLA-4 and PD-1 more than doubled the rate of tumor rejection and increased tumor-infiltrating T-cells while reducing Tregs and MDSCs in the TME [82]. Synergism has also been described between antibodies targeting PD-1 and TIM-3 [61], and PD-1 and LAG-3 [58] in solid tumor models, leading to current clinical trials evaluating these combinations in patients with advanced solid tumors (NCT02608268, NCT01968109, NCT02460224).

A phase I trial of combined nivolumab (anti-PD-1) and ipilimumab (anti-CTLA-4) in advanced melanoma showed an overall response of 40 % and objective responses in 53 % of patients treated with the maximal tolerated dose [83]. These outcomes exceed responses seen with either drug as a monotherapy. Preliminary results from another phase I trial combining durvalumab (anti-PD-L1) and tremelimumab (anti-CTLA-4) in NSCLC patients showed an overall response rate of 25 %, and the interesting finding that this efficacy did not depend on PD-L1 expression in the tumor [84]. Many further studies combining checkpoint inhibitors with one another and with co-stimulatory molecules are currently underway and summarized in Table 1.

In addition, simultaneous agonism of co-stimulatory pathways and antagonism of inhibitory checkpoints allows one to "step on the gas while taking the foot off the brakes." In solid tumor models, combined treatment with agonistic anti-OX40 mAb and anti-CTLA-4 mAb improved survival and induced tumor regression through expansion of effector CD8 T-cells [85]. Combined targeting of OX40 and PD-L1 or OX40 and CTLA-4 is currently under study in early phase trials in advanced solid tumors (NCT02221960 & NCT02205333). Studies in solid tumor models also demonstrated synergy between mAbs targeting CD137, PD-1, and CTLA-4 [86]. Based on these data, two current phase I/II trials are evaluating the combination of anti-CD137 and anti-PD-1/PD-L1 mAb in advanced solid tumors (NCT02554812 & NCT02179918).

Combination of immunotherapies with standard or targeted therapies

In addition to combination immunotherapies for HNSCC, other promising strategies under investigation include the combination of these agents with standard-of-care or targeted therapies. Studies in HNSCC and other cancer types suggest that radiotherapy, cisplatin chemotherapy, and other cytotoxic drugs may enhance anti-tumor adaptive immunity in the TME [87–90]. As a result, radiation and cisplatin may also increase immune checkpoint expression [89–92]. These findings suggest a strong rationale for combining radiation and/or chemotherapy with checkpoint inhibitors and other immune therapies, and such combinations are currently under study in multiple clinical trials.

The Cancer Genome Atlas and other studies have revealed specific genomic alterations in HNSCC that may be targeted by specific therapies [93]. Although cetuximab is so far the only targeted agent that is FDA-approved for HNSCC, a myriad of targeted agents are under investigation in preclinical and clinical studies of HNSCC. Future treatment strategies are likely to utilize combinations of targeted agents with immune and standard therapies.

HPV-specific immunotherapies

As mentioned above, HPV-associated HNSCC represents distinct mechanisms of antiviral immune escape, and this disease entity also may benefit from specific antiviral immunotherapies. Since patients with HPV-associated disease generally have an excellent prognosis and high cure rates, newer therapeutic strategies have focused on improving upon long-term toxicities seen with current therapies. Therapeutic vaccines and adoptive transfer of immune cells have been studied in HPV-associated HNSCC [2] and will be combined with surgery, chemoradiation, targeted therapies or other immune therapies in ongoing and future trials. Trials of combination immunotherapies specific to patients with HPV-associated disease are detailed in Table 1.

Conclusions

Recent advances in understanding the balance between costimulatory and inhibitory immune pathways at the immune synapse have encouraged interest in re-directing these signals from tumor-promoting immunosuppression towards tumor-fighting immunity. With the development of an array of costimulatory agonists and checkpoint inhibitors, these immune-based strategies have become a focal point for research in many cancers, including HNSCC. In addition to focusing on clinical application of these novel immunotherapies, much work is underway to investigate mechanisms of resistance in those patients who do not achieve durable responses. Rational design of combination strategies represents a promising approach to target resistance, while care must be taken to avoid immune over-activation and serious autoimmune consequences.

Acknowledgements
Not applicable.

Funding
This work was supported by NIH, National Institute on Deafness and Other Communication Disorders intramural project number ZIA-DC-DC000090. The NIH had no direct role in the writing of this manuscript.

Authors' contributions
RJD drafted the manuscript and carried out a literature review, NCS carried out the primary literature review and helped to draft the manuscript, RLF conceived of the review and helped to draft the manuscript. All authors read and approved the final manuscript.

Competing interests
RLF serves as a paid member of committees, panels or boards for Merck, Celgene, Bristol Myers Squibb, and AstraZeneca/Medimmune, and receives research funding from VentiRx, Bristol Myers Squibb, and AstraZeneca/Medimmune.

Author details
[1]Tumor Biology Section, Head and Neck Surgery Branch, National Institute on Deafness and Other Communication Disorders, National Institutes of Health, 10 Center Drive, Room 5B-39, Bethesda, MD 20892, USA. [2]Department of Otolaryngology, Hillman Cancer Center Research Pavilion, University of Pittsburgh, 5117 Centre Avenue, Room 2.26b, Pittsburgh, PA 15213-1863, USA. [3]Department of Immunology, Hillman Cancer Center Research Pavilion, University of Pittsburgh, 5117 Centre Avenue, Room 2.26b, Pittsburgh, PA 15213-1863, USA. [4]Cancer Immunology Programm, Hillman Cancer Center Research Pavilion, University of Pittsburgh Cancer Institute, 5117 Centre Avenue, Room 2.26b, Pittsburgh, PA 15213-1863, USA. [5]Department of Otolaryngology-Head and Neck Surgery, Johns Hopkins School of Medicine, 6420 Rockledge Drive, Suite 4920, Bethesda, MD 20817, USA.

References
1.   Ferlay J, Soerjomataram I, Dikshit R, Eser S, Mathers C, Rebelo M, et al. Cancer incidence and mortality worldwide: sources, methods and major patterns in GLOBOCAN 2012. Int J Cancer. 2015;136:E359–86.
2.   Ferris RL. Immunology and Immunotherapy of Head and Neck Cancer. J Clin Oncol. 2015;33:3293–304.
3.   Champiat S, Ferte C, Lebel-Binay S, Eggermont A, Soria JC. Exomics and immunogenics: Bridging mutational load and immune checkpoints efficacy. Oncoimmunology. 2014;3:e27817.
4.   Keck MK, Zuo Z, Khattri A, Stricker TP, Brown CD, Imanguli M, et al. Integrative analysis of head and neck cancer identifies two biologically distinct HPV and three non-HPV subtypes. Clin Cancer Res. 2015;21:870–81.
5.   Lawrence MS, Stojanov P, Polak P, Kryukov GV, Cibulskis K, Sivachenko A, et al. Mutational heterogeneity in cancer and the search for new cancer-associated genes. Nature. 2013;499:214–8.
6.   Balermpas P, Michel Y, Wagenblast J, Seitz O, Weiss C, Rodel F, et al. Tumour-infiltrating lymphocytes predict response to definitive chemoradiotherapy in head and neck cancer. Br J Cancer. 2014;110:501–9.
7.   Schantz SP, Shillitoe EJ, Brown B, Campbell B. Natural killer cell activity and head and neck cancer: a clinical assessment. J Natl Cancer Inst. 1986;77:869–75.
8.   Gajewski TF, Schreiber H, Fu YX. Innate and adaptive immune cells in the tumor microenvironment. Nat Immunol. 2013;14:1014–22.
9.   Ressing ME, Sette A, Brandt RM, Ruppert J, Wentworth PA, Hartman M, et al. Human CTL epitopes encoded by human papillomavirus type 16 E6 and E7 identified through in vivo and in vitro immunogenicity studies of HLA-A*0201-binding peptides. J Immunol. 1995;154:5934–43.
10. Sckisel GD, Bouchlaka MN, Monjazeb AM, Crittenden M, Curti BD, Wilkins DE, et al. Out-of-Sequence Signal 3 Paralyzes Primary CD4(+) T-Cell-Dependent Immunity. Immunity. 2015;43:240–50.
11. Curtsinger JM, Mescher MF. Inflammatory cytokines as a third signal for T cell activation. Curr Opin Immunol. 2010;22:333–40.
12. Bauman JE, Ferris RL. Integrating novel therapeutic monoclonal antibodies into the management of head and neck cancer. Cancer. 2014;120:624–32.
13. Allen CT, Clavijo PE, Van Waes C, Chen Z. Anti-Tumor Immunity in Head and Neck Cancer: Understanding the Evidence, How Tumors Escape and Immunotherapeutic Approaches. Cancers (Basel). 2015;7:2397–414.
14. Baruah P, Lee M, Odutoye T, Williamson P, Hyde N, Kaski JC, et al. Decreased levels of alternative co-stimulatory receptors OX40 and 4-1BB characterise T cells from head and neck cancer patients. Immunobiology. 2012;217:669–75.
15. Kuss I, Donnenberg AD, Gooding W, Whiteside TL. Effector CD8 + CD45RO-CD27-T cells have signalling defects in patients with squamous cell carcinoma of the head and neck. Br J Cancer. 2003;88:223–30.
16. Tsukishiro T, Donnenberg AD, Whiteside TL. Rapid turnover of the CD8(+)CD28(–) T-cell subset of effector cells in the circulation of patients with head and neck cancer. Cancer Immunol Immunother. 2003;52:599–607.
17. Ryan JM, Wasser JS, Adler AJ, Vella AT. Enhancing the safety of antibody-based immunomodulatory cancer therapy without compromising therapeutic benefit: Can we have our cake and eat it too? Expert Opin Biol Ther. 2016;16:655–74.
18. Lynch DH. The promise of 4-1BB (CD137)-mediated immunomodulation and the immunotherapy of cancer. Immunol Rev. 2008;222:277–86.
19. Melero I, Shuford WW, Newby SA, Aruffo A, Ledbetter JA, Hellstrom KE, et al. Monoclonal antibodies against the 4-1BB T-cell activation molecule eradicate established tumors. Nat Med. 1997;3:682–5.

20. Vahle AK, Hermann S, Schafers M, Wildner M, Kerem A, Ozturk E, et al. Multimodal imaging analysis of an orthotopic head and neck cancer mouse model and application of anti-CD137 tumor immune therapy. Head Neck. 2016;38:542–9.

21. Lucido CT, Vermeer PD, Wieking BG, Vermeer DW, Lee JH. CD137 enhancement of HPV positive head and neck squamous cell carcinoma tumor clearance. Vaccines (Basel). 2014;2:841–53.

22. Vonderheide RH, Glennie MJ. Agonistic CD40 antibodies and cancer therapy. Clin Cancer Res. 2013;19:1035–43.

23. Sathawane D, Kharat RS, Halder S, Roy S, Swami R, Patel R, et al. Monocyte CD40 expression in head and neck squamous cell carcinoma (HNSCC). Hum Immunol. 2013;74:1–5.

24. Cao W, Cavacini LA, Tillman KC, Posner MR. CD40 function in squamous cell cancer of the head and neck. Oral Oncol. 2005;41:462–9.

25. Posner MR, Cavacini LA, Upton MP, Tillman KC, Gornstein ER, Norris Jr CM. Surface membrane-expressed CD40 is present on tumor cells from squamous cell cancer of the head and neck in vitro and in vivo and regulates cell growth in tumor cell lines. Clin Cancer Res. 1999;5:2261–70.

26. Bergstrom RT, Silverman DA, Chambers K, Kim JA. CD40 monoclonal antibody activation of antigen-presenting cells improves therapeutic efficacy of tumor-specific T cells. Otolaryngol Head Neck Surg. 2004;130: 94–103.

27. Hoffmann TK, Meidenbauer N, Muller-Berghaus J, Storkus WJ, Whiteside TL. Proinflammatory cytokines and CD40 ligand enhance cross-presentation and cross-priming capability of human dendritic cells internalizing apoptotic cancer cells. J Immunother. 2001;24:162–71.

28. Diehl L, den Boer AT, Schoenberger SP, van der Voort EI, Schumacher TN, Melief CJ, et al. CD40 activation in vivo overcomes peptide-induced peripheral cytotoxic T-lymphocyte tolerance and augments anti-tumor vaccine efficacy. Nat Med. 1999;5:774–9.

29. Vonderheide RH, Dutcher JP, Anderson JE, Eckhardt SG, Stephans KF, Razvillas B, et al. Phase I study of recombinant human CD40 ligand in cancer patients. J Clin Oncol. 2001;19:3280–7.

30. Beatty GL, Torigian DA, Chiorean EG, Saboury B, Brothers A, Alavi A, et al. A phase I study of an agonist CD40 monoclonal antibody (CP-870,893) in combination with gemcitabine in patients with advanced pancreatic ductal adenocarcinoma. Clin Cancer Res. 2013;19:6286–95.

31. Johnson P, Challis R, Chowdhury F, Gao Y, Harvey M, Geldart T, et al. Clinical and biological effects of an agonist anti-CD40 antibody a cancer research UK phase I study. Clin Cancer Res. 2015;21:1321–8.

32. Vonderheide RH, Burg JM, Mick R, Trosko JA, Li D, Shaik MN, et al. Phase I study of the CD40 agonist antibody CP-870,893 combined with carboplatin and paclitaxel in patients with advanced solid tumors. Oncoimmunology. 2013;2:e23033.

33. Vetto JT, Lum S, Morris A, Sicotte M, Davis J, Lemon M, et al. Presence of the T-cell activation marker OX-40 on tumor infiltrating lymphocytes and draining lymph node cells from patients with melanoma and head and neck cancers. Am J Surg. 1997;174:258–65.

34. Weinberg AD, Rivera MM, Prell R, Morris A, Ramstad T, Vetto JT, et al. Engagement of the OX-40 receptor in vivo enhances antitumor immunity. J Immunol. 2000;164:2160–9.

35. Hirschhorn-Cymerman D, Rizzuto GA, Merghoub T, Cohen AD, Avogadri F, Lesokhin AM, et al. OX40 engagement and chemotherapy combination provides potent antitumor immunity with concomitant regulatory T cell apoptosis. J Exp Med. 2009;206:1103–16.

36. Gough MJ, Crittenden MR, Sarff M, Pang P, Seung SK, Vetto JT, et al. Adjuvant therapy with agonistic antibodies to CD134 (OX40) increases local control after surgical or radiation therapy of cancer in mice. J Immunother. 2010;33:798–809.

37. Curti BD, Kovacsovics-Bankowski M, Morris N, Walker E, Chisholm L, Floyd K, et al. OX40 is a potent immune-stimulating target in late-stage cancer patients. Cancer Res. 2013;73:7189–98.

38. Boutros C, Tarhini A, Routier E, Lambotte O, Ladurie FL, Carbonnel F, et al. Safety profiles of anti-CTLA-4 and anti-PD-1 antibodies alone and in combination. Nat Rev Clin Oncol. 2016;13:473–86.

39. Ferris R. PD-1 targeting in cancer immunotherapy. Cancer. 2013;119:E1–3.

40. Strome SE, Dong H, Tamura H, Voss SG, Flies DB, Tamada K, et al. B7-H1 blockade augments adoptive T-cell immunotherapy for squamous cell carcinoma. Cancer Res. 2003;63:6501–5.

41. Lyford-Pike S, Peng S, Young GD, Taube JM, Westra WH, Akpeng B, et al. Evidence for a role of the PD-1:PD-L1 pathway in immune resistance of

HPV-associated head and neck squamous cell carcinoma. Cancer Res. 2013; 73:1733–41.

42. Badoual C, Hans S, Merillon N, Van Ryswick C, Ravel P, Benhamouda N, et al. PD-1-expressing tumor-infiltrating T cells are a favorable prognostic biomarker in HPV-associated head and neck cancer. Cancer Res. 2013;73: 128–38.

43. Schoppy DW, Sunwoo JB. Immunotherapy for Head and Neck Squamous Cell Carcinoma. Hematol Oncol Clin North Am. 2015;29:1033–43.

44. Mehra R, Seiwert TY, Mahipal A, Weiss J, Berger R, Eder JP, et al. Efficacy and safety of pembrolizumab in recurrent/metastatic head and neck squamous cell carcinoma (R/M HNSCC): Pooled analyses after long-term follow-up in KEYNOTE-012. J Clin Oncol. 34;2016 (suppl; abstr 6012)

45. Gillison ML, Blumenschein GJ, Fayette J, Guigay J, Colevas AD, Licitra L, et al. Nivolumab (nivo) vs investigator's choice (IC) for recurrent or metastatic (R/M) head and neck squamous cell carcinoma (HNSCC): CheckMate-141 [abstract]. In: Proceedings of the Annual Meeting of the American Association for Cancer Research. New Orleans: AACR; 2016 Abstract nr CT099; 2016.

46. Ferris RL, Blumenschein GR, Fayette J, Guigay J, Colevas AD, Licitra LF, et al. Further evaluations of nivolumab (nivo) versus investigator's choice (IC) chemotherapy for recurrent or metastatic (R/M) squamous cell carcinoma of the head and neck (SCCHN): CheckMate 141. J Clin Oncol. 34, 2016 (suppl; abstr 6009).

47. Honeychurch J, Cheadle EJ, Dovedi SJ, Illidge TM. Immuno-regulatory antibodies for the treatment of cancer. Expert Opin Biol Ther. 2015;15:787–801.

48. Strauss L, Bergmann C, Gooding W, Johnson J. T., Whiteside, T. L. The frequency and suppressor function of CD4 + CD25highFoxp3+ T cells in the circulation of patients with squamous cell carcinoma of the head and neck. Clin Cancer Res. 2007;13:6301–11.

49. Wing K, Onishi Y, Prieto-Martin P, Yamaguchi T, Miyara M, Fehervari Z, Nomura T, Sakaguchi S. CTLA-4 control over Foxp3+ regulatory T cell function. Science (80-). 2008;322:271–5.

50. Leach DR, Krummel MF, Allison JP. Enhancement of antitumor immunity by CTLA-4 blockade. Science (80-). 1996;271:1734–6.

51. Hodi FS, O'Day SJ, McDermott DF, Weber RW, Sosman JA, Haanen JB, Gonzalez R, Robert C, Schadendorf D, Hassel JC, Akerley W, van den Eertwegh AJ, Lutzky J, Lorigan P, Vaubel JM, Linette GP, Hogg D, Ottensmeier CH, Lebbe C, Peschel C, Quirt I, Clark JI, Wolchok JD, Weber JS, Tian J, Yellin MJ, Nichol GM, Hoos A, Urba WJ. Improved survival with ipilimumab in patients with metastatic melanoma. N Engl J Med. 2010; 363:711–23.

52. Robert C, Thomas L, Bondarenko I, O'Day S, Weber J, Garbe C, Lebbe C, Baurain JF, Testori A, Grob JJ, Davidson N, Richards J, Maio M, Hauschild A, Miller Jr WH, Gascon P, Lotem M, Harmankaya K, Ibrahim R, Francis S, Chen TT, Humphrey R, Hoos A, Wolchok JD. Ipilimumab plus dacarbazine for previously untreated metastatic melanoma. N Engl J Med. 2011;364:2517–26.

53. Jie HB, Gildener-Leapman N, Li J, Srivastava RM, Gibson SP, Whiteside TL, Ferris RL. Intratumoral regulatory T cells upregulate immunosuppressive molecules in head and neck cancer patients. Br J Cancer. 2013;109:2629–35.

54. Sega EI, Leveson-Gower DB, Florek M, Schneidawind D, Luong RH, Negrin RS. Role of lymphocyte activation gene-3 (Lag-3) in conventional and regulatory T cell function in allogeneic transplantation. PLoS One. 2014;9:e86551.

55. Grosso JF, Kelleher CC, Harris TJ, Maris CH, Hipkiss EL, De Marzo A, Anders R, Netto G, Getnet D, Bruno TC, Goldberg MV, Pardoll DM, Drake CG. LAG-3 regulates CD8+ T cell accumulation and effector function in murine self- and tumor-tolerance systems. J Clin Invest. 2007;117:3383–92.

56. Huang C-T, Workman CJ, Flies D, Pan X, Marson AL, Zhou G, Hipkiss EL, Ravi S, Kowalski J, Levitsky HI, Powell JD, Pardoll DM, Drake CG, Vignali DAA. Role of LAG-3 in regulatory T cells. Immunity. 2004;21:503–13.

57. Huang R-Y, Eppolito C, Lele S, Shrikant P, Matsuzaki J, Odunsi K. LAG3 and PD1 co-inhibitory molecules collaborate to limit CD8+ T cell signaling and dampen antitumor immunity in a murine ovarian cancer model. Oncotarget. 2015;6:27359–77.

58. Woo SR, Turnis ME, Goldberg MV, Bankoti J, Selby M, Nirschl CJ, et al. Immune inhibitory molecules LAG-3 and PD-1 synergistically regulate T-cell function to promote tumoral immune escape. Cancer Res. 2012;72:917–27.

59. Gao X, Zhu Y, Li G, Huang H, Zhang G, Wang F, et al. TIM-3 expression characterizes regulatory T cells in tumor tissues and is associated with lung cancer progression. PLoS One. 2012;7:e30676.

60. Ferris RL, Lu B, Kane LP. Too much of a good thing? Tim-3 and TCR signaling in T cell exhaustion. J Immunol. 2014;193:1525–30.

61. Sakuishi K, Apetoh L, Sullivan JM, Blazar BR, Kuchroo VK, Anderson AC. Targeting Tim-3 and PD-1 pathways to reverse T cell exhaustion and restore anti-tumor immunity. J Exp Med. 2010;207:2187–94.

62. Ngiow SF, von Scheidt B, Akiba H, Yagita H, Teng MWL, Smyth MJ. Anti-TIM3 antibody promotes T cell IFN-γ-mediated antitumor immunity and suppresses established tumors. Cancer Res. 2011;71:3540–51.

63. Chapoval AI, Ni J, Lau JS, Wilcox RA, Flies DB, Liu D, et al. B7-H3: a costimulatory molecule for T cell activation and IFN-gamma production. Nat Immunol. 2001;2:269–74.

64. Suh W-K, Gajewska BU, Okada H, Gronski MA, Bertram EM, Dawicki W, et al. The B7 family member B7-H3 preferentially down-regulates T helper type 1-mediated immune responses. Nat Immunol. 2003;4:899–906.

65. Prasad DVR, Nguyen T, Li Z, Yang Y, Duong J, Wang Y, et al. Murine B7-H3 is a negative regulator of T cells. J Immunol. 2004;173:2500–6.

66. Katayama A, Takahara M, Kishibe K, Nagato T, Kunibe I, Katada A, et al. Expression of B7-H3 in hypopharyngeal squamous cell carcinoma as a predictive indicator for tumor metastasis and prognosis. Int J Oncol. 2011;38:1219–26.

67. Loo D, Alderson RF, Chen FZ, Huang L, Zhang W, Gorlatov S, et al. Development of an Fc-enhanced anti-B7-H3 monoclonal antibody with potent antitumor activity. Clin Cancer Res. 2012;18:3834–45.

68. Srivastava RM, Lee SC, Andrade Filho PA, Lord CA, Jie HB, Davidson HC, et al. Cetuximab-activated natural killer and dendritic cells collaborate to trigger tumor antigen-specific T-cell immunity in head and neck cancer patients. Clin Cancer Res. 2013;19:1858–72.

69. Lopez-Albaitero A, Lee SC, Morgan S, Grandis JR, Gooding WE, Ferrone S, et al. Role of polymorphic Fc gamma receptor IIIa and EGFR expression level in cetuximab mediated, NK cell dependent in vitro cytotoxicity of head and neck squamous cell carcinoma cells. Cancer Immunol Immunother. 2009;58:1853–64.

70. Li J, Srivastava RM, Ettyreddy A, Ferris RL. Cetuximab ameliorates suppressive phenotypes of myeloid antigen presenting cells in head and neck cancer patients. J Immunother Cancer. 2015;3:54.

71. Kohrt HE, Colevas AD, Houot R, Weiskopf K, Goldstein MJ, Lund P, Mueller A, et al. Targeting CD137 enhances the efficacy of cetuximab. J Clin Invest. 2014;124:2668–82.

72. Houot R, Kohrt H. CD137 stimulation enhances the vaccinal effect of anti-tumor antibodies. Oncoimmunology. 2014;3:e941740.

73. Jie HB, Schuler PJ, Lee SC, Srivastava RM, Argiris A, Ferrone S, et al. CTLA-4(+) Regulatory T Cells Increased in Cetuximab-Treated Head and Neck Cancer Patients Suppress NK Cell Cytotoxicity and Correlate with Poor Prognosis. Cancer Res. 2015;75:2200–10.

74. Schon MP, Schon M. TLR7 and TLR8 as targets in cancer therapy. Oncogene. 2008;27:190–9.

75. Lan T, Kandimalla ER, Yu D, Bhagat L, Li Y, Wang D, et al. Stabilized immune modulatory RNA compounds as agonists of Toll-like receptors 7 and 8. Proc Natl Acad Sci U S A. 2007;104:13750–5.

76. Peng G, Guo Z, Kiniwa Y, Voo KS, Peng W, Fu T, et al. Toll-like receptor 8-mediated reversal of CD4+ regulatory T cell function. Science. 2005;309:1380–4.

77. Lu H, Dietsch GN, Matthews MA, Yang Y, Ghanekar S, Inokuma M, et al. VTX-2337 is a novel TLR8 agonist that activates NK cells and augments ADCC. Clin Cancer Res. 2012;18:499–509.

78. Stephenson RM, Lim CM, Matthews M, Dietsch G, Hershberg R, Ferris RL. TLR8 stimulation enhances cetuximab-mediated natural killer cell lysis of head and neck cancer cells and dendritic cell cross-priming of EGFR-specific CD8+ T cells. Cancer Immunol Immunother. 2013;62:1347–57.

79. Northfelt DW, Ramanathan RK, Cohen PA, Von Hoff DD, Weiss GJ, Dietsch GN, et al. A phase I dose-finding study of the novel Toll-like receptor 8 agonist VTX-2337 in adult subjects with advanced solid tumors or lymphoma. Clin Cancer Res. 2014;20:3683–91.

80. Seiwert TY, Haddad RI, Gupta S, Mehra R, Tahara M, Berger R, et al. Antitumor activity and safety of pembrolizumab in patients (pts) with advanced squamous cell carcinoma of the head and neck (SCCHN): Preliminary results from KEYNOTE-012 expansion cohort. J Clin Oncol. 33, 2015 (suppl; abstr LBA6008)

81. Twyman-Saint Victor C, Rech AJ, Maity A, Rengan R, Pauken KE, Stelekati E, et al. Radiation and dual checkpoint blockade activate non-redundant immune mechanisms in cancer. Nature. 2015;520:373–7.

82. Curran MA, Montalvo W, Yagita H, Allison JP. PD-1 and CTLA-4 combination blockade expands infiltrating T cells and reduces regulatory T and myeloid cells within B16 melanoma tumors. Proc Natl Acad Sci. 2010;107:4275–80.

83. Wolchok JD, Kluger H, Callahan MK, Postow MA, Rizvi NA, Lesokhin AM, et al. Nivolumab plus ipilimumab in advanced melanoma. N Engl J Med. 2013;369:122–33.

84. Rizvi N, Chaft J, Balmanoukian A, Goldberg SB, Sanborn RE, Steele KE, et al. Tumor response from durvalumab (MEDI4736) + tremelimumab treatment in patients with advanced non-small cell lung cancer (NSCLC) is observed regardless of PD-L1 status. J Immunother Cancer. 2015;3:193.

85. Redmond WL, Linch SN, Kasiewicz MJ. Combined targeting of costimulatory (OX40) and coinhibitory (CTLA-4) pathways elicits potent effector T cells capable of driving robust antitumor immunity. Cancer Immunol Res. 2014;2:142–53.

86. Dai M, Wei H, Yip YY, Feng Q, He K, Popov V, et al. Long-lasting complete regression of established mouse tumors by counteracting Th2 inflammation. J Immunother. 2013;36:248–57.

87. de Biasi AR, Villena-Vargas J, Adusumilli PS. Cisplatin-induced antitumor immunomodulation: a review of preclinical and clinical evidence. Clin Cancer Res. 2014;20:5384–91.

88. Hato SV, Khong A, de Vries IJM, Lesterhuis WJ. Molecular pathways: the immunogenic effects of platinum-based chemotherapeutics. Clin Cancer Res. 2014;20:2831–7.

89. Dovedi SJ, Illidge TM. The antitumor immune response generated by fractionated radiation therapy may be limited by tumor cell adaptive resistance and can be circumvented by PD-L1 blockade. Oncoimmunology. 2015;4:e1016709.

90. Schmitt NC, Cash H, Ferris RL, Van Waes C, Allen CT. Cisplatin Increases Expression of Antigen Presentation Machinery and Programmed Death Ligand 1 in Head and Neck Squamous Cell Carcinoma Cells. Abstract for 9th International Conference on Head and Neck Cancer, American Head and Neck Society, 2016.

91. Sridharan V, Margalit DN, Curreri SA, Severgnini M, Hodi FS, Haddad RI, et al. Systemic Immunologic Effects of Definitive Radiation in Head and Neck Cancer. Int J Radiat Oncol. 2016;94:864.

92. Parikh F, Duluc D, Imai N, Clark A, Misiukiewicz K, Bonomi M, et al. Chemoradiotherapy-induced upregulation of PD-1 antagonizes immunity to HPV-related oropharyngeal cancer. Cancer Res. 2014;74:7205–16.

93. Cancer Genome Atlas Network. Comprehensive genomic characterization of head and neck squamous cell carcinomas. Nature. 2015;517:576–82.

11

Genomically personalized therapy in head and neck cancer

Kyaw L. Aung and Lillian L. Siu[*]

Abstract

The current treatment paradigm in head and neck cancer does not adequately address its clinical and biological heterogeneity. Data from genomic profiling studies in head and neck squamous cell carcinoma (HNSCC) have revealed the molecular features that are unique to HNSCC subgroups. This progress in the understanding of HNSCC biology provides an opportunity to develop personalized therapies for patients with distinct molecular subtypes to achieve better clinical outcomes including survival. However there are several well-recognized challenges that need to be overcome before genotype-matched therapies make precision medicine a reality for patients with HNSCC. Selection of appropriate patients for biomarker directed clinical trials based on sound scientific rationale will be critical in making cancer genomics more applicable in this malignancy.

Background

Head and neck cancer is a heterogeneous disease comprising epithelial tumors of the upper aerodigestive tract. The majority (~90 %) are squamous cell carcinomas arising from the oral cavity, oropharynx, hypopharynx and larynx classed together as head and neck squamous cell carcinomas (HNSCC) [1]. The main risk factors for developing HNSCC are tobacco smoking, alcohol drinking [2] and human papillomavirus (HPV) infection [3]. HPV-positive HNSCC, which is usually found in oropharynx, is a sexually transmitted disease with a rising incidence in many developed countries [4]. It is biologically and clinically distinct from HPV-negative HNSCC that is classically associated with tobacco and alcohol exposure. Patients with HPV-positive disease have a better prognosis compared to those with HPV-negative disease [5].

The standard treatment paradigm for HNSCC is based on anatomical location and stage of the disease. The biological heterogeneity of HNSCC, however, is not routinely incorporated in the current clinical management algorithms. In general, surgery and/or radiotherapy represent the treatment of choice for early stage disease. Surgery is usually preferred for oral cavity tumors, with the need for post-operative adjuvant radiotherapy typically based on recurrence risks that are determined by stage and tumor pathology. Radiotherapy is generally given as primary treatment in oropharyngeal, hypopharyngeal and laryngeal tumors due to the interest in organ preservation, with salvage surgery considered for local recurrences after primary radiotherapy. Concurrent cisplatin-based chemo-radiotherapy is the standard of care for locoregionally advanced disease. For those patients who are deemed inappropriate candidates for platinum-based chemoradiotherapy, radiotherapy combined with the anti-epidermal growth factor receptor (EGFR) monoclonal antibody cetuximab, may be an alternative. The ideal risk-adapted therapeutic strategies aiming to optimize disease control with minimal long-term toxicities in favorable risk early stage disease, and to maximize survival outcomes with acceptable toxicities in poor risk disease, are still evolving.

For recurrent and metastatic HNSCC, platinum-based chemotherapy remains the mainstay of treatment, and addition of cetuximab to first line chemotherapy (cisplatin or carboplatin plus 5-fluorouracil) offers modest survival benefit [6]. Currently, there is no universally agreed second line therapy.

So far, the search for personalized therapy in patients with HNSCC remains elusive. Cetuximab is the only targeted biological agent approved for use in HNSCC and neither *EGFR* copy number nor level of EGFR expression was shown to predict its response [7, 8]. The hope, however, has been that as we sequence broader and deeper into HNSCC genomes, biological

* Correspondence: Lillian.Siu@uhn.ca

Drug Development Program, Princess Margaret Cancer Centre, University Health Network, 610 University Avenue, Suite 5-718, Toronto, ON M5G 2M9, Canada

drivers in individual HNSCC will be identified with a high precision allowing development of genotype-matching therapy. The emerging data from HNSCC genome sequencing studies [9–13], including recent results from The Cancer Genome Atlas (TCGA) initiative [14], now provide an opportunity to develop genomically personalized therapy for patients with HNSCC.

Genomic landscape of HNSCC
Structural alterations
Genomic structural alterations are commonly seen in HNSCC regardless of HPV status. Both HPV-positive and HPV-negative tumors harbor amplifications of 1q, 3q, 5p and 8q and deletions of 3p, 5q, and 11q [9, 10, 12–14]. The amplification of 3q26/28 region containing squamous lineage transcription factors, *TP63* and *SOX2*, and *PIK3CA* oncogene is seen in both, but more frequently in HPV-positive subtype [9, 10, 12–14]. In HPV-positive tumors, recurrent deletions in *TRAF3* and 11q including *ATM1* and focal amplification of *E2F1* are also seen but 9p21.3 containing *CDKN2A* is usually intact [14]. In contrast, in HPV-negative tumors, 9p21.3 is commonly deleted while 11q13 containing *CCND1*, *FADD* and *CTTN*, and 11q22 containing *BIRC2* and *YAP1* are amplified [14]. It is noteworthy that 7p region that includes *EGFR* is less amplified in HPV-positive tumors [14].

From a biological perspective, recurrent *CDKN2A* deletions and *CCND1* amplification seen in HPV-negative tumors and *E2F1* amplifications in HPV-positive tumors indicate that loss of cell cycle regulation is the fundamental event in HNSCC carcinogenesis. The importance of mitogen activated protein kinase (MAPK) pathway in HPV-negative HNSCC is highlighted by *EGFR* amplification and PI3K-PTEN-AKT-mTOR pathway in both HPV-positive and HPV-negative tumors by *PI3KCA* amplification. Recurrent deletions in *TRAF3* in HPV-positive tumors and amplification of *FADD* and *BIRC2* in HPV-negative tumors showed that NF-kB pathway activation is an important biological driver in HNSCC. *TRAF3* deletions also indicate defective innate immunity response in HPV-positive HNSCC.

Somatic mutations
Genes in cell cycle regulation
Alterations in genes that regulate cell cycle are commonly seen in HNSCC. In HPV-negative tumors, *TP53* is mutated in 80–87 % and *CDKN2A* gene alterations are seen in 32–57 % [11, 12, 14]. *CDKN2A* can also be silenced by promoter hypermethylation in HPV-negative HNSCC [15] and it is noteworthy that CDKN2A expression is lost in almost all HPV-negative HNSCC [16]. On the other hand, *TP53* and *CDKN2A* gene alterations are infrequent in HPV-positive tumors. A small subset of HPV-

negative oral cavity squamous cell carcinoma do not have *TP53* mutations but harbor activating *HRAS* mutations and inactivating *CASP8* mutations constituting a distinct subset with a favorable prognosis [14]. *RB1* mutations, although rare at <10 %, are seen predominantly in HPV-positive tumors [11]. *MYC*, in contrast, is amplified in 5–15 % of HPV-negative tumors [11, 14].

PIK3CA & PTEN
PIK3CA is the most commonly altered oncogene in HNSCC [11, 12, 14]. The presence of hotspot mutations in *PIK3CA* helical domain is a unique feature of HPV-positive tumors, whereas, in HPV-negative tumors, mutations occur throughout the gene despite helical and kinase domain mutations are still common [11, 12, 14]. Twenty one percent of patients in the TCGA cohort had a *PIK3CA* mutation and of those, 25 % also had concurrent *PIK3CA* amplification [14]. An additional 20 % of tumors had *PIK3CA* amplification without mutations [14]. In addition to *PIK3CA* alterations, *PTEN* mutations or deletions are seen in ~11 % of HPV-positive HNSCC and 5 % of HPV-negative HNSCC [11, 17, 18].

Genes encoding receptor tyrosine kinase (RTK) and MAPK pathways
HPV-positive and HPV-negative HNSCC have alterations in genes encoding RTK and MAPK pathways at differing frequencies. While alterations in *EGFR*, *FGFR1*, and *IGF1R* are predominantly seen in HPV-negative tumors, *FGFR2 and FGFR3* alterations including *FGFR3* fusions are more frequent in HPV-positive tumors [12, 14]. *MET* amplification occurs in 2–13 % of HNSCC predominantly in the HPV-negative subtype [19]. *ERBB2* alterations are seen in both subtypes at a low frequency (3–4 %) [14]. Mutations in MAPK pathway, mainly *HRAS* mutations in HPV-negative tumors and *KRAS* mutation in HPV-positive tumors, are seen in ~6 % of HNSCC [12, 14].

DNA damage response genes
Mutations in *BRCA1*, *BRCA2* and *ATR* are seen in 6 %, 7 % and 4–10 % of HNSCC respectively [11]. *ATM* mutations are also seen in 1–16 % of HPV-positive HNSCC across studies [11, 12, 14].

NOTCH1
NOTCH1 is one of the most commonly mutated genes in HNSCC (11- 19 %) [9, 10, 14]. Inactivating mutations are predominantly found in HNSCC cases of the TCGA cohort whereas activating gain of function mutations with overexpression of downstream effectors are found predominantly in Chinese HNSCC cases [20–22]. It is well recognized that the biological role of NOTCH could be contextual [23] and NOTCH undoubtedly plays a

complex biological role in HNSCC making it challenging to target without further biological insight.

Patterns of gene expression

In 2002, Belbin et al. first reported that HNSCC could be classified by gene expression patterns ($N = 17$) [24]. Four main subtypes of HNSCC (Group 1–4) based on expression pattern of 12814 genes were subsequently described by Chung et al. ($N = 60$) [25]. These four subtypes were validated independently in the University of North Carolina cohort ($N = 138$) and subtypes 1–4 were named as basal, mesenchymal, atypical and classical respectively [26]. The basal subtype is characterized by activation of EGFR pathway. The mesenchymal subtype has epithelial to mesenchymal transition (EMT) gene expression signature. The atypical subtype mainly consisted of HPV-positive tumors with high expression of *CDKN2A*, *LIG1* and *RPA2*. The classical subtype showed tobacco-induced gene expression signature.

TCGA also independently validated these four signatures ($N = 278$) [14]. Integrated analysis of DNA alterations and RNA expression patterns in TCGA cohort showed that basal subtype tumors had *NOTCH1* inactivation with intact oxidative stress signaling. This subtype also included tumors with *CASP8* and *HRAS* mutations. In contrast, high expression of CD56, a natural killer cell marker, and HLA class I mutations were seen in the mesenchymal subtype. The atypical subtype again consisted mainly of HPV-positive tumors characterized by activating mutations in *PIK3CA* helical domain and a lack of chromosome 7 amplifications indicating a low level of *EGFR* amplification. In contrast, the classical subtype was seen in heavy smokers and at laryngeal site, characterized by *TP53* mutation, *CDKN2A* loss, chromosome 3q amplification and alteration of oxidative stress genes.

These studies, however, suffer from underrepresentation of HPV-positive tumors. Gene expression analysis

of a cohort enriched with HPV-positive HNSCC by et al. demonstrated that such tumors could be classified into classical-HPV and mesenchymal-HPV [27]. While both subtypes were characterized by enriched cell cycle genes, classical-HPV also had activation of putrescine (polyamine) degradation pathway possibly related to detoxification of tobacco use and mesenchymal-HPV had enrichment of immune response genes related to the tumoral CD8$^+$ T lymphocytes infiltration [27]. HPV-negative mesenchymal tumors in this study also had enrichment of similar immune related genes [27] inferring mesenchymal tumors might respond better to immunotherapy.

Genomically driven dysregulated pathways and personalized therapies

The gene alterations found in HNSCC across studies [9–14] perturb multiple biological pathways. Herein, these pathways are discussed in the context of rationally matched therapies (summarized in Fig. 1).

TP53 and cell cycle regulation

TP53 is the most commonly mutated tumor suppressor in HNSCC and almost all HNSCC displayed a dysregulated cell cycle [14]. Loss of cell cycle regulation at G1 to S phase checkpoint is the dominant biological feature in HNSCC. *TP53* and *CDKN2A* loss of function alterations and *CCND1* amplification are the main driving mechanisms of this dysregulation in HPV-negative tumors [11, 12, 14]. In HPV-positive tumors, degradation of TP53 and RB1 by E6 and E7 viral proteins and focal amplification of *E2F1* are the main culprits [12, 14].

To exploit cell cycle dysregulation as a drug target in HNSCC, cyclin dependent kinase (CDK) inhibitors are of particular interest for patients with *CCND1* amplified tumors. CDK4/6 inhibitors, ribociclib (LEE011) and palbociclib, which prolong progression free survival of patients with hormone receptor positive, HER2-negative

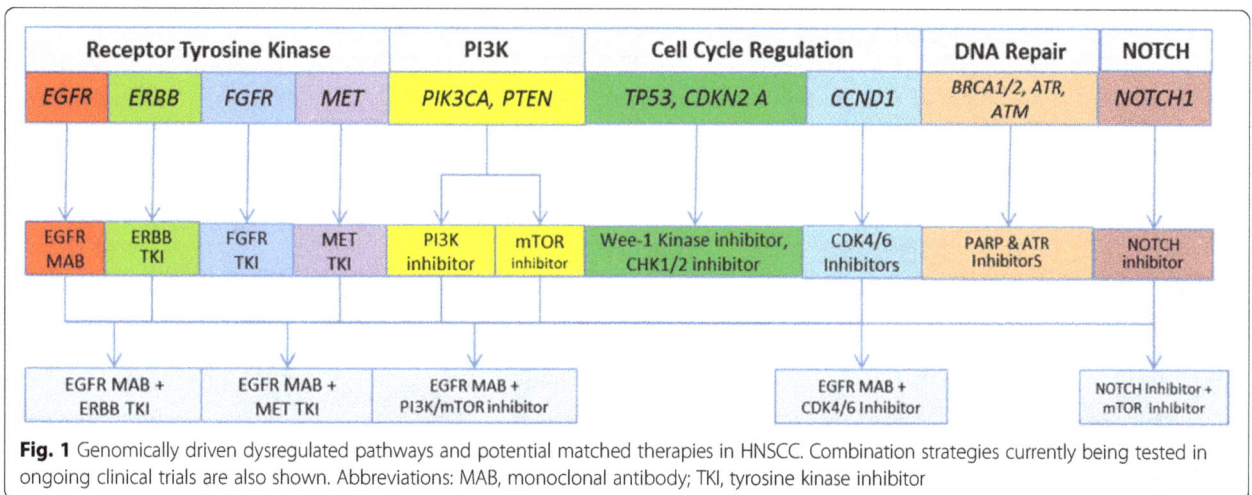

Receptor Tyrosine Kinase				PI3K		Cell Cycle Regulation		DNA Repair	NOTCH
EGFR	ERBB	FGFR	MET	PIK3CA, PTEN		TP53, CDKN2 A	CCND1	BRCA1/2, ATR, ATM	NOTCH1
EGFR MAB	ERBB TKI	FGFR TKI	MET TKI	PI3K inhibitor	mTOR inhibitor	Wee-1 Kinase inhibitor, CHK1/2 inhibitor	CDK4/6 Inhibitors	PARP & ATR InhibitorS	NOTCH inhibitor
EGFR MAB + ERBB TKI	EGFR MAB + MET TKI	EGFR MAB + PI3K/mTOR inhibitor					EGFR MAB + CDK4/6 Inhibitor		NOTCH Inhibitor + mTOR Inhibitor

Fig. 1 Genomically driven dysregulated pathways and potential matched therapies in HNSCC. Combination strategies currently being tested in ongoing clinical trials are also shown. Abbreviations: MAB, monoclonal antibody; TKI, tyrosine kinase inhibitor

advanced breast cancer [28, 29], are currently in early phase development in HNSCC (Tables 1 and 2).

In vitro inhibition of G2 to M phase checkpoint enhances apoptosis induced by DNA damaging agents in TP53 mutant HNSCC [30]. A WEE-1 kinase inhibitor, AZD1775, which disrupts G2 checkpoint by inhibiting CDK1 phosphorylation, is currently being tested in HNSCC in the neo-adjuvant setting in combination with chemotherapy (NCT02508246) and in the locoregionally advanced setting combined with chemoradiotherapy (NCT02585973). Inhibition of checkpoint kinase 1/2 (CHK1/2) also induces mitotic catastrophe followed by cell death in TP53 mutant HNSCC in vitro [31]. As such combining CHK1/2 inhibitors with radiotherapy or DNA damaging agents seems a rational strategy in HNSCC with TP53 loss of function mutations. On the other hand, in breast, ovarian, colon and prostate cancer cells, WEE-1 was found to be a synthetic lethal partner of CHK1 and combined inhibition of WEE-1 and CHK-1 results in tumor growth inhibition in vitro and in vivo regardless of TP53 status [32]. Interestingly, in HPV-positive HNSCC, combining radiotherapy with WEE-1 kinase inhibition increases apoptosis in vitro that is caspase mediated but independent of TP53 [33]. Currently, the role of TP53 mutation status in predicting response to WEE-1 and CHK1/2 inhibition remains unclear in HNSCC.

PI3K-PTEN-AKT-mTOR pathway

PIK3CA is the most commonly mutated oncogene in HNSCC and, combined with other gene alterations, PI3K-PTEN-AKT-mTOR pathway is dysregulated in ~30 % of HNSCC [11, 14, 34]. One of the most "actionable" target in this pathway is the activating gain of function PIK3CA mutations, as PI3K inhibitors of different classes, either alone or in combination with other targeted agents, are in active development in HNSCC (Tables 1 and 2). On the other hand, loss of function gene alterations in PTEN is a challenge to target directly, since the restoration of its tumor suppressive function is not straightforward.

In in vitro studies and patient derived xenografts, PIK3CA mutations sensitized response to PI3K and mTOR inhibitors [34, 35]. However, no significant improvement in clinical outcomes was seen with PX-866, an irreversible PI3K inhibitor, in unselected population of HNSCC when combined with doxcetaxel or cetuximab [36, 37]. In particular, 8 patients with PIK3CA mutant tumors did not respond to the PX-866 and cetuximab combination raising doubts over the role of PIK3CA mutations in predicting response to PI3K pathway inhibition. On the other hand, promising tumor activity was seen with BYL719, a PI3K class I α isoform inhibitor, when combined with cetuximab in a phase Ib study [38] suggesting that efficacy of isoform specific PI3K inhibitors may be different from that of pan-PI3K inhibitors in HNSCC. It is plausible that mutations causing different amino acid substitutions at different positions might have different biological functions with variable sensitivities to PI3K inhibitors [39]. BYL719 is also currently being evaluated with cisplatin-based chemoradiotherapy in locoregionally advanced setting in a phase I study (NCT02537223).

Previous studies demonstrated that mTOR inhibitors, temsirolimus and everolimus, have limited antitumor activity in platinum-refractory recurrent or metastatic HNSCC [40, 41]. Although response rates were higher in platinum naïve setting [42, 43], these studies were performed in non-selected populations and as such the role

Table 1 Current active trials in HNSCC with novel single agents[a]

Trial Number	Trial phase	Drug	Pathway targeted	Molecular selection	Setting	Status
NCT02429089	1	LEE011	Cell cycle	No	Recurrent, metastatic	Recruiting
NCT02264678	1, 2	AZD6738	DNA repair	No	Recurrent, metastatic, in combination with chemotherapy or MEDI4736 or olaparib	Recruiting
NCT02567396	1	Talazoparib	DNA repair	No	Recurrent, metastatic	Not yet recruiting
NCT01711541	1, 2	Veliparib	DNA repair	No	Recurrent, metastatic, in combination with chemotherapy	
NCT02365662	1	ABBV-221	EGFR	No	Recurrent, metastatic	Recruiting
NCT01345669	3	Afatinib	ERBB	No	Placebo controlled post-chemoradiotherapy	Recruiting
NCT01415674	2	Afatinib	ERBB	No	Neoadjuvant	Active, not recruiting
NCT01427478	3	Afatinib	ERBB	No	Placebo controlled randomised phase 3, maintenance therapy after post-operative chemoradiotherapy	Recruiting
NCT02131155	3	Afatinib	ERBB	No	Placebo controlled adjuvant trial	Recruiting
NCT02216916	2	HM781-36B	ERBB	No	Recurrent, metastatic	Recruiting
NCT02145312	2	BYL719	PI3K	No	Recurrent, metaststic	Not yet recruiting
NCT02540928	2a	AMG319	PI3K	HPV-negative	Placebo controlled neoadjuvant therapy	Recruiting

[a]Clinical trials with immune checkpoint inhibitors are not included in this Table

Table 2 Current active trials in HNSCC testing the safety and efficacy of novel drug combinations

Trials	Trial phase	Drug 1	Drug 2	Pathway 1	Pathway 2	Setting	Status
NCT01716416	1	Pazopanib	Cetuximab	Angiogenesis	EGFR	Recurrent, metastatic	Recruiting
NCT02499120	2	Palbociclib	Cetuximab	Cell cycle	EGFR	Plcebo controlled randomized phase II, recurrent, metastatic	Recruiting
NCT02101034	1,2	Palbociclib	Cetuximab	Cell cycle	EGFR	Recurrent, metastatic	Recruiting
NCT01711541	1, 2	Veliparib	Chemotherapy	DNA repair	EGFR	Recurrent, metastatic	Recruiting
NCT02538627	1	MM-151	MM-121	EGFR	ERBB	Recurrent, metastatic	Recruiting
NCT02501096	1, 2	Pembrolizumab	Lenvatinib	Immune	Angiogenesis	Recurrent, metastatic	Recruiting
NCT02454179	2	Pembrolizumab	ACP-196	Immune	Bruton Tyrosine Kinase	Recurrent, metastatic	Recruiting
NCT02646748	1	Pembrolizumab	INCB039110/ INCB050465	Immune	JAK/PI3K	Recurrent, metastatic	Recruiting
NCT01468896	1, 2	Recombinant interleukin-2	Cetuximab	Immune	EGFR	Recurrent, metastatic	Active, not recruiting
NCT02507154	1, 2	NK cells	Cetuximab	Immune	EGFR	Recurrent, metastatic	Recruiting
NCT02643550	1, 2	Monalizumab	Cetuximab	Immune	EGFR	Recurrent, metastatic	Recruiting
NCT02110082	1	Urelumab	Cetuximab	Immune	EGFR	Recurrent, metastatic	Active, not recruiting
NCT02124850	1	Motolimod/ Nivolumab	Cetuximab	Immune	EGFR	Stage II-IVA, neoadjuvant	Recruiting
NCT02586987	1	MEDI4736	Selumetinib	Immune	MEK	Recurrent, metastatic	Recruiting
NCT01871311	1	Nilotinib	Cetuximab	Kit	EGFR	Recurrent, metastatic	Recruiting
NCT02277197	1	Ficlatuzumab	Cetuximab	MET	EGFR	Recurrent, metastatic	Recruiting
NCT01332266	1, 2	E7050	Cetuximab	MET	EGFR	Recurrent, metastatic	Recruiting
NCT02205398	1	INC280	Cetuximab	MET	EGFR	Recurrent, metastatic	Recruiting
NCT01285037	1	LY2801653	Cetuximab	MET	EGFR	Recurrent, metastatic	Recruiting
NCT01602315	1b, 2	BYL719	Cetuximab	PI3K	EGFR	Recurrent, metastatic	Active, not recruiting
NCT01488318	2	Dasatinib	Cetuximab	Scr	EGFR	Recurrent, metastatic	Recruiting

of *PIK3CA* or *PTEN* alterations in predicting response to mTOR inhibitors in HNSCC is not clearly known.

Receptor tyrosine kinase pathways
EGFR

Overexpression of EGFR was seen in >90 % of HNSCC and associated with a poor prognosis [44–48]. Cetuximab improves survival of patients in both locoregionally advanced setting and recurrent or metastatic setting when combined with radiotherapy and chemotherapy respectively [6, 49]. However, single agent response to cetuximab in recurrent or metastatic HNSCC is 13 % at best indicating there is primary resistance to EGFR inhibition [50].

EGFR alterations are found in ~15 % of patients with HNSCC predominantly in HPV-negative tumors [12, 14]. Neither *EGFR* copy number nor level of EGFR expression was shown to predict cetuximab response [7, 8]. *EGFR* mutations including *EGFRvIII* are also extremely rare in HNSCC and unlikely to be useful

as predictive biomarkers for EGFR targeted therapy [14, 47, 51–53]. However, alterations in *ERBB2*, *MET*, *PIK3CA*, *PTEN* and *HRAS* can co-occur with *EGFR* alterations and may explain mechanisms of EGFR inhibitor resistance in individual HNSCC [14]. Combined inhibition of EGFR and other RTK and/or downstream pathways based on genotype of tumors might overcome primary and secondary resistance to EGFR inhibition leading to improved clinical outcomes. Currently, the safety and efficacy of cetuximab combined with multiple molecular targeted therapies are being tested in various phase 1 and 2 clinical trials (Table 2).

ERBB

ERBB2 alteration (amplification plus mutation) is seen in ~4 % of HPV-negative HNSCC and ~3 % of HPV-positive HNSCC [14]. Afatinib, an irreversible pan-ERBB inhibitor, was recently shown to improve progression-free-survival in a non-selected population of recurrent or metastatic HNSCC when compared to methotrexate in the second line setting, indicating that targeting ERBB pathway is a valid therapeutic strategy in HNSCC [54]. Dacomitinib, another irreversible pan-ERBB inhibitor, also demonstrated a single agent response rate of ~13 % in a phase 2 study [55]. Presence of mutations in *PIK3CA* or *PTEN* seems to predict poor PFS in patients treated with dacomitinib in a separate study [56] indicating dual inhibition of ERBB and PI3K pathways might produce better clinical benefit in patients with *PIK3CA* or *PTEN* alterations. A recent phase Ib study has already established maximum tolerated dose of the combination of cetuximab and afitinib [57]. From a genomic perspective, patients with *EGFR* and *ERBB* aberrations are likely to derive better clinical benefit from this novel combination. ERBB targeted agents are currently in active clinical development in HNSCC (Tables 1 and 2).

FGFR

FGFR1 alterations (amplification or mutations) are seen in ~12 % of HPV-negative HNSCC and *FGFR3* alterations (mutations or fusions) in ~11 % of HPV-positive HNSCC [14]. In a preclinical study *FGFR1* mRNA and protein expression level but not *FGFR1* copy number was found to be associated with response to a pan-FGFR inhibitor BGJ398 [58]. Data from squamous cell lung cancer suggest that *FGFR1*-amplified tumor cells with co-expression of MYC are more sensitive to FGFR inhibition [59]. Currently there is no clinical data to indicate the efficacy of FGFR inhibitors in HNSCC as they are still in early stages of drug development.

MET

MET amplification is found in 2–13 % of HNSCC and it is mutated in ~6 % [19]. Acquired *MET* amplification is a well-recognized biological mechanism of resistance to EGFR inhibition [60–62] and MET overexpression is frequently seen in HNSCC [19]. However, in a phase II study of foretinib, an oral multikinase inhibitor of MET and VEGFR2, in an unselected HNSCC population, no partial or complete response was seen [63]. Despite this disappointing result, combination treatment of MET inhibitors with cetuximab or other RTK inhibitors in selected population is biologically rational and still worth investigating.

Immune related pathways and genomic predictors for immunotherapy

HNSCC is an immunosuppressive disease and immune checkpoint inhibitors (ICI) are emerging as a promising therapy for patients with HNSCC. Low frequency mutations of *HLA-A*, *HLA-B* and *B2M* are seen in both HPV-positive and HPV-negative tumors implicating that tumor antigen presentation may be disrupted in tumors harboring these genetic alterations [14]. Early data indicate that single agent response to PD-1/PD-L1 pathway inhibition in HNSCC is ~12–20 % [64, 65]. Although objective response rates are higher in patients with PD-L1 positive tumors, PD-L1 expression was not a binary predictive biomarker as PD-L1 negative tumors can demonstrate meaningful tumor shrinkage or clinical benefit [64, 65]. No definite difference in response rate to ICI between HPV-positive and HPV-negative subtypes has been observed [64, 65]. CheckMate 141 (NCT02105636), a phase III study that is comparing the efficacy of nivolumab, an anti-PD-1 inhibitor, in the platinum-resistant recurrent or metastatic setting with investigator's choice of therapy has been stopped early because it met the primary overall survival endpoint at a preplanned interim analysis [66].

In squamous cell lung cancer, response to nivolumab was shown to associate with tumor mutation burden, neo-antigen load and smoking mutation signature [67]. Although hypermutated phenotype is rare in HNSCC, neo-antigen landscape and smoking signature may be relevant in predicting immunotherapy response in HNSCC. Seventy five percent of HPV-positive HNSCC and 23 % of HPV-negative HNSCC in the combined University of Chicago and TCGA cohort ($N = 134 + 424 = 558$) have an inflamed tumor phenotype [62]. This phenotype is characterized by enrichment of immune response genes related to intra-tumoral $CD8^+$ T lymphocyte infiltration, PD-L1 expression and expression of CTLA-4, LAG3, PD-L2 and IDO [68]. There is also a strong correlation between inflamed tumor phenotype and mesenchymal subtype [68]. Considering these emerging data, it is tempting to speculate that HNSCC with this gene expression signature may respond better to ICI. This hypothesis, however, needs further prospective clinical validation.

DNA damage response and homologous recombination (HR) deficiency

Interestingly somatic mutations in genes involved in DNA damage response including HR are seen in HNSCC at various frequencies [11]. Somatic mutations in *BRCA1* (~6 %), *BRCA2* (~7 %), *ATR* (4–10 %) and *ATM* (1-16 %) are all reported providing the rationale for targeting DNA repair pathway in these tumors [12]. Inactivation of Fanconi anemia/BRCA pathway via promoter hypermethylation of *FANCF* was also seen in 15 % of patients with HNSCC in a previous study [69]. PARP inhibitors and ATR inhibitors, in combination with radiotherapy or cisplatin, are of particular interest for patients with HR deficient genotype. Currently ATR inhibitors, AZD6738 and VX-970, are in early phase of development in HNSCC (NCT02264678; NCT02567422). Furthermore, in a phase I study of AZD1775, a wee-1 kinase inhibitor, a HNSCC patient with a *BRCA* mutation achieved a partial response [70] supporting that DNA repair pathway might be a valid therapeutic target in selected HNSCC population.

Notch pathway

NOTCH1 is one of the most commonly mutated genes in HNSCC (~10–15 %) [9, 10, 14] and associated with a poor prognosis [21]. NOTCH pathway plays complex biological roles including cell differentiation, proliferation, angiogenesis and survival [71–73]. As such NOTCH pathway inhibition could be a valid therapeutic strategy in HNSCC. A recent phase I study reported that 2 out of 15 HNSCC patients (13 %) treated with combination of NOTCH inhibitor MK-0752 and mTOR inhibitor ridaforolimus achieved partial response [74]. However, considering the fact that both activating and inactivating NOTCH mutations are seen in HNSCC and the increased risk of squamous cell carcinoma of skin observed with gamma-secretase inhibitors in patients with Alzheimer's disease [75, 76], targeting NOTCH pathway in HNSCC in the right biological context with minimal risk will be challenging. Further biological insight will be necessary before NOTCH pathway inhibition can be optimally exploited for treatment of patients with HNSCC.

Challenges & future directions

The recent genomic profiling studies identified biologically distinct HNSCC subgroups providing rationale for developing genomically directed personalized therapies. However, there are well-recognized challenges. Currently available genomic data in HNSCC is limiting as they were mostly derived from early stage resectable and locally advanced tumors with gross underrepresentation of recurrent/metastatic disease (Table 3) and do not truly inform the biological drivers of recurrent and metastatic HNSCC in which most novel targeted agents are currently being tested. Most studies also included only small number of HPV-positive cases (Table 3). Moreover, they were conducted in heterogeneous patient populations without detailed clinical annotation and as such lack power to determine prognostic and predictive value of genetic alterations identified.

From a biological point of view, the main challenges are those posed by spatial and temporal tumor heterogeneity. Considering profound intra-tumor genetic heterogeneity found in multiple solid tumor types [77–79]

including HNSCC [80, 81], it will be difficult to make accurate assessment of tumor genetic characteristics from a single tumor biopsy. To address this in patients with multiple metastatic sites, ideally multiple tumor biopsies from all disease sites will be necessary to assess tumor genomic profile accurately. Cleary, this is not logistically feasible in current oncology practice and innovative tumor sampling methods will be necessary to overcome this challenge. One potential method is mutation profiling of plasma-derived circulating tumor DNA (ctDNA) using next generation sequencing (NGS). As tumor DNA from different metastatic sites are shed into circulation, it could be argued that ctDNA contains mutations or genetic alterations derived from all sub-clones of tumors. With rapid advances in NGS technologies, several groups have demonstrated that molecular characterization of ctDNA is feasible [82–87]. Analysis of serial ctDNA samples could reveal clonal evolution of tumors highlighting the future potential of ctDNA mutation profiling in addressing both spatial and temporal intra-tumor genetic heterogeneity. In appropriate HNSCC cases, it might also be possible to study tumor mutations from DNA isolated from saliva. The feasibility of tumor specific mutation testing from ctDNA and saliva in patients with HNSCC has been explored in a recent study [88].

The obvious drug targets in cancer genomes are activating mutations in driver oncogenes. In HNSCC *PIK3CA* is the most frequently mutated oncogene (~20 %) and PI3K inhibitors are in active development. However, despite the preclinical evidence showing *PIK3CA* mutations sensitize response to PIK3A inhibitors, clinical results so far have been disappointing except possibly for BYL719, a PI3K class I α isoform inhibitor, in combination with cetuximab where some signals of activity have been observed. Further biological insight will be needed to advance development of PI3K inhibitors in HNSCC. Beyond *PIK3CA*, actionable mutations in other oncogenic driver genes such as *ERBB*, *FGFR*, and *MET* are relatively rare making it challenging to conduct biomarker directed clinical trials. Future trials with innovative designs will be needed to address this issue.

Table 3 Summary of head and neck cancer clinical samples in genome sequencing studies

Study	Total samples	Oral cavity	Oropharynx	Hypopharynx	Larynx	Other primary sites	Lymph nodes	Metastatic samples	HPV-Positive	HPV-Negative
Stransky et al. [9]	92	51 (55 %)	15 (16 %)	7 (8 %)	15 (16 %)	2 (2 %)	–	–	13 (14 %)	79 (86 %)
Agrawal et al. [10]	32	NK	NK	NK	NK	NK	–	–	4 (12 %)	28 (88 %)
Chung et al. [11]	252	53 (21 %)	12 (5 %)	–	7 (3 %)	103 (41 %)	25 (10 %)	80 (32 %)	84 (33 %)	168 (67 %)
Seiwert et al. [12]	120	23 (19 %)	67 (56 %)	8 (7 %)	19 (16 %)	3 (2 %)	–	–	51 (42 %)	69 (58 %)
Pickering et al. [13]	38	38 (100 %)	–	–	–	–	–	–	NK	NK
TCGA [14]	279	172 (62 %)	33 (12 %)	–	72 (26 %)	–	–	–	36 (13 %)	243 (87 %)

Abbreviation: *NK* not known, *TCGA* The Cancer Genome Atlas

Although genetic alterations in tumor suppressor genes *TP53* and *CDKN2A* are common in HNSCC, these alterations are notoriously difficult to exploit for targeted therapeutics at present. Again, mutations in other tumor suppressor genes are seen at low frequencies. Further studies will be needed to elucidate synthetic lethal interactions between these genetic events using computational algorithms such as DAISY (data mining synthetic lethality identification pipeline) [89] or using si-RNA, sh-RNA or CRISPR (clustered regularly interspaced short palindromic repeats) screens so that rational treatment strategies could be developed based on tumor genomic profiles [90]. Currently, one of the most exciting synthetic lethality opportunities involves the use of DNA damaging agents such as PARP inhibitors or ATR inhibitors in patients with HR deficient tumors.

From a genomic perspective, it will be necessary to understand the clonal composition and progression of tumors to develop effective genotype-matched therapy. As clonal selection and progression would have occurred that led to the development of clinically detectable recurrent or metastatic disease, actual clonal composition of advanced HNSCC could be different from that of primary tumors and arguably might contain more genetic driver events that are actionable. Accurate charting of clonal and sub-clonal genetic events in recurrent and metastatic HNSCC based on absolute quantification of somatic mutation events will be critical in finding the relevant therapeutic targets in individual tumors [91, 92]. It is plausible that some genetic alterations are present only in minor sub-clones and targeting those might not produce meaningful clinical benefits.

Considering different biological pathways are active in different subtypes of HNSCC, single agent activity of targeted agents in non-selected population is likely to be modest. To significantly improve clinical outcomes, rational combination treatment strategies should be tested prospectively in selected populations enriched by unique tumor molecular features present in the recurrent or metastatic tumors. Currently, based on available genomic data mainly derived from early stage tumors, the proportion of HNSCC patients who could benefit from personalized therapy remains relatively small considering the most common genetic events in HNSCC occur in tumor suppressor genes. However, concerted large scale genomic profiling programs such as SPECTA (Screening Patients for Efficient Clinical Trial Access) of EORTC (European Organization for Research and Treatment of Cancer) that aims to profile advanced solid tumors to offer genotype-matched therapies could more accurately inform targetable genetic events in recurrent/metastatic HNSCC. These initiatives may also shed insight on the proportion of patients who truly benefit from personalized treatment strategies with acceptable toxicity profiles.

Beyond targeted therapy, ICI are now emerging as a promising new therapy in HNSCC. The genomic predictors of response to ICI clearly exist in other cancer types [67, 93] and it would be prudent to identify genomic and immune mechanisms that underlie tumor immune escape and ICI resistance in HNSCC. As future therapeutic opportunities arise with advances in our understanding of HNSCC biology, there will also be new challenges of translating these advances to personalized therapies. The vision for precision medicine in HNSCC requires concerted interest and continuous effort in the conduct of innovative but complex biomarker directed multidisciplinary trials.

Conclusion

New treatment paradigms for patients with HNSCC are currently evolving. At present the two main subtypes of HNSCC classified by HPV status remains the most clinically relevant. Development of personalized therapy in HNSCC is still in early stage and results from ongoing preclinical and clinical studies will provide further insight into future novel therapeutic strategies. It is, however, critical that future studies select appropriate patients for potential matched therapies based on sound biological rationale to realize precision medicine in head and neck cancer.

Abbreviations

CDK, Cyclin Dependent Kinase; CRISPR, Clustered Regularly Interspaced Short Palindromic Repeats; ctDNA, circulating tumor DNA; DAISY, Data Mining Synthetic Lethality Identification Pipeline; EGFR, Epidermal Growth Factor Receptor; EMT, Epithelial Mesenchymal Transition; EORTC, European Organization for Research and Treatment of Cancer; HNSCC, Head and Neck Squamous Cell Carcinoma; HPV, Human Papillomavirus; HR, Homologous Recombination; ICI, Immune Checkpoint Inhibitors; MAPK, Mitogen Activated Protein Kinase; NGS, Next Generation DNA Sequencing; RTK, Receptor Tyrosine Kinase; SPECTA, Screening Patients for Efficient Clinical Trial Access; TCGA, The Cancer Genome Atlas.

Funding

Both authors are employees of the University Health Network, Toronto, Canada and there is no other source of funding directly related to this manuscript.

Authors' contributions

KA drafted the manuscript. LS corrected and finalized the manuscript. Both authors read and approved the final manuscript.

Competing interests

The authors declare that they have no competing interests.

References

1. Pai SI, Westra WH. Molecular pathology of head and neck cancer: implications for diagnosis, prognosis, and treatment. Annu Rev Pathol. 2009;4:49–70.

2. Maier H, Dietz A, Gewelke U, Heller WD, Weidauer H. Tobacco and alcohol and the risk of head and neck cancer. Clin Investig. 1992;70:320–7.

3. Mork J, Lie AK, Glattre E, et al. Human papillomavirus infection as a risk factor for squamous-cell carcinoma of the head and neck. N Engl J Med. 2001;344:1125–31.

4. Chaturvedi AK, Engels EA, Pfeiffer RM, et al. Human papillomavirus and rising oropharyngeal cancer incidence in the United States. J Clin Oncol. 2011;29:4294–301.

5. Ang KK, Harris J, Wheeler R, et al. Human papillomavirus and survival of patients with oropharyngeal cancer. N Engl J Med. 2010;363:24–35.

6. Vermorken JB, Mesia R, Rivera F, et al. Platinum-based chemotherapy plus cetuximab in head and neck cancer. N Engl J Med. 2008;359:1116–27.

7. Licitra L, Mesia R, Rivera F, et al. Evaluation of EGFR gene copy number as a predictive biomarker for the efficacy of cetuximab in combination with chemotherapy in the first-line treatment of recurrent and/or metastatic squamous cell carcinoma of the head and neck: EXTREME study. Ann Oncol. 2011;22:1078–87.

8. Licitra L, Storkel S, Kerr KM, et al. Predictive value of epidermal growth factor receptor expression for first-line chemotherapy plus cetuximab in patients with head and neck and colorectal cancer: analysis of data from the EXTREME and CRYSTAL studies. Eur J Cancer. 2013;49:1161–8.

9. Stransky N, Egloff AM, Tward AD, et al. The mutational landscape of head and neck squamous cell carcinoma. Science. 2011;333:1157–60.

10. Agrawal N, Frederick MJ, Pickering CR, et al. Exome sequencing of head and neck squamous cell carcinoma reveals inactivating mutations in NOTCH1. Science. 2011;333:1154–7.

11. Chung CH, Guthrie VB, Masica DL, et al. Genomic alterations in head and neck squamous cell carcinoma determined by cancer gene-targeted sequencing. Ann Oncol. 2015;26:1216–23.

12. Seiwert TY, Zuo Z, Keck MK, et al. Integrative and comparative genomic analysis of HPV-positive and HPV-negative head and neck squamous cell carcinomas. Clin Cancer Res. 2015;21:632–41.

13. Pickering CR, Zhang J, Yoo SY, et al. Integrative genomic characterization of oral squamous cell carcinoma identifies frequent somatic drivers. Cancer Discov. 2013;3:770–81.

14. Cancer Genome Atlas N. Comprehensive genomic characterization of head and neck squamous cell carcinomas. Nature. 2015;517:576–82.

15. Guerrero-Preston R, Michailidi C, Marchionni L, et al. Key tumor suppressor genes inactivated by "greater promoter" methylation and somatic mutations in head and neck cancer. Epigenetics. 2014;9:1031–46.

16. Lim AM, Do H, Young RJ, et al. Differential mechanisms of CDKN2A (p16) alteration in oral tongue squamous cell carcinomas and correlation with patient outcome. Int J Cancer. 2014;135:887–95.

17. Shao X, Tandon R, Samara G, et al. Mutational analysis of the PTEN gene in head and neck squamous cell carcinoma. Int J Cancer. 1998;77:684–8.

18. Pedrero JM, Carracedo DG, Pinto CM, et al. Frequent genetic and biochemical alterations of the PI 3-K/AKT/PTEN pathway in head and neck squamous cell carcinoma. Int J Cancer. 2005;114:242–8.

19. Seiwert TY, Jagadeeswaran R, Faoro L, et al. The MET receptor tyrosine kinase is a potential novel therapeutic target for head and neck squamous cell carcinoma. Cancer Res. 2009;69:3021–31.

20. Izumchenko E, Sun K, Jones S, et al. Notch1 mutations are drivers of oral tumorigenesis. Cancer Prev Res (Phila). 2015;8:277–86.

21. Song X, Xia R, Li J, et al. Common and complex Notch1 mutations in Chinese oral squamous cell carcinoma. Clin Cancer Res. 2014;20:701–10.

22. Sun W, Gaykalova DA, Ochs MF, et al. Activation of the NOTCH pathway in head and neck cancer. Cancer Res. 2014;74:1091–104.

23. Bolos V, Grego-Bessa J, de la Pompa JL. Notch signaling in development and cancer. Endocr Rev. 2007;28:339–63.

24. Belbin TJ, Singh B, Barber I, et al. Molecular classification of head and neck squamous cell carcinoma using cDNA microarrays. Cancer Res. 2002;62:1184–90.

25. Chung CH, Parker JS, Karaca G, et al. Molecular classification of head and neck squamous cell carcinomas using patterns of gene expression. Cancer Cell. 2004;5:489–500.

26. Walter V, Yin X, Wilkerson MD, et al. Molecular subtypes in head and neck cancer exhibit distinct patterns of chromosomal gain and loss of canonical cancer genes. PLoS One. 2013;8, e56823.

27. Keck MK, Zuo Z, Khattri A, et al. Integrative analysis of head and neck cancer identifies two biologically distinct HPV and three non-HPV subtypes. Clin Cancer Res. 2015;21:870–81.

28. Finn RS, Crown JP, Lang I, et al. The cyclin-dependent kinase 4/6 inhibitor palbociclib in combination with letrozole versus letrozole alone as first-line treatment of oestrogen receptor-positive, HER2-negative, advanced breast cancer (PALOMA-1/TRIO-18): a randomised phase 2 study. Lancet Oncol. 2015;16:25–35.

29. Turner NC, Ro J, Andre F, et al. Palbociclib in Hormone-Receptor-Positive Advanced Breast Cancer. N Engl J Med. 2015;373:209–19.

30. Osman AA, Monroe MM, Ortega Alves MV, et al. Wee-1 kinase inhibition overcomes cisplatin resistance associated with high-risk TP53 mutations in head and neck cancer through mitotic arrest followed by senescence. Mol Cancer Ther. 2015;14:608–19.

31. Gadhikar MA, Sciuto MR, Alves MV, et al. Chk1/2 inhibition overcomes the cisplatin resistance of head and neck cancer cells secondary to the loss of functional p53. Mol Cancer Ther. 2013;12:1860–73.

32. Carrassa L, Chila R, Lupi M, et al. Combined inhibition of Chk1 and Wee1: in vitro synergistic effect translates to tumor growth inhibition in vivo. Cell Cycle. 2012;11:2507–17.

33. Tanaka N, Patel AA, Wang J, et al. Wee-1 Kinase Inhibition Sensitizes High-Risk HPV+ HNSCC to Apoptosis Accompanied by Downregulation of MCl-1 and XIAP Antiapoptotic Proteins. Clin Cancer Res. 2015;21:4831–44.

34. Lui VW, Hedberg ML, Li H, et al. Frequent mutation of the PI3K pathway in head and neck cancer defines predictive biomarkers. Cancer Discov. 2013;3: 761–9.

35. Mazumdar T, Byers LA, Ng PK, et al. A comprehensive evaluation of biomarkers predictive of response to PI3K inhibitors and of resistance mechanisms in head and neck squamous cell carcinoma. Mol Cancer Ther. 2014;13:2738–50.

36. Jimeno A, Bauman JE, Weissman C, et al. A randomized, phase 2 trial of docetaxel with or without PX-866, an irreversible oral phosphatidylinositol 3-kinase inhibitor, in patients with relapsed or metastatic head and neck squamous cell cancer. Oral Oncol. 2015;51:383–8.

37. Jimeno A, Shirai K, Choi M, et al. A randomized, phase II trial of cetuximab with or without PX-866, an irreversible oral phosphatidylinositol 3-kinase inhibitor, in patients with relapsed or metastatic head and neck squamous cell cancer. Ann Oncol. 2015;26:556–61.

38. Gonzalez-Angulo AM, Juric D, Argiles G, et al. Safety, pharmacokinetics, and preliminary activity of the alpha specific PI3K inhibitor: Results from the first-in-human study. J Clin Oncol 31, 2013 (suppl; abstr 2531).

39. Barbareschi M, Buttitta F, Felicioni L, et al. Different prognostic roles of mutations in the helical and kinase domains of the PIK3CA gene in breast carcinomas. Clin Cancer Res. 2007;13:6064–9.

40. Grunwald V, Keilholz U, Boehm A, et al. TEMHEAD: a single-arm multicentre phase II study of temsirolimus in platin- and cetuximab refractory recurrent and/or metastatic squamous cell carcinoma of the head and neck (SCCHN) of the German SCCHN Group (AIO). Ann Oncol. 2015;26:561–7.

41. Massarelli E, Lin H, Ginsberg LE, et al. Phase II trial of everolimus and erlotinib in patients with platinum-resistant recurrent and/or metastatic head and neck squamous cell carcinoma. Ann Oncol. 2015;26:1476–80.

42. Fury MG, Sherman E, Ho A, et al. A phase I study of temsirolimus plus carboplatin plus paclitaxel for patients with recurrent or metastatic (R/M) head and neck squamous cell cancer (HNSCC). Cancer Chemother Pharmacol. 2012;70:121–8.

43. Saba NF, Hurwitz SJ, Magliocca K, et al. Phase 1 and pharmacokinetic study of everolimus in combination with cetuximab and carboplatin for recurrent/metastatic squamous cell carcinoma of the head and neck. Cancer. 2014;120:3940–51.

44. Ozanne B, Richards CS, Hendler F, Burns D, Gusterson B. Over-expression of the EGF receptor is a hallmark of squamous cell carcinomas. J Pathol. 1986;149:9–14.

45. Grandis JR, Tweardy DJ. Elevated levels of transforming growth factor alpha and epidermal growth factor receptor messenger RNA are early markers of carcinogenesis in head and neck cancer. Cancer Res. 1993;53:3579–84.

46. Ang KK, Berkey BA, Tu X, et al. Impact of epidermal growth factor receptor expression on survival and pattern of relapse in patients with advanced head and neck carcinoma. Cancer Res. 2002;62:7350–6.

47. Hama T, Yuza Y, Saito Y, et al. Prognostic significance of epidermal growth factor receptor phosphorylation and mutation in head and neck squamous cell carcinoma. Oncologist. 2009;14:900–8.

48. Keren S, Shoude Z, Lu Z, Beibei Y. Role of EGFR as a prognostic factor for survival in head and neck cancer: a meta-analysis. Tumour Biol. 2014;35:2285–95.

49. Bonner JA, Harari PM, Giralt J, et al. Radiotherapy plus cetuximab for squamous-cell carcinoma of the head and neck. N Engl J Med. 2006;354:567–78.

50. Vermorken JB, Trigo J, Hitt R, et al. Open-label, uncontrolled, multicenter phase II study to evaluate the efficacy and toxicity of cetuximab as a single agent in patients with recurrent and/or metastatic squamous cell carcinoma of the head and neck who failed to respond to platinum-based therapy. J Clin Oncol. 2007;25:2171–7.

51. Lee JW, Soung YH, Kim SY, et al. Somatic mutations of EGFR gene in squamous cell carcinoma of the head and neck. Clin Cancer Res. 2005;11:2879–82.

52. Loeffler-Ragg J, Witsch-Baumgartner M, Tzankov A, et al. Low incidence of mutations in EGFR kinase domain in Caucasian patients with head and neck squamous cell carcinoma. Eur J Cancer. 2006;42:109–11.

53. Khattri A, Zuo Z, Bragelmann J, et al. Rare occurrence of EGFRvIII deletion in head and neck squamous cell carcinoma. Oral Oncol. 2015;51:53–8.

54. Machiels JP, Haddad RI, Fayette J, et al. Afatinib versus methotrexate as second-line treatment in patients with recurrent or metastatic squamous-cell carcinoma of the head and neck progressing on or after platinum-based therapy (LUX-Head & Neck 1): an open-label, randomised phase 3 trial. Lancet Oncol. 2015;16:583–94.

55. Abdul Razak AR, Soulieres D, Laurie SA, et al. A phase II trial of dacomitinib, an oral pan-human EGF receptor (HER) inhibitor, as first-line treatment in recurrent and/or metastatic squamous-cell carcinoma of the head and neck. Ann Oncol. 2013;24:761–9.

56. Kim HS, Kwon HJ, Jung I, et al. Phase II clinical and exploratory biomarker study of dacomitinib in patients with recurrent and/or metastatic squamous cell carcinoma of head and neck. Clin Cancer Res. 2015;21:544–52.

57. Janjigian YY, Smit EF, Groen HJ, et al. Dual inhibition of EGFR with afatinib and cetuximab in kinase inhibitor-resistant EGFR-mutant lung cancer with and without T790M mutations. Cancer Discov. 2014;4:1036–45.

58. Goke F, Franzen A, Hinz TK, et al. FGFR1 Expression Levels Predict BGJ398 Sensitivity of FGFR1-Dependent Head and Neck Squamous Cell Cancers. Clin Cancer Res. 2015;21:4356–64.

59. Malchers F, Dietlein F, Schottle J, et al. Cell-autonomous and non-cell-autonomous mechanisms of transformation by amplified FGFR1 in lung cancer. Cancer Discov. 2014;4:246–57.

60. Engelman JA, Zejnullahu K, Mitsudomi T, et al. MET amplification leads to gefitinib resistance in lung cancer by activating ERBB3 signaling. Science. 2007;316:1039–43.

61. Chau NG, Perez-Ordonez B, Zhang K, et al. The association between EGFR variant III, HPV, p16, c-MET, EGFR gene copy number and response to EGFR inhibitors in patients with recurrent or metastatic squamous cell carcinoma of the head and neck. Head Neck Oncol. 2011;3:11.

62. Rabinowits G, Haddad RI. Overcoming resistance to EGFR inhibitor in head and neck cancer: a review of the literature. Oral Oncol. 2012;48:1085–9.

63. Seiwert T, Sarantopoulos J, Kallender H, McCallum S, Keer HN, Blumenschein Jr G. Phase II trial of single-agent foretinib (GSK1363089) in patients with recurrent or metastatic squamous cell carcinoma of the head and neck. Invest New Drugs. 2013;31:417–24.

64. Seiwert TY, Haddad RI, Gupta S, et al. Antitumor activity and safety of pembrolizumab in patients with advanced squamous carcinoma of head and neck: Preliminary results from KEYNOTE-012 expansion cohort. J Clin Oncol 2015;33:suppl: abstr LBA6008.

65. Segal NH, Ou SI, Balmanoukian AS, et al. Safety and effecacy of MEDI4736, an anti-PD-L1 antibody, in patients from a squamous cell carcinoma of the head and neck (SCCHN) expansion cohort. J Clin Oncol. 2015;33.

66. Gillison ML, Blumenschein G, Fayette J, et al. Nivolumab Versus Investigator's Choice (IC) for Recurrent or Metastatic (R/M) Head and Neck Squamous Cell Carcinoma (SCCHN): CheckMate-141. Presented at: AACR 2016 Annual Meeting, New Orleans; April 16–20, 2016. Abstract CT099.

67. Rizvi NA, Hellmann MD, Snyder A, et al. Cancer immunology. Mutational landscape determines sensitivity to PD-1 blockade in non-small cell lung cancer. Science. 2015;348:124–8.

68. Saloura V, Zuo Z, Koeppen H, et al. Correlation of T-cell inflamed phenotype with mesenchymal sutype, PD-L1 and other immune checkpoints in head and neck cancer. J Clin Oncol. 2014;32(suppl; abstr 6009):5s.

69. Marsit CJ, Liu M, Nelson HH, Posner M, Suzuki M, Kelsey KT. Inactivation of the Fanconi anemia/BRCA pathway in lung and oral cancers: implications for treatment and survival. Oncogene. 2004;23:1000–4.

70. Do K, Wilsker D, Ji J, et al. Phase I Study of Single-Agent AZD1775 (MK-1775), a Wee1 Kinase Inhibitor, in Patients With Refractory Solid Tumors. J Clin Oncol. 2015;33:3409–15.

71. Hori K, Sen A, Artavanis-Tsakonas S. Notch signaling at a glance. J Cell Sci. 2013;126:2135–40.

72. Kerbel RS. Tumor angiogenesis. N Engl J Med. 2008;358:2039–49.

73. Struhl G, Adachi A. Nuclear access and action of notch in vivo. Cell. 1998;93:649–60.

74. Piha-Paul SA, Munster PN, Hollebecque A, et al. Results of a phase 1 trial combining ridaforolimus and MK-0752 in patients with advanced solid tumours. Eur J Cancer. 2015;51:1865–73.

75. Coric V, Salloway S, van Dyck CH, et al. Targeting Prodromal Alzheimer Disease With Avagacestat: A Randomized Clinical Trial. JAMA Neurol. 2015;72:1324–33.

76. Henley DB, Sundell KL, Sethuraman G, Dowsett SA, May PC. Safety profile of semagacestat, a gamma-secretase inhibitor: IDENTITY trial findings. Curr Med Res Opin. 2014;30:2021–32.

77. Gerlinger M, Rowan AJ, Horswell S, et al. Intratumor heterogeneity and branched evolution revealed by multiregion sequencing. N Engl J Med. 2012;366:883–92.

78. Gerlinger M, Catto JW, Orntoft TF, Real FX, Zwarthoff EC, Swanton C. Intratumour heterogeneity in urologic cancers: from molecular evidence to clinical implications. Eur Urol. 2015;67:729–37.

79. de Bruin EC, McGranahan N, Mitter R, et al. Spatial and temporal diversity in genomic instability processes defines lung cancer evolution. Science. 2014;346:251–6.

80. Mroz EA, Tward AD, Pickering CR, Myers JN, Ferris RL, Rocco JW. High intratumor genetic heterogeneity is related to worse outcome in patients with head and neck squamous cell carcinoma. Cancer. 2013;119:3034–42.

81. Mroz EA, Tward AD, Hammon RJ, Ren Y, Rocco JW. Intra-tumor genetic heterogeneity and mortality in head and neck cancer: analysis of data from the Cancer Genome Atlas. PLoS Med. 2015;12, e1001786.

82. Forshew T, Murtaza M, Parkinson C, et al. Noninvasive identification and monitoring of cancer mutations by targeted deep sequencing of plasma DNA. Sci Transl Med. 2012;4:136ra68.

83. Murtaza M, Dawson SJ, Tsui DW, et al. Non-invasive analysis of acquired resistance to cancer therapy by sequencing of plasma DNA. Nature. 2013;497:108–12.

84. Dawson SJ, Tsui DW, Murtaza M, et al. Analysis of circulating tumor DNA to monitor metastatic breast cancer. N Engl J Med. 2013;368:1199–209.

85. Hong MK, Macintyre G, Wedge DC, et al. Tracking the origins and drivers of subclonal metastatic expansion in prostate cancer. Nat Commun. 2015;6:6605.

86. Murtaza M, Dawson SJ, Pogrebniak K, et al. Multifocal clonal evolution characterized using circulating tumour DNA in a case of metastatic breast cancer. Nat Commun. 2015;6:8760.

87. Girotti MR, Gremel G, Lee R, et al. Application of Sequencing, Liquid Biopsies, and Patient-Derived Xenografts for Personalized Medicine in Melanoma. Cancer Discov. 2016;6:286–99.

88. Wang Y, Springer S, Mulvey CL, et al. Detection of somatic mutations and HPV in the saliva and plasma of patients with head and neck squamous cell carcinomas. Sci Transl Med. 2015;7:293ra104.

89. Jerby-Arnon L, Pfetzer N, Waldman YY, et al. Predicting cancer-specific vulnerability via data-driven detection of synthetic lethality. Cell. 2014; 158:1199–209.

90. Thompson JM, Nguyen QH, Singh M, Razorenova OV. Approaches to identifying synthetic lethal interactions in cancer. Yale J Biol Med. 2015;88:145–55.

91. Carter SL, Cibulskis K, Helman E, et al. Absolute quantification of somatic DNA alterations in human cancer. Nat Biotechnol. 2012;30:413–21.

92. Van Loo P, Campbell PJ. ABSOLUTE cancer genomics. Nat Biotechnol. 2012;30:620–1.

93. Snyder A, Wolchok JD, Chan TA. Genetic basis for clinical response to CTLA-4 blockade. N Engl J Med. 2015;372:783.

12

Predictors of circulating INTERLEUKIN-6 levels in head and neck cancer patients

Sylvine Carrondo Cottin[1,2]* ⓘ, Stéphane Turcotte[1,2], Pierre Douville[1,2], François Meyer[1,2] and Isabelle Bairati[1,2]

Abstract

Background: Circulating interleukin-6 (IL-6) improves outcome prediction for second primary cancer (SPC) in head and neck cancer (HNC) patients. This study aimed to identify factors associated with IL-6 serum levels in HNC patients.

Methods: This study was conducted as part of a phase III chemoprevention trial. IL-6 was measured using chemiluminescent immunometric assay on pretreatment serum sample obtained from 527 stage I-II HNC patients. Patients' lifestyle habits, sociodemographic, medical and tumor characteristics were evaluated before radiation therapy (RT). Factors independently associated with IL-6 levels before RT were identified using multiple linear regression.

Results: The median IL-6 serum level was 3.1 ng/L. In the multivariate analysis, eight factors were significantly associated ($p < 0.05$) with IL-6: age, gender, marital status, body mass index, tobacco consumption, comorbidities, Karnofsky Performance Status and HNC site. Smoking duration and lifetime pack-years were positively associated with IL-6 serum levels in a dose-response relationship (p-value for trend ≤ 0.03).

Conclusions: Circulating IL-6 is a strong predictor of the occurrence of SPC in HNC patients. We identified eight factors independently associated with serum IL-6 levels in 527 stage I-II HNC patients.
The dose-response relationship between lifetime smoking and IL-6 serum levels suggested a causal role of tobacco exposure on IL-6 production. Further studies are needed to establish whether the effect of tobacco exposure on SPC could be partly mediated by IL-6, a pro-inflammatory cytokine.

Keywords: Head and neck cancer, Interleukin-6, Tobacco use, Alcohol consumption

Background

Head and neck cancers (HNC) are the seventh most common cancer worldwide with an annual incidence of 15 per 100,000 [1]. Due to modern surgery and radiation therapy, locoregional control of early-stage HNC has improved to reach 50 to 95% at 5 years depending on the cancer site [2]. In particular, early-stage glottic cancer has an excellent prognosis with cause-specific survival varying between 88 and 97% at 5 years [3]. However, patients with a history of HNC are at high risk for developing second primary cancers (SPC) [4] as, within 5 years, about 20% will be diagnosed with one or more multiple primary cancers, which strongly compromises their survival.

Interleukin-6 (IL-6) is a pro-inflammatory cytokine that has been described as being involved in many tumorigenesis processes [5], particularly angiogenesis [6, 7], tumor cell migration and invasion [8] and cell growth and proliferation [9, 10]. In a recent cohort study conducted among 6545 middle-aged adults, IL-6 serum level was able to predict all-causes and cancer-related mortalities over a period of 17 years [11]. In addition, when the three promising inflammatory biomarkers (α1-acid glycoprotein, C-reactive protein and IL-6) were considered together, IL-6 was the only one that remained associated with mortality by cancer. Strong evidence from a meta-analysis also showed that higher IL-6 serum levels were associated with poor prognosis in non-small cell lung cancer patients [12]. In HNC, IL-6 was identified as a predictor of recurrence and overall survival in a cohort of 444 HNC patients, most of whom had pharyngeal and advanced cancers [13]. We also reported that higher pre-treatment IL-6 serum levels were significantly

* Correspondence: sylvine.cottin-carrondo@crchudequebec.ulaval.ca
[1]Centre de recherche sur le cancer, Université Laval, 6, rue McMahon, 1899-2, Quebec City, QC G1R 2J6, Canada
[2]Centre de recherche du CHU de Québec - Université Laval, Quebec City, QC, Canada

associated with the occurrence of SPC [14] and death by SPC in 527 early-stage HNC patients.

Heavy smoking and alcohol consumption are standard risk factors for HNC [15]. In addition, smoking status affects SPC risk and site [16]. Associations between IL-6 serum levels and both tobacco and alcohol consumption have been described in various populations [17, 18]. A cross-sectional study conducted on 444 HNC patients at the time of their diagnosis suggested that only two health behaviors (smoking and decreased sleep) were independently associated with IL-6 serum levels [19]. As IL-6 appears to be a valid predictor in cancer prognosis, it would be useful to further examine the effects of cumulative past exposure to various health behaviors on IL-6 serum levels. The objective of this study was to identify the predictors of IL-6 serum levels in HNC patients. In addition, we specifically examined the influence of long-term tobacco and alcohol consumption on IL-6 serum levels.

Methods
Study population
This study was conducted as part of a randomized controlled chemoprevention trial (NCT00169845) [20] evaluating the efficacy of α-tocopherol and β-carotene supplementation in reducing the incidence of SPC. The ethics review board of the five radiotherapy centers participating in the trial approved the protocol. All patients gave their written informed consent prior to randomization.

Eligible patients were aged 18 years and over, had received a first diagnosis of stage I or II squamous cell carcinoma of the head and neck area (tongue, gums or mouth, oropharynx, hypopharynx and larynx) and were treated by radiation therapy (RT) between October 1, 1994 and June 6, 2000 in one of five radiotherapy centers in the province of Quebec, Canada. A total of 527 patients among the 540 HNC randomized patients (97. 6%) with available pretreatment serum samples were included in the analyses.

Baseline data collection
All the baseline data were collected before the patients were randomized in the trial and before they started their RT. Trained research nurses administered a structured general questionnaire to evaluate patients' characteristics, including their demographic and socioeconomic data, Karnofsky Performance Status (KPS) [21] and medical history. The Charlson Comorbidity Index, a comorbidity score, was calculated based on the medical history [22]. Sleep disturbance was assessed using the item 11 of the EORTC QLQ-C30 instrument [23]. The study nurses weighed and measured the patients during the visit and asked patients

about their weight at 20 years of age. Current body mass index (BMI) and BMI at 20 years of age were calculated.

A validated food frequency questionnaire [24] assessing dietary intake over the year preceding randomization was used to evaluate the self-reported consumption of beer, wine, aperitifs and spirits. A standard drink was predefined for beverages (beer: 1 bottle; wine: 4 oz; aperitif: 2 oz; spirits: 1 oz) and 10 profiles of consumption were proposed (number of drinks per day, week or month). Average daily intake of alcohol (g per day) was then calculated. The same method was used to assess the average daily intake of alcohol over the past 10 years. In addition, a question assessed whether patients had a history of alcohol abuse.

Lifetime smoking habits were recorded for all tobacco products (cigarette, cigar, pipe, chewing) using a structured questionnaire. For all products and for all smoking periods, we assessed the mean consumption per day, week or month and the duration. In addition, age at first cigarette, time since quitting cigarette smoking and patients' current cigarette smoking status were recorded. The number of pack-years, the duration and intensity of cigarette smoking as well as the number of years since quitting cigarette smoking were calculated.

The radiation oncologists provided detailed information on the primary tumor: precise site, dimensions and clinical stage according to the TNM classification [25].

IL-6 measurement
Baseline serum samples were obtained at the time of randomisation before any trial intervention and before RT. Samples were kept frozen at −80 °C and then thawed shortly before determination of IL-6 levels. In order to avoid any influence of the trial intervention, IL-6 was measured on baseline samples using an IMMULITE®1000 immunoassay analyzer with chemiluminescent immunometric assay (Siemens Healthcare Diagnostics).

Statistics
IL-6 serum level was the outcome and was treated as a continuous variable. Given the skewed distribution of IL-6, IL-6 was log transformed (natural log) for all analyses. The selected sociodemographic factors were sex, age (≤ 50, 51–60, 61–70 and > 70), marital status (not married vs. married) and household income (< $40,000 vs. ≥ $40,000). Clinical variables considered were KPS (60–80 vs. ≥ 90), Charlson Comorbidity Index (0, 1, ≥ 2), diabetes (yes vs. no), cancer site (glottis vs. other) and TNM stage (stage I vs. II). The selected health behavior variables were BMI, past and current tobacco and alcohol consumption. Current BMI and BMI at 20 years of age were classified according to the WHO categories (< 18.5: underweight; ≥ 18.5 to < 30: normal weight and overweight;

≥ 30: obesity) [26]. History of cigarette smoking was considered using variables measuring the duration of cigarette smoking, the average number of cigarettes smoked and the average number of pack-years consumed. These variables were categorized according to the quartiles in those exposed to cigarette smoking. Alcohol consumption during the preceding year (g/day in quartiles), alcohol consumption in the past 10 years (g/day in quartiles) as well as a history of alcohol abuse (yes vs. no) were considered.

Student t-test or analysis of variance were performed to examine all the associations between IL-6 serum levels and the selected factors. All the variables associated with IL-6 serum levels in the bivariate analyses ($P \le 0.20$) were considered for inclusion in a multivariate linear regression model. The final model was constructed using a backward elimination procedure. Before fitting the final model, tests for collinearity among the variables were done. The regression diagnostics methods used on the final model showed the appropriateness of the regression assumptions (linearity, variance homogeneity, Gaussian distribution of the residuals). A non-parametric bootstrap resampling method was performed on the residuals to assess the reliability of the regression model [27]. The bootstrap validation process began by forming 2000 bootstrap samples of equal size ($n = 527$) with replacement. Each bootstrap sample was used as a training sample. Regression coefficients were estimated by the bootstrapping method and their 95% confidence intervals were calculated using the method of bias-corrected accelerated percentile intervals.

For all variables describing lifetime cigarette smoking, the associations with IL-6 were tested using a multivariate linear regression adjusting for all factors retained in the final model. Tests for linear trend were done to verify whether IL-6 serum levels tended to increase with cumulative past exposure to cigarette consumption. For trend tests, exposures were considered as linear for ordered categorical variables.

All statistical analyses were performed using SAS (version 9.4; SAS Institute Inc.) and R (version 3.4.0; R development Core Team) statistical software. All statistical tests were 2-sided ($\alpha = 0.05$).

Results

The median baseline IL-6 serum level was 3.1 ng/L (interquartile range: 2.2–4.4). Characteristics of the 527 HNC patients are presented in Table 1. The mean age was 62. 5 years old (SD = 9.8) and most of the patients were male (78.8%). Patients' HNC were predominantly stage I (61.7%) glottic cancer (64.5%). Only 3.4% of patients were underweight, while 17.8% were obese. Use of tobacco products during the previous year was reported by 70.6% of the HNC patients, while 4.9% reported never having consumed tobacco products during their life. Daily alcohol

Table 1 Sociodemographic, clinical and health behavior characteristics of patients with head and neck cancer ($N = 527$)

Factors	Categories	N (%)
Age (years)	≤ 50	55 (10.4)
	> 50 ≤ 60	155 (29.4)
	> 60 ≤ 70	197 (37.4)
	> 70	120 (22.8)
Sex	Female	112 (21.3)
	Male	415 (78.8)
Current body mass index (kg/m²)	< 18.5	18 (3.4)
	≥ 18.5 < 30	415 (78.8)
	≥ 30	94 (17.8)
Body mass index at 20 years (kg/m²)	< 18.5	47 (8.9)
	≥ 18.5 < 30	462 (87.7)
	≥ 30	18 (3.4)
Marital status	Not married	137 (26.0)
	Married	390 (74.0)
Household income (per year)	< $40,000	388 (73.6)
	≥ $40,000	139 (26.4)
Karnofsky Performance Status (%)	90–100	485 (92.0)
	60–80	42 (8.0)
Charlson Comorbidity Index	0	323 (61.3)
	1	128 (24.3)
	≥ 2	76 (14.4)
Diabetes	No	488 (92.6)
	Yes	39 (7.4)
Glottic cancer	No	187 (35.5)
	Yes	340 (64.5)
TNM clinical stage	I	325 (61.7)
	II	202 (38.3)
Tobacco consumption (all tobacco products)	Never	26 (4.9)
	Former	372 (70.6)
	Current	129 (24.5)
History of alcohol abuse	No	439 (83.3)
	Yes	88 (16.7)
Sleep disturbance	Not at all	285 (54.1)
	A little	132 (25.0)
	Quite a bit	62 (11.8)
	Very much	48 (9.1)

consumption during the previous year was low (the median value was 2.32 g/day) and 16.7% reported having a history of alcohol abuse.

Unadjusted associations between IL-6 levels and the selected factors are presented in Table 2. In these analyses, 14 factors were associated with IL-6 (P-value ≤0.20): age ($P < 0.0001$), sex ($P = 0.04$), current BMI and BMI at 20 years of age ($P = 0.02$ and 0.04, respectively), marital status ($P = 0$.

02), household income ($P = 0.02$), KPS ($P < 0.0001$), Charlson Comorbidity Index ($P < 0.0001$), diabetes ($P = 0.06$), cancer site ($P = 0.0004$), TNM stage ($P = 0.007$), tobacco consumption ($P = 0.0008$), history of alcohol abuse ($P = 0.03$) and sleep disturbance ($P = 0.20$).

For the final multivariate linear regression (Table 3), two factors (diabetes, household income) were excluded because of high collinearity with other variables. In addition, BMI at 20 years of age, TNM stage, alcohol abuse and sleep disturbance were no longer associated with IL-6. The remaining eight factors independently associated with IL-6 explained 18% of the variability of IL-6 serum level ($R^2 = 0.18$). Sociodemographic characteristics positively associated with IL-6 were age ($\beta = +0.01$, $P < 0.0001$) and male gender ($\beta = +0.26$, $P < 0.0005$), while married patients ($\beta = -0.16$, $P = 0.02$) had lower IL-6 levels. Three factors characterizing the patients' medical condition were independently associated with IL-6 serum levels. Higher IL-6 serum levels were observed in patients with a lower KPS ($\beta = +0.38$, $P = 0.0004$) and in those with a higher Charlson Comorbidity Index ($\beta = +0.23$, $P = 0.006$ for an index of 2 or more), while IL-6 levels were lower in patients with glottic cancer ($\beta = -0.28$, $P < 0.0001$). Two health behavior variables were positively and independently associated with IL-6 levels: current obesity ($\beta = +0.27$, $P = 0.0003$) and tobacco consumption ($\beta = +0.43$, $P = 0.001$ for former users; $\beta = +0.51$, $P = 0.0004$ for current users). The bootstrap model confirmed the reliability of the final model in that the estimates of the regression coefficients and their 95% confidence intervals were very similar.

Associations and tests for linear trend between lifetime cigarette consumption and IL-6 serum levels are shown in Table 4. IL-6 serum levels increased with longer duration of cigarette smoking (P-value for trend = 0.03) and the number of pack-years consumed (P-value for trend = 0.03). Among former cigarette smokers, IL-6 levels decreased with the number of years since quitting (P-value for trend = 0.02).

Discussion

This study showed that eight factors were independently associated with circulating IL-6, a marker of HNC patients' prognosis. IL-6 serum levels were higher with increasing age, in males, in unmarried patients, in patients with lower KPS or higher Charlson Comorbidity Indexes, and in those with HNC at a site other than the glottis. Two health behavior factors, obesity and smoking status, were independently associated with IL-6. In addition, we showed that lifetime cigarette consumption was a strong predictor of pro-inflammatory IL-6 serum levels in HNC patients with a dose-response relationship.

This cross-sectional study, based on baseline data collected at the time of randomization in a clinical trial, has several strengths and limitations. Our study population was derived from a representative population of patients with stage I and II HNC treated by radiation therapy, since 85% of the eligible HNC patients agreed to participate in this multicenter trial conducted in the province of Quebec. Only 2.4% of the participants were not included in these analyses because no serum samples were available. The bootstrapping method used for validation of the model identifying eight independent factors showed that the model was reliable in predicting circulating IL-6. To corroborate our findings, we also examined the relationships between IL-6 and long-term alcohol and tobacco exposure. To our knowledge, this is the first study conducted on HNC patients that has examined the associations between long-term exposure to alcohol and tobacco and IL-6. In cross-sectional studies, associations with lifetime exposure could be affected to some extent by patients' ability to recall their past exposure. This potential source of bias was probably minimized in our study, since past exposure was assessed independently of the patients' IL-6 status using a well-structured interview conducted by trained research nurses. In addition, the associations with long-term exposure to tobacco or alcohol corroborated well with those found with their respective current exposure.

High IL-6 serum levels have consistently been reported with advancing age [28] and, to a lesser extent, in middle-aged subjects selected from general populations [29, 30]. IL-6 serum levels might reflect a dysregulation of the immune system in older people but could also act as a disease marker. Ferrucci et al. [30] reported that IL-6 serum levels increased linearly with age in 367 men and 731 women aged 20–102 years from a general population. However, when cardiovascular disease, cancers and other conditions were taken into account, the magnitude of the association between age and circulating IL-6 decreased substantially but remained statistically significant in men. A recent study conducted among 987 healthy and non-obese subjects aged 20 to 80 showed that after adjusting for sex, BMI, tobacco and alcohol status, IL-6 levels in both serum and peripheral blood mononuclear cells were higher only in subjects aged 65 to 80 [31]. In our HNC population that consisted mostly of middle-aged and older people as well as in Duffy et al.'s HNC study population [19], age remained positively associated with IL-6 serum levels after adjustment for comorbidities and several risk factors, suggesting a true association with age. However, residual confounding could have occurred in these studies, since part of the age association with IL-6 in HNC patients could be due to the presence of occult second primary cancer at the time of HNC diagnosis, a condition associated with increased IL-6 serum levels [14].

Recent studies, using Mendelian randomization analyses, conducted among thousands of people, have established a causal relationship between genetic markers of adiposity

Table 2 Associations between selected factors and IL-6 serum levels (N = 527)

Factors	Categories	Median IL-6 (ng/L) (IQR)	Crude β (SE)	P-value
Age (years)	≤ 50	2.4 (1.0–3.7)	Reference	
	> 50 ≤ 60	2.9 (2.0–3.9)	0.15 (0.11)	
	> 60 ≤ 70	3.2 (2.4–4.4)	0.34 (0.11)	
	> 70	3.5 (2.6–5.1)	0.48 (0.11)	< 0.0001
Sex	Female	3.0 (2.2–3.9)	Reference	
	Male	3.1 (2.2–4.6)	0.15 (0.07)	0.04
Current body mass index (kg/m^2)	< 18.5	3.5 (2.5–5.1)	0.13 (0.17)	
	≥ 18.5 < 30	2.9 (2.1–4.1)	Reference	
	≥ 30	3.8 (2.7–4.9)	0.22 (0.08)	0.02
Body mass index at 20 years (kg/m^2)	< 18.5	3.0 (2.0–4.9)	−0.06 (0.11)	
	≥ 18.5 < 30	3.1 (2.2–4.4)	Reference	
	≥ 30	4.1 (2.7–7.0)	0.43 (0.17)	0.04
Marital status	Not married	3.3 (2.5–4.6)	Reference	
	Married	3.0 (2.1–4.4)	−0.16 (0.07)	0.02
Household income (per year)	< $40,000	3.3 (2.3–4.6)	Reference	
	≥ $40,000	2.7 (2.0–3.7)	−0.22 (0.07)	0.02
Karnofsky Performance Status (%)	90–100	3.0 (2.2–4.3)	Reference	
	60–80	4.9 (2.9–5.8)	0.46 (0.11)	< 0.0001
Charlson Comorbidity Index	0	2.9 (2.1–3.9)	Reference	
	1	3.4 (2.1–5.1)	0.24 (0.07)	
	≥ 2	3.7 (2.8–5.2)	0.38 (0.09)	< 0.0001
Diabetes	No	3.0 (2.2–4.4)	Reference	
	Yes	3.6 (2.8–5.0)	0.22 (0.12)	0.06
Glottic cancer	No	3.5 (2.5–5.0)	Reference	
	Yes	2.9 (2.1–4.1)	−0.22 (0.06)	0.0004
TNM clinical stage	I	2.9 (2.1–4.2)	Reference	
	II	3.4 (2.4–4.9)	0.17 (0.06)	0.007
Tobacco consumption (all tobacco products)	Never	2.2 (1.0–3.3)	Reference	
	Former	3.0 (2.2–4.4)	0.48 (0.14)	
	Current	3.5 (2.4–5.1)	0.57 (0.15)	0.0008
History of alcohol abuse	No	3.0 (2.2–4.3)	Reference	
	Yes	3.6 (2.5–5.3)	0.18 (0.08)	0.03
Alcohol consumption during the preceding year (g/d)	0	3.4 (2.3–4.6)	Reference	
	≤ 2.32	3.0 (2.1–4.3)	−0.03 (0.09)	0.31
	> 2.32 ≤ 12.48	2.9 (2.2–4.2)	−0.13 (0.09)	
	> 12.48	3.1 (2.4–5.0)	0.02 (0.09)	
Alcohol consumption during the past 10 years (g/d)	≤ 0.39	3.3 (2.1–4.3)	Reference	
	> 0.39 ≤ 10.49	3.1 (2.2–4.4)	−0.05 (0.09)	
	> 10.49 ≤ 42.88	2.8 (2.1–4.1)	−0.08 (0.09)	
	> 42.88	3.3 (2.5–5.1)	0.04 (0.09)	0.50
Sleep disturbance	Not at all	3.0 (2.1–4.4)	Reference	
	A little	3.0 (2.2–4.0)	−0.004 (0.07)	
	Quite a bit	3.5 (2.5–4.9)	0.16 (0.10)	
	Very much	3.1 (2.5–5.0)	0.17 (0.11)	0.20

β is the parameter estimate associated with the increment of one unit of ln IL-6; *IQR* Interquartile range, *SE* Standard error

and circulating IL-6 levels [32–34]. The BMI-genetic scores were consistently and positively associated with IL-6, but the associations were attenuated in younger subjects and in men [32]. Among HNC patients, we also found a positive association between IL-6 and obesity, as defined by a BMI ≥ 30 kg/m². Adipose tissue contains multiple types of cells, including adipocytes, macrophages and immune active cells, all metabolically active in producing IL-6, especially in the context of obesity [35, 36]. Studies have suggested that IL-6 could be released differentially according to body fat distribution patterns [37]. Adipose tissue biopsies done in 47 healthy overweight or obese subjects showed that pro-inflammatory T-helper (Th)-1, Th17 and CD8 T-cells were significantly more frequent in visceral adipose tissue (VAT) than in subcutaneous adipose tissue (SAT) [38]. Concurrently, IL-6 expression, a marker of Th1 and M1 macrophage activation, was twofold greater in VAT than in SAT. In 97 subjects aged 22–69, randomly selected from the general population, VAT and SAT were quantified using a two-dimensional ultrasound image [39]. IL-6 serum levels were positively associated with VAT in overweight/obese participants, while there was no association with SAT. This differential expression of IL-6 according to the VAT and SAT compartments might partly explain the discordance between studies of the effect of sex on circulating IL-6 [29,

30, 40]. Large studies conducted in general populations in the United States showed that, compared with women, men have a higher volume of VAT [41] and a lower volume of SAT [42].

In our study population of early-stage HNC, site was a stronger predictor of IL-6 serum levels than TNM stage. This is explained well by other studies. Elevated serum levels of IL-6 are consistently observed among patients with advanced-stage HNC, in particular in those with positive lymph nodes [19, 43]. In patients with early-stage (T1-T2, N0, M0) laryngeal cancer, those with glottic cancer have significantly lower IL-6 serum levels compared with those with supraglottic cancer, while there was no difference between laryngeal subsites in advanced stages [44]. In our study, 50% of the patients had stage I glottic cancer, which is an infiltrating tumor limited to the vocal cords and frequently no more than a few millimeters in size. Using high throughput technologies, several gene signatures and protein networks have been identified in HNC [45]. The IL-6/IL-6R/JAK/STAT3 is one of these pathways, which contributes to the development and progression of HNC cancers [45, 46]. The IL-6 gene is also a target of nuclear factor–kappa B (NF-kB) [45, 47]. NF-kB inhibition downregulates IL-6 gene and protein expression and decreases the release of several cytokines. In addition,

Table 3 Factors independently associated with IL-6 serum levels in the multivariate linear regression and in the bootstrapping regression model (N = 527)

Factors	Categories	Multivariate linear regression			Bootstrapping regression model		
		β (SE)	95% CI	P-value	β (SE)	95% CI	P-value
Age (years)	Continuous	0.01 (0.003)	0.01; 0.02	< 0.0001	0.01 (0.003)	0.01; 0.02	< 0.0001
Sex	Female	Reference			Reference		
	Male	0.26 (0.07)	0.12; 0.41	0.0005	0.26 (0.07)	0.12; 0.40	0.0005
Current body mass index (kg/m²)	< 18.5	0.08 (0.16)	−0.23; 0.38	0.63	0.07 (0.14)	−0.21; 0.38	0.63
	≥ 18.5 < 30	Reference			Reference		
	≥ 30	0.27 (0.07)	0.12; 0.41	0.0003	0.27 (0.07)	0.14; 0.40	0.0003
Marital status	Not married	Reference			Reference		
	Married	- 0.16 (0.07)	−0.29; −0.03	0.02	−0.16 (0.07)	−0.29; − 0.02	0.02
Karnofsky Performance Status (%)	90–100	Reference			Reference		
	60–80	0.38 (0.11)	0.17; 0.58	0.0004	0.37 (0.12)	0.16; 0.64	0.0004
Charlson Comorbidity Index	0	Reference			Reference		
	1	0.15 (0.07)	0.01; 0.28	0.03	0.15 (0.08)	0.01; 0.31	0.03
	≥ 2	0.23 (0.08)	0.07; 0.40	0.006	0.23 (0.07)	0.10; 0.39	0.006
Glottic cancer	No	Reference			Reference		
	Yes	−0.28 (0.06)	−0.40; −0.16	< 0.0001	− 0.28 (0.06)	− 0.41; − 0.16	< 0.0001
Tobacco consumption (all tobacco products)	Never	Reference			Reference		
	Former	0.43 (0.13)	0.17; 0.69	0.001	0.43 (0.11)	0.21; 0.63	0.001
	Current	0.51 (0.14)	0.23; 0.79	0.0004	0.51 (0.12)	0.26; 0.74	0.0004

β is the parameter estimate associated with the increment of one unit of ln IL-6; *CI* Confidence interval, *SE* Standard error

Table 4 Multivariate analyses showing lifetime cigarette consumption variables associated with IL-6 serum levels ($N = 527$)

Factors	Categories	N (%)	Median IL–6 (ng/L) (IQR)	Adjusted β^* (SE)	P-value
Duration of cigarette smoking (years)	Never smokers	30 (5.7)	2.2 (1.0–3.3)	Reference	
	Ever smokers				
	< 32	120 (22.8)	2.6 (1.5–3.7)	0.36 (0.13)	0.008
	≥ 32 < 40	116 (22.0)	3.0 (2.2–4.6)	0.48 (0.13)	0.0004
	≥ 40 < 47	131 (24.9)	3.3 (2.5–4.3)	0.50 (0.13)	0.0001
	≥ 47	130 (24.7)	3.7 (2.7–5.4)	0.57 (0.13)	< 0.0001
			P-trend < 0.0001		
			P-trend 0.03 (excluding never smokers)		
Average number of cigarettes per day	Never smokers	30 (5.7)	2.2 (1.0–3.3)	Reference	
	Ever smokers				
	< 20	119 (22.6)	2.9 (2.2–4.3)	0.40 (0.13)	0.003
	≥ 20 < 25	70 (13.3)	3.0 (2.1–4.3)	0.52 (0.14)	0.0003
	≥ 25 < 30	167 (31.7)	3.3 (2.4–4.6)	0.54 (0.13)	< 0.0001
	≥ 30	141 (26.8)	3.2 (2.3–4.9)	0.49 (0.13)	0.0002
			P-trend 0.003		
			P-trend 0.25 (excluding never smokers)		
Pack-years of cigarettes	Never smokers	30 (5.7)	2.2 (1.0–3.3)	Reference	
	Ever smokers				
	< 32	123 (23.3)	2.7 (2.0–4.0)	0.35 (0.13)	0.008
	≥ 32 < 47	125 (23.7)	3.0 (2.3–4.3)	0.52 (0.13)	< 0.0001
	≥ 47 < 67	123 (23.3)	3.3 (2.4–4.7)	0.55 (0.13)	< 0.0001
	≥ 67	126 (23.9)	3.5 (2.5–5.2)	0.52 (0.13)	< 0.0001
			P-trend 0.0002		
			P-trend 0.03 (excluding never smokers)		
Years since cigarette smoking cessation	≥ 10	107 (20.3)	2.8 (2.0–4.3)	Reference	
	≥ 1 < 10	60 (11.4)	3.2 (2.4–4.9)	0.21 (0.08)	0.010
	< 1	201 (38.1)	3.0 (2.3–4.4)	0.20 (0.11)	0.060
			P-trend 0.02		

β is the parameter estimate associated with the increment of one unit of ln IL-6; *IQR* Interquartile range, *SE* Standard error. * β ajusted for all factors in Table 3, except for tobacco consumption

there is a cross-talk between NF-kB and STAT3 signaling pathways in HNC cell lines. Experimental studies are currently being conducted to identify selective inhibitors of IL-6 induced STAT3 in the treatment of HNC [46, 48, 49].

Human Papilloma Virus (HPV) infection is recognized to be a risk factor for specific HNC sites, in particular for oropharyngeal cancer [50]. In our cohort of early HNC, most of the patients had laryngeal cancer (83.0%), while 11.7% had oral cancer and only 3.2% had oropharyngeal cancer. A large international study using 3680 samples, estimated that the prevalence of HPV-DNA, targeting 25 HPV types, was only 5.7% in laryngeal cancer, which represents the majority of our study population [51]. For oral cavity cancer, the HPV-DNA prevalence was 7.4%, while for oropharyngeal cancers, the prevalence increased over calendar time. During the time-period 1995–1999,

corresponding to the recruitment of the majority of our HNC cohort, HPV-DNA prevalence was 10.1%. We could reasonably conclude that a small number of patients in our cohort were HPV-positive. In HNC, few studies have evaluated the association between HPV infection and circulating IL-6. These studies, conducted among small series of HNC patients, gave conflicting results. Guerrera et al. [52] found that IL-6 serum levels were significantly higher among HPV-negative patients compared to HPV-positive patients, while Argiris et al. [53] reported no difference in serum IL-6 levels between HPV-positive and negative patients.

In our study, married patients showed lower IL-6 levels compared to non-married patients. It is doubtful that this relationship could be attributable to HPV infection since the opposite would be expected, according to the findings of Guerrera et al. [52]. One plausible explanation is that married people have better dietary and other health behaviours associated with lower levels of circulating cytokines [54]. Overall, these data suggest that HPV status probably had little impact on IL-6 status in this HNC cohort.

Modifiable health behaviors have been reported to influence systemic IL-6 levels [17–19]. Some authors have hypothesized that IL-6 levels might differ according to sex because of different health behaviors [29]. Large studies conducted in general populations have consistently reported a U- or J-shaped association between alcohol intake and IL-6 serum levels with a nadir for moderate consumption (1–2 drinks per day) [55–58]. In particular, a recent prospective cohort study conducted among 8209 British civil servants showed that moderate drinkers (8 to 168 g of ethanol per week for men and 8 to 112 g for women) stable over a period of 10 years had lower serum levels of IL-6 compared with stable non-drinkers and stable heavy drinkers [55]. Current and past alcohol consumption were not predictors of IL-6 serum levels in our study, but most of the patients had low and moderate alcohol consumption. As reported by Duffy et al. [19], we found that only patients with a history of alcohol abuse had higher IL-6 serum levels, but this association was no longer statistically significant after adjustment for other covariates, including tobacco.

Activated monocytes/macrophages [59–61] and epithelial cells [62] have been described as producing pro-inflammatory cytokines, including IL-6. These cell types can be activated by carcinogens found in tobacco products [63, 64]. In a mouse model, cigarette smoke has been shown to upregulate IL-6, leading to the differentiation of T-helper cells in IL-17-producing T-cells [65]. In addition, tobacco-induced oxidative stress also activates the NF-kB family of transcription factors, which upregulates the expression of pro-inflammatory cytokines [66, 67]. In our study, current smoking status was a health behavior independently associated with IL-6 serum levels. This corroborates well with the findings of the only cross-sectional study previously conducted on HNC patients [19] as well as with studies conducted on healthy people [68]. In addition, our study showed that cumulative exposure to cigarette smoking was significantly associated in a dose-dependent manner with IL-6 serum levels. This supports a causality link between smoking and IL-6 status in HNC patients. Due to the impact of tobacco on IL-6 serum levels found in this HNC population and our previous findings showing that IL-6 serum level was a strong predictor of SPC in HNC patients [14], further analyses will be conducted to examine whether the association between tobacco and SPC is partly mediated by IL-6. This will contribute to a better understanding of the role of inflammation in the occurrence of cancer.

Funding

This study was supported by grants from the Canadian Cancer Society Research Institute. The funding body did not take part in the design of the study and collection, analysis, and interpretation of data or in writing the manuscript.

Authors' contributions

All authors have read and approved the submitted manuscript. The manuscript is not under consideration elsewhere nor published elsewhere in whole or in part. All authors participated in the conception, design and development of methodology of this study. They also participated in the acquisition, analysis and interpretation of the data and in the writing and revision of the manuscript.

IB and FM, MDs and cancer epidemiologists, were the principal investigators of the study, which was supported by the Canadian Cancer Society Research Institute. Serum IL-6 dosages were done under the supervision of PD, MD (Biochemistry). ST, MSc (Biostatistics), conducted the statistical analyses under the principal investigators' supervision. SCC, PhD, also performed statistical analyses, data interpretation and was in charge of writing the manuscript.

Competing interests

The authors declare that they have no competing interests.

References

1. Howlader N NA, Krapcho M, Miller D, Bishop K, Altekruse SF, Kosary CL, Yu M, Ruhl J, Tatalovich Z, Mariotto A, Lewis DR, Chen HS, Feuer EJ, Cronin KA (eds). : SEER Cancer Statistics Review, 1975–2013, National Cancer Institute.. In., Based on November 2015 SEER data submission, posted to the SEER web site. edn. Bethesda, MD, http://seer.cancer.gov/csr/1975_2013/; April 2016.
2. Bernier J. 1950- éditeur intellectuel SpringerLink (service en ligne): head and neck cancer : multimodality management. Switzerland: Springer; 2016.
3. Halperin ECP, Carlos A, 1934- Ovid Technologies, Inc. Perez and Brady's principles and practice of radiation oncology. Philadelphia: Wolters Kluwer/ Lippincott Williams & Wilkins; 2013.
4. Morris LG, Sikora AG, Hayes RB, Patel SG, Ganly I. Anatomic sites at elevated risk of second primary cancer after an index head and neck cancer. Cancer Causes Control. 2011;22(5):671–9.
5. Kumari N, Dwarakanath BS, Das A, Bhatt AN. Role of interleukin-6 in cancer progression and therapeutic resistance. Tumour Biol. 2016;
6. Nilsson MB, Langley RR, Fidler IJ. Interleukin-6, secreted by human ovarian carcinoma cells, is a potent proangiogenic cytokine. Cancer Res. 2005;65(23): 10794–800.
7. Gopinathan G, Milagre C, Pearce OM, Reynolds LE, Hodivala-Dilke K, Leinster DA, Zhong H, Hollingsworth RE, Thompson R, Whiteford JR, et al. Interleukin-6 stimulates defective angiogenesis. Cancer Res. 2015;75(15):3098–107.
8. Sun W, Liu DB, Li WW, Zhang LL, Long GX, Wang JF, Mei Q, Hu GQ. Interleukin-6 promotes the migration and invasion of nasopharyngeal carcinoma cell lines and upregulates the expression of MMP-2 and MMP-9. Int J Oncol. 2014;44(5):1551–60.
9. Calo V, Migliavacca M, Bazan V, Macaluso M, Buscemi M, Gebbia N, Russo A. STAT proteins: from normal control of cellular events to tumorigenesis. J Cell Physiol. 2003;197(2):157–68.

10. Wei LH, Kuo ML, Chen CA, Chou CH, Lai KB, Lee CN, Hsieh CY. Interleukin-6 promotes cervical tumor growth by VEGF-dependent angiogenesis via a STAT3 pathway. Oncogene. 2003;22(10):1517–27.

11. Singh-Manoux A, Shipley MJ, Bell JA, Canonico M, Elbaz A, Kivimaki M. Association between inflammatory biomarkers and all-cause, cardiovascular and cancer-related mortality. CMAJ. 2017;189(10):E384–90.

12. Liao C, Yu Z, Guo W, Liu Q, Wu Y, Li Y, Bai L. Prognostic value of circulating inflammatory factors in non-small cell lung cancer: a systematic review and meta-analysis. Cancer Biomark. 2014;14(6):469–81.

13. Duffy SA, Taylor JM, Terrell JE, Islam M, Li Y, Fowler KE, Wolf GT, Teknos TN. Interleukin-6 predicts recurrence and survival among head and neck cancer patients. Cancer. 2008;113(4):750–7.

14. Meyer F, Samson E, Douville P, Duchesne T, Liu G, Bairati I. Serum prognostic markers in head and neck cancer. Clin Cancer Res. 2010;16(3):1008–15.

15. Maasland DH, van den Brandt PA, Kremer B, Goldbohm RA, Schouten LJ. Alcohol consumption, cigarette smoking and the risk of subtypes of head-neck cancer: results from the Netherlands cohort study. BMC Cancer. 2014;14:187.

16. Gan SJ, Dahlstrom KR, Peck BW, Caywood W, Li G, Wei Q, Zafereo ME, Sturgis EM. Incidence and pattern of second primary malignancies in patients with index oropharyngeal cancers versus index nonoropharyngeal head and neck cancers. Cancer. 2013;119(14):2593–601.

17. Mukamal KJ, Jenny NS, Tracy RP, Siscovick DS. Alcohol consumption, interleukin-6 and apolipoprotein E genotypes, and concentrations of interleukin-6 and serum amyloid P in older adults. Am J Clin Nutr. 2007;86(2):444–50.

18. Lu B, Solomon DH, Costenbader KH, Keenan BT, Chibnik LB, Karlson EW. Alcohol consumption and markers of inflammation in women with preclinical rheumatoid arthritis. Arthritis Rheum. 2010;62(12):3554–9.

19. Duffy SA, Teknos T, Taylor JM, Fowler KE, Islam M, Wolf GT, Ghanem TA, Terrell JE. Health behaviors predict higher interleukin-6 levels among patients newly diagnosed with head and neck squamous cell carcinoma. Can Epidemiol Biomarkers Prev. 2013;22(3):374–81.

20. Bairati I, Meyer F, Gelinas M, Fortin A, Nabid A, Brochet F, Mercier JP, Tetu B, Harel F, Masse B, et al. A randomized trial of antioxidant vitamins to prevent second primary cancers in head and neck cancer patients. J Natl Cancer Inst. 2005;97(7):481–8.

21. Schag CC, Heinrich RL, Ganz PA. Karnofsky performance status revisited: reliability, validity, and guidelines. J Clin Oncol. 1984;2(3):187–93.

22. Charlson M, Szatrowski TP, Peterson J, Gold J. Validation of a combined comorbidity index. J Clin Epidemiol. 1994;47(11):1245–51.

23. Aaronson NK, Ahmedzai S, Bergman B, Bullinger M, Cull A, Duez NJ, Filiberti A, Flechtner H, Fleishman SB, de Haes JC, et al. The European Organization for Research and Treatment of Cancer QLQ-C30: a quality-of-life instrument for use in international clinical trials in oncology. J Natl Cancer Inst. 1993;85(5):365–76.

24. Meyer F, Bairati I, Fradet Y, Moore L. Dietary energy and nutrients in relation to preclinical prostate cancer. Nutr Cancer. 1997;29(2):120–6.

25. Cancer. AJCo: Manual for staging of cancer. 4th ed. Philadelphia: Lippincott-Raven; 1993.

26. Body mass index - BMI [http://www.euro.who.int/en/health-topics/disease-prevention/nutrition/a-healthy-lifestyle/body-mass-index-bmi].

27. Fox J: Bootstrapping regression models: an R and S-plus companion to applied regression. 2002.

28. Krabbe KS, Pedersen M, Bruunsgaard H. Inflammatory mediators in the elderly. Exp Gerontol. 2004;39(5):687–99.

29. Navarro SL, Kantor ED, Song X, Milne GL, Lampe JW, Kratz M, White E. Factors associated with multiple biomarkers of systemic inflammation. Cancer Epidemiol Biomarkers Prev. 2016;25(3):521–31.

30. Ferrucci L, Corsi A, Lauretani F, Bandinelli S, Bartali B, Taub DD, Guralnik JM, Longo DL. The origins of age-related proinflammatory state. Blood. 2005;105(6):2294–9.

31. Lee DH, Kim M, Kim M, Lee YJ, Yoo HJ, Lee SH, Lee JH: Age-dependent alterations in serum cytokines, peripheral blood mononuclear cell cytokine production, natural killer cell activity, and prostaglandin F2alpha. Immunol Res. 2017;65(5):1009–16.

32. Fall T, Hagg S, Ploner A, Magi R, Fischer K, Draisma HH, Sarin AP, Benyamin B, Ladenvall C, Akerlund M, et al. Age- and sex-specific causal effects of adiposity on cardiovascular risk factors. Diabetes. 2015;64(5):1841–52.

33. Dale CE, Fatemifar G, Palmer TM, White J, Prieto-Merino D, Zabaneh D, Engmann JEL, Shah T, Wong A, Warren HR, et al. Causal associations of adiposity and body fat distribution with coronary heart disease, stroke subtypes, and type 2 diabetes mellitus: a Mendelian randomization analysis. Circulation. 2017;135(24):2373–88.

34. Holmes MV, Lange LA, Palmer T, Lanktree MB, North KE, Almoguera B, Buxbaum S, Chandrupatla HR, Elbers CC, Guo Y, et al. Causal effects of body mass index on cardiometabolic traits and events: a Mendelian randomization analysis. Am J Hum Genet. 2014;94(2):198–208.

35. Jung UJ, Choi MS. Obesity and its metabolic complications: the role of adipokines and the relationship between obesity, inflammation, insulin resistance, dyslipidemia and nonalcoholic fatty liver disease. Int J Mol Sci. 2014;15(4):6184–223.

36. Engin A. The pathogenesis of obesity-associated adipose tissue inflammation. Adv Exp Med Biol. 2017;960:221–45.

37. Fain JN. Release of inflammatory mediators by human adipose tissue is enhanced in obesity and primarily by the nonfat cells: a review. Mediat Inflamm. 2010;2010:513948.

38. McLaughlin T, Liu LF, Lamendola C, Shen L, Morton J, Rivas H, Winer D, Tolentino L, Choi O, Zhang H, et al. T-cell profile in adipose tissue is associated with insulin resistance and systemic inflammation in humans. Arterioscler Thromb Vasc Biol. 2014;34(12):2637–43.

39. Schlecht I, Fischer B, Behrens G, Leitzmann MF. Relations of visceral and abdominal subcutaneous adipose tissue, body mass index, and waist circumference to serum concentrations of parameters of chronic inflammation. Obesity facts. 2016;9(3):144–57.

40. Seyed-Sadjadi N, Berg J, Bilgin AA, Grant R. Visceral fat mass: is it the link between uric acid and diabetes risk? Lipids Health Dis. 2017;16(1):142.

41. Bidulescu A, Liu J, Hickson DA, Hairston KG, Fox ER, Arnett DK, Sumner AE, Taylor HA, Gibbons GH. Gender differences in the association of visceral and subcutaneous adiposity with adiponectin in African Americans: the Jackson heart study. BMC Cardiovasc Disord. 2013;13:9.

42. Camhi SM, Bray GA, Bouchard C, Greenway FL, Johnson WD, Newton RL, Ravussin E, Ryan DH, Smith SR. The relationship of waist circumference and BMI to visceral, subcutaneous, and total body fat: sex and race differences. Obesity (Silver Spring, Md). 2011;19(2):402–8.

43. Riedel F, Zaiss I, Herzog D, Gotte K, Naim R, Hormann K. Serum levels of interleukin-6 in patients with primary head and neck squamous cell carcinoma. Anticancer Res. 2005;25(4):2761–5.

44. Sotirovic J, Peric A, Vojvodic D, Baletic N, Zaletel I, Stanojevic I, Erdoglija M, Milojevic M. Serum cytokine profile of laryngeal squamous cell carcinoma patients. J Laryngol Otol. 2017;131(5):455–61.

45. Yan B, Broek RV, Saleh AD, Mehta A, Van Waes C, Chen Z. Signaling networks of activated oncogenic and altered tumor suppressor genes in head and neck cancer. J Carcinog Mutagen. 2013;Suppl 7:4.

46. Sen M, Johnston PA, Pollock NI, DeGrave K, Joyce SC, Freilino ML, Hua Y, Camarco DP, Close DA, Huryn DM, et al. Mechanism of action of selective inhibitors of IL-6 induced STAT3 pathway in head and neck cancer cell lines. J Chem Biol. 2017;10(3):129–41.

47. Squarize CH, Castilho RM, Sriuranpong V, Pinto DS Jr, Gutkind JS. Molecular cross-talk between the NFkappaB and STAT3 signaling pathways in head and neck squamous cell carcinoma. Neoplasia. 2006;8(9):733–46.

48. Mihara M, Hashizume M, Yoshida H, Suzuki M, Shiina M. IL-6/IL-6 receptor system and its role in physiological and pathological conditions. Clinical science (Lond). 2012;122(4):143–59.

49. Finkel KA, Warner KA, Kerk S, Bradford CR, McLean SA, Prince ME, Zhong H, Hurt EM, Hollingsworth RE, Wicha MS, et al. IL-6 inhibition with MEDI5117 decreases the fraction of head and neck cancer stem cells and prevents tumor recurrence. Neoplasia. 2016;18(5):273–81.

50. Anantharaman D, Gheit T, Waterboer T, Abedi-Ardekani B, Carreira C, McKay-Chopin S, Gaborieau V, Marron M, Lagiou P, Ahrens W, et al. Human papillomavirus infections and upper aero-digestive tract cancers: the ARCAGE study. J Natl Cancer Inst. 2013;105(8):536–45.

51. Castellsague X, Alemany L, Quer M, Halec G, Quiros B, Tous S, Clavero O, Alos L, Biegner T, Szafarowski T, et al. HPV involvement in head and neck cancers: comprehensive assessment of biomarkers in 3680 patients. J Natl Cancer Inst. 2016;108(6):djv403.

52. Guerrera IC, Quetier I, Fetouchi R, Moreau F, Vauloup-Fellous C, Lekbaby B, Rousselot C, Chhuon C, Edelman A, Lefevre M, et al. Regulation of interleukin-6 in head and neck squamous cell carcinoma is related to papillomavirus infection. J Proteome Res. 2014;13(2):1002–11.

53. Argiris A, Lee SC, Feinstein T, Thomas S, Branstetter BF, Seethala R, Wang L, Gooding W, Grandis JR, Ferris RL. Serum biomarkers as potential predictors of antitumor activity of cetuximab-containing therapy for locally advanced head and neck cancer. Oral Oncol. 2011;47(10):961–6.

54. Eng PM, Kawachi I, Fitzmaurice G, Rimm EB. Effects of marital transitions on changes in dietary and other health behaviours in US male health professionals. J Epidemiol Community Health. 2005;59(1):56–62.

55. Bell S, Mehta G, Moore K, Britton A. Ten-year alcohol consumption typologies and trajectories of C-reactive protein, interleukin-6 and interleukin-1 receptor antagonist over the following 12 years: a prospective cohort study. J Intern Med. 2017;281(1):75–85.

56. Marques-Vidal P, Bochud M, Bastardot F, von Kanel R, Ferrero F, Gaspoz JM, Paccaud F, Urwyler A, Luscher T, Hock C, et al. Associations between alcohol consumption and selected cytokines in a Swiss population-based sample (CoLaus study). Atherosclerosis. 2012;222(1):245–50.

57. Volpato S, Pahor M, Ferrucci L, Simonsick EM, Guralnik JM, Kritchevsky SB, Fellin R, Harris TB. Relationship of alcohol intake with inflammatory markers and plasminogen activator inhibitor-1 in well-functioning older adults: the health, aging, and body composition study. Circulation. 2004;109(5):607–12.

58. Pai JK, Hankinson SE, Thadhani R, Rifai N, Pischon T, Rimm EB. Moderate alcohol consumption and lower levels of inflammatory markers in US men and women. Atherosclerosis. 2006;186(1):113–20.

59. Li YY, Hsieh LL, Tang RP, Liao SK, Yeh KY. Interleukin-6 (IL-6) released by macrophages induces IL-6 secretion in the human colon cancer HT-29 cell line. Hum Immunol. 2009;70(3):151–8.

60. Del Corno M, Donninelli G, Varano B, Da Sacco L, Masotti A, Gessani S. HIV-1 gp120 activates the STAT3/interleukin-6 axis in primary human monocyte-derived dendritic cells. J Virol. 2014;88(19):11045–55.

61. Aarstad HJ, Aarstad HH, Vintermyr OK, Kross KW, Lybak S, Heimdal JH. In vitro monocyte IL-6 secretion levels following stimulation with autologous spheroids derived from tumour or benign mucosa predict long-term survival in head and neck squamous cell carcinoma patients. Scand J Immunol. 2017;85(3):211–9.

62. Shi L, Dong N, Ji D, Huang X, Ying Z, Wang X, Chen C. Lipopolysaccharide-induced CCN1 production enhances interleukin-6 secretion in bronchial epithelial cells. Cell Biol Toxicol. 2017;

63. Walters MJ, Paul-Clark MJ, McMaster SK, Ito K, Adcock IM, Mitchell JA. Cigarette smoke activates human monocytes by an oxidant-AP-1 signaling pathway: implications for steroid resistance. Mol Pharmacol. 2005;68(5):1343–53.

64. Lee J, Taneja V, Vassallo R. Cigarette smoking and inflammation: cellular and molecular mechanisms. J Dent Res. 2012;91(2):142–9.

65. Zhou H, Hua W, Jin Y, Zhang C, Che L, Xia L, Zhou J, Chen Z, Li W, Shen H. Tc17 cells are associated with cigarette smoke-induced lung inflammation and emphysema. Respirology. 2015;20(3):426–33.

66. Yeon JY, Suh YJ, Kim SW, Baik HW, Sung CJ, Kim HS, Sung MK. Evaluation of dietary factors in relation to the biomarkers of oxidative stress and inflammation in breast cancer risk. Nutrition. 2011;27(9):912–8.

67. Karin M. Nuclear factor-kappaB in cancer development and progression. Nature. 2006;441(7092):431–6.

68. Fernandez-Real JM, Vayreda M, Richart C, Gutierrez C, Broch M, Vendrell J, Ricart W. Circulating interleukin 6 levels, blood pressure, and insulin sensitivity in apparently healthy men and women. J Clin Endocrinol Metab. 2001;86(3):1154–9.

13

Venous thromboembolism in head and neck cancer surgery

Faisal I. Ahmad and Daniel R. Clayburgh*[iD]

Abstract

Background: Venous thromboembolism (VTE) is a major cause of perioperative morbidity and mortality. Historically, otolaryngology surgery has been seen as very low risk of VTE, given the relatively short procedures and healthy patient population. However, head and neck surgery patients have multiple additional risk factors for VTE compared to general otolaryngology patients, and only recently has research been directed at examining this population of patients regarding VTE risk.

Review: VTE has long been recognized as a major issue in other surgical specialties, with VTE rates of 15–60 % in some specialties in the absence of prophylaxis with either mechanical compression or anticoagulation. Multiple large-scale retrospective studies have shown that the incidence of VTE in otolaryngology patients is quite low, ranging between 0.1 and 1.6 %. However, these studies indicated that head and neck cancer patients may have an increased risk of VTE. Further retrospective studies focusing on head and neck cancer patients found a VTE rate of approximately 2 %, but one study also found a suspected VTE rate of 5.6 % based on clinical symptoms, indicating that retrospective studies may underreport the true incidence. A single prospective study found a 13 % risk of VTE after major head and neck surgery. Furthermore, risk stratification using the Caprini risk assessment model demonstrates that the highest risk patients may have a VTE risk of 18.3 %, although this may be lowered (but not eliminated) through the use of appropriate prophylactic anticoagulation.

Conclusion: VTE is likely a more significant concern in head and neck surgery patients than previously realized. Appropriate prophylaxis with mechanical compression and anticoagulation is essential; risk stratification may serve as a useful tool to identify head and neck cancer patients at highest risk for VTE.

Background

Venous thromboembolism (VTE), which includes deep vein thrombosis (DVT) and pulmonary embolism (PE), is a common problem in hospitalized patients and can cause significant morbidity and mortality. This condition is responsible for 5 to 10 % of all hospital deaths, and is estimated to affect as many as 600,000 patients a year in the United States [1]. Surgery increases the risk of VTE nearly 20-fold [2]. In the absence of prophylaxis, the estimated incidence of VTE among general surgery patients is 15 to 40 % and is notably higher at 40 to 60 % in orthopedic surgery patients [3]. In the setting of cancer, surgery further doubles this risk compared to patients

without cancer [4]. The incidence of VTE also varies depending on the type of cancer, with malignancies of the bone, ovary, brain and liver/pancreas associated with the highest incidences [5, 6].

In a 2003 study including over 7 million patients in 944 hospitals in the United States [7], VTE was the second most common serious post-operative complication. On average, a post-operative episode of VTE increases the patient length of stay by over 5 days, resulting in excess charges of $21,000, and has a 6.56 % excess mortality rate. Furthermore, outpatient anticoagulation after VTE is expensive, with 1 year of therapeutic anticoagulation and monitoring costing approximately $33,000 [8]. Nevertheless, post-operative VTEs are highly preventable and represent the most common cause of preventable 30-day surgical mortality in patients undergoing cancer resection [6, 9]. Consequently, chemoprophylaxis with anticoagulants such as low-

* Correspondence: clayburg@ohsu.edu
Department of Otolaryngology- Head & Neck Surgery, Oregon Health and Science University, 3181 SW Sam Jackson Park Road, PV01, Portland, OR 97239, USA

molecular-weight heparin or fondaparinux is frequently recommended in post-operative patients [3].

The risk of VTE in general otolaryngology has been considered to be very low, as procedures are often done on an outpatient basis and there is no associated immobilization or impairment of ambulation. Prior retrospective studies of general otolaryngology patients have demonstrated a low risk of VTE, between 0.1 and 2.4 % [10–13]. The bleeding risk associated with VTE chemoprophylaxis also presents a unique set of complications in head and neck surgery, including airway compromise, wound complications, and failure of microvascular reconstruction. As such, compliance with VTE chemoprophylaxis guidelines has been low among head and neck surgeons [14]. However, patients with head and neck cancer are intrinsically different than otherwise healthy general otolaryngology patients, and often have multiple risk factors for VTE development, including malignancy, pulmonary comorbidity, large, complex surgeries, and other medical problems. More recent studies have indicated that head and neck surgery patients demonstrate substantially higher rates of VTE, reaching nearly 20 % in the highest-risk subgroups [12]. The purpose of this review is to examine the literature on incidence and prophylaxis of VTE in head and neck surgery patients.

Venous thromboembolism pathophysiology and prophylaxis

In the 1800s, multiple pathologic factors—abnormal blood flow or stasis, endothelial injury, and hypercoagulability—were described as the etiologic agents for venous thrombosis. Dubbed Virchow's triad, this provides a framework for understanding thrombus formation. Although an extensive list of risk factors are known for VTE (Table 1), all these risk factors can be distilled down to affecting one or more of these central principles of Virchow's Triad. A review of the molecule underpinnings of coagulation are outside the scope of this paper, but have been reviewed extensively in other publications [15–19].

Nevertheless, while the inciting mechanisms in situations of vascular injury are relatively well known, it is somewhat less clear how thrombus formation may occur in the setting of an intact endothelium, as occurs with venous thromboembolism. In this setting, thrombus formation is likely much more dependent upon inflammation, stasis, and/or hypercoagulability. Both cancer and surgery are well-known to induce pro-inflammatory states and thus induce hypercoagulability, putting post-surgical patients, and oncologic surgical patients in particular, at much higher risk for VTE development. Given the significant morbidity and mortality that may be caused by VTE, prophylaxis against VTE has been

Table 1 Risk factors for venous thromboembolism

Surgery
Trauma
Immobility/paresis
Cancer
Cancer therapy
Venous compression
Previous VTE
Increasing age
Pregnancy/postpartum
Oral contraceptive/HRT
Estrogen receptor modulators
Erythropoiesis-stimulating agents
Acute medical illness
Inflammatory bowel disease
Nephrotic syndrome
Myeloproliferative disorders
Paroxysmal nocturnal hemoglobinuria
Obesity
Central venous catheterization
Inherited/acquired thrombophilia

widely studied. Methods of VTE prophylaxis can generally be divided into two broad categories: mechanical and pharmacologic. Pharmacologic prophylaxis includes anticoagulants such as unfractionated heparin, low-molecular weight heparin, fondaparinux, and warfarin. While these drugs increase bleeding risk after surgery, they to do provide significant protection from the development of VTE. There is no evidence to support the use of inferior vena cava filters in VTE prophylaxis; in fact, not only do these filters increase the total procedure cost, they may actually raise the risk of DVT [20]. The American College of Chest Physicians was created guidelines for the use of thromboprophylaxis, and this article provides a thorough review of VTE prophylaxis modalities and their relative risks and benefits [9].

VTE in cancer patients

The association between thromboembolism and malignancy has been recognized for over 150 years. In 1865 Armand Trousseau described cancer-associated thrombosis and a unique alteration of the blood, thereby recognizing the hypercoagulable state induced by malignancy [21]. Approximately 20 % of cancer patients experience thrombosis at some point, and thrombosis may be found on autopsy in up to 60 % of patients that die of cancer [22, 23]. In a retrospective study from the Netherlands, Blom et al. [5] found that the risk of VTE was 12.3 per 1000 in cancer patients compared to 2 per

1000 for the general population. Specifically, the cumulative incidence of VTE was highest for cancers of bone, ovary, brain and pancreas. Interestingly, they also found patients with distant metastases had a nearly two-fold increase in relative risk VTE compared to those without metastatic disease. Unfortunately, data for head and neck cancer was not available in sub-group analysis, likely due to the rarity of head and neck cancer compared to more common types.

The six-fold increased incidence of venous thrombosis in cancer patients can be attributed to baseline patient characteristics, tumor factors, and factors relating to oncologic treatment. Risk factors and comorbid conditions that are associated with head and neck cancer also play a role in VTE formation and include older age, tobacco use, obesity, and abnormal pulmonary function (e.g. COPD) [3, 24]. Although the exact mechanisms by which malignancy increases the incidence of VTE formation have not been completely elucidated, it is believed that inflammatory cytokines may induce endothelial injury and promote a hypercoagulable state. These procoagulants may be directly released by the tumor, or through induction of procoagulant production by native cells.

Venous thromboembolism in other surgical specialties

Data regarding the incidence of VTE in other surgical specialties and evidence for chemoprophylaxis is abundant, and an exhaustive review of this literature is beyond the scope of this paper. Historically, prospective screening studies have demonstrated that the incidence of asymptomatic VTE is 15–40 % in abdominal surgery and 40–60 % in orthopedic surgery in the absence of VTE prophylaxis [3]. However, multiple recent studies have demonstrated an overall incidence of 1–2 % with modern prophylaxis regimens among a heterogeneous mix of surgical procedures [25–27]. A recent retrospective study using the American College of Surgeons National Surgical Quality Improvement Program examined VTE after cancer surgery [6]. This study found a 1.6 % incidence of VTE in over 44,000 patients with 33.4 % of these occurring after discharge. Furthermore, patients who experienced a VTE had a statistically significant 6-fold (8.0 vs 1.3 %) increase in mortality. Though this study could not attribute causality between VTE and mortality, other studies have demonstrated that VTE is the most-common cause of 30-day postoperative mortality in cancer surgery patients [27]. In a systematic review of 25 randomized trials comparing combined chemoprophylaxis and compression devices with compression alone, Zereba et al. [28] demonstrated a 44 % reduction in the risk of DVT with combined therapy. However, the use of chemoprophylaxis also increased the relative risk of bleeding by 74 %. Thus,

current clinical practice guidelines recommend the use of anticoagulation (either heparin or low molecular weight heparin) along with compression devices in all patients with malignancy undergoing major surgery, unless a high risk of bleeding exists [29].

Although prophylaxis is often considered for patients during the acute inpatient hospitalization, there is data to suggest that anticoagulation after discharge may also be beneficial. A prospective, placebo-controlled, double-blind trial in which patients undergoing abdominal surgery for cancer were randomized to therapy with enoxaparin for 4 weeks versus only 1 week showed a 60 % decrease in venographically demonstrated thrombosis with longer therapy [30]. Furthermore, this risk reduction in thromboembolic events was durable even 3 months after surgery. Accordingly, the American Society of Clinical Oncology in their 2014 Clinical Practice Guideline recommends chemoprophylaxis in patients with active cancer undergoing major surgery starting preoperatively and continuing at least 7–10 days with consideration of extending therapy for up to 4 weeks [29].

Venous thromboembolism in head and neck cancer surgery

Although it is well known that the incidence of VTE for cancer patients is increased compared patients without cancer, data for the incidence of VTE in head and neck cancer patients and the need for chemoprophylaxis is extremely limited. As previously mentioned, early assumptions regarding VTE in surgical head and neck cancer patients was extrapolated from general otolaryngology patients. In a study from 1998, Moreano et al. [31] examined almost 13,000 patients at a tertiary care center and found a VTE rate of 0.3 % in general otolaryngology patients and 0.6 % in head and neck surgery patients. In another more recent retrospective study [11], approximately 6000 otolaryngology patients at a tertiary care center were examined and only six cases (0.1 %) of symptomatic VTE were discovered. However, all observed VTE occurred in head and neck surgery patients; 824 total patients had surgery for malignancy and the 6 observed VTE yielded a rate of 0.6 %.

Although these studies hinted that head and neck surgery patients may be at higher risk for VTE than general otolaryngology patients, many previously felt that head and neck surgery patients may be at substantially lower risk for VTE than standard surgical oncology patients. Unlike surgery of the chest, abdomen, pelvis, or lower extremities that may severely limit patient mobility for an extended period of time, head and neck surgery patients are often able to get out of bed and ambulate quite soon after surgery. Furthermore, the risks of anticoagulation in these patients may be higher, as bleeding complications in the head and neck may have more profound consequences. Hemorrhage into the airway can rapidly prove life-threatening, and a hematoma in the confines of the neck may easily compromise vascular anastomoses for microvascular reconstructions. Thus, there is concern that the risk/benefit ratio for postoperative anticoagulation may not be as favorable in head and neck surgery patients as that seen in other surgical fields. Accordingly, the use of VTE prophylaxis by head and neck surgeons has been exceedingly variable. In a survey of over 600 practicing otolaryngologists, significant variability was seen in the use of VTE prophylaxis, with 74 % of respondents routinely prescribing postop SCD use, 38 % using postop compression stockings, 36 % using low molecular weight heparin, and 16 % using heparin [32].

Despite these concerns regarding VTE prophylaxis in head and neck cancer patients, in many areas guidelines developed in other specialties regarding the need for VTE prophylaxis have been applied to head and neck surgery patients. However, there is very little high-quality data that specifically addresses VTE in head and neck surgery patients; most studies are retrospective in nature. A retrospective study from Australia [33] examined the incidence of VTE in 1018 patients undergoing oncologic head and neck surgery. In this cohort, 56 % of patients received VTE chemoprophylaxis, while the remainder did not. Although the rate of VTE was 0 % in both groups, the group receiving chemoprophylaxis had a six-fold increase in bleeding and hematoma rate. Garritano et al. [13] assessed 268 patients undergoing inpatient procedures for head and neck cancer and found an incidence 1.1 % (3/268). A study from Pakistan [34] examined rates of VTE in 413 patients undergoing surgery for head and neck cancer. Their overall rate of VTE was 2.9 % despite routine prophylaxis with low molecular weight heparin. They also found that patients who developed VTE typically had longer cases (10.8 versus 6.9 h), and involved reconstruction with a pedicled or free flap.

However, there is an inherent issue with these retrospective studies, in that they may underreport the true incidence of venous thromboembolism. These studies would necessarily only detect those VTE that became clinically evident around the time of surgery, and may miss patients with either clinically silent VTE, unrecognized/misdiagnosed VTE, or those that did not manifest clinical symptoms until after hospital discharge. The possibility of significant underreporting of VTE in retrospective studies was raised by the study by Thai et al. [35], which retrospectively examined 134 head and neck cancer patients undergoing resection and microvascular reconstruction. They found a 1.4 % (2/134) rate of confirmed VTE as documented in the chart. However, when other clinical symptoms were assessed that could

be the result of VTE (i.e. leg swelling, sudden death, or other possible sequelae of VTE without evidence of VTE assessment in the medical record), the rate of possible VTE rose to 5.8 % (8/134). Additionally, they showed that strong predictors of a patient developing a VTE included prior VTE, blood transfusion, high body mass index, and older age. This study highlights the difficulty with retrospective data for VTE assessment, as it suggests that in certain high-risk groups (i.e. major ablative surgery with microvascular reconstruction) the rate of VTE may be higher than initially assumed.

The clear next step required to better understand VTE risk in head and neck surgery is high-quality prospective studies. To date, only a single prospective study has been conducted to assess VTE incidence in head and neck cancer surgery [24]. This study enrolled 100 consecutive patients undergoing major surgery to treat head and neck cancer (defined as anticipated postoperative length of hospital stay >4 days, typically involving microvascular reconstruction or other large procedures such as total laryngectomy). Patients received routine clinical examination for VTE, as well as lower extremity Doppler ultrasound evaluation on postoperative day 2 or 3. Patients were also followed clinically for 30 days after surgery. This demonstrated a 13 % overall rate of VTE in this patient population – much higher than that seen in previous retrospective studies. More specifically, eight patients had clinically significant VTE (7 DVT and 1 PE) and 5 patients had asymptomatic lower extremity superficial VTE. Although routine chemoprophylaxis was not part of the study protocol, 14 patients received anticoagulation for other indications and had a higher rate of bleeding complications (30.1 versus 5.6 %) compared to those without anticoagulation. While this study was designed as a pilot study rather than a full assessment of VTE risk, and is not adequately powered to provide further detail on VTE risk based on tumor type, surgical procedure, or other factors, it does suggest that the true incidence of VTE in high-risk head and neck surgery patients is higher than previously reported and may be more similar to other high-risk surgery groups. Further work will be needed to define the risks and benefits of routine chemoprophylaxis on the incidence of VTE in surgical head and neck cancer patients, and provide further granularity regarding VTE risk in the head and neck surgery population, such as differences between tumor histology, subsites, procedures, and other factors.

Risk stratification in head and neck cancer patients

Given the potential risks of VTE chemoprophylaxis in head and neck surgery patients, alongside the wide variation in reported VTE incidence rates, the optimal strategy for VTE prevention in head and neck patients may be to specifically target chemoprophylaxis towards the patients at highest risk of VTE, and spare patients at low risk from the potential bleeding complications associated with anticoagulation. Thus, there is significant interest in risk stratifying patients for VTE. In 2001 Caprini et al. [36] proposed a risk assessment model (RAM) for stratifying the risk of VTE in both surgical and non-surgical patients. The Caprini RAM predicts the risk of VTE by adding together points for various VTE risk factors (Table 2). In this model, the points for each risk factor are weighted based on their association with developing VTE. The Caprini RAM has been validated in a retrospective cohort of approximately 8000 general, vascular, and urologic surgery inpatients [37]. The risk of developing a VTE was strongly associated with the Caprini score and is demonstrated in Table 3. Risk factors that are particularly germane to surgical head and neck cancer patients include obesity (BMI > 25), serious lung disease or abnormal pulmonary function, advancing age, malignancy and major surgery (>45 min). It is important to note that with this tool, the difference between major and minor surgery is defined only by time of greater than or less than 45 min, rather than by specific procedure. Based on this definition, nearly all ablative head and neck procedures would meet the definition of major surgery.

While the Caprini RAM was not developed specifically for surgery, it has actually been studied most extensively as a risk stratification tool in head and neck surgery. Shuman et al. [12] retrospectively assigned Caprini scores to 2016 otolaryngology inpatients and then examined their 30-day rate of VTE. Notably, none of these patients received thromboprophylaxis with heparin or low molecular weight heparin. In this study, 88 % of patients were assigned as having high (total score 3–4) or highest (total score >5) risk, which likely reflects in-patient status of this population. Although the overall 30-day rate of VTE was only 1.3 %, patients with a Caprini score of <5 had a 0.5 % incidence of VTE compared to 2.4 % for patients with a score of 7–8 and 18.3 % for patients with a score >8. Evaluation of specific risk factors revealed that patients with higher scores were those with cancer, chronic obstructive pulmonary disease, recent stroke, central access, and infections. The same group later compared the above results to a cohort of 1482 otolaryngology patients that had received chemoprophylaxis for VTE [38]. In the cohort that received chemoprophylaxis, the rate of overall VTE was similar at 1.2 %. However, when patients were stratified by Caprini score, a non-statistically significant reduction in VTE rate was seen with chemoprophylaxis in patients with scores between 7–8 (1.9 versus 2.4 %), and >8 (10.7 versus 18.3 %).

In another study, Yarlagadda et al. [39] retrospectively reviewed 704 otolaryngology patients that received

Table 2 Caprini Risk Assessment Model

Each Risk Factor Represents 1 Point	Each Risk Factor Represents 2 Points
• Age 41–60 years	• Age 61–74 years
• Swollen legs	• Arthroscopic surgery
• Varicose veins	• Malignancy (present or previous)
• Obesity (BMI > 25)	• Laparoscopic surgery (>45 min)
• Minor surgery planned	• Patient confined to bed (>72 h)
• Sepsis (<1 month)	• Immobilizing plaster cast (<1 month)
• Serious lung disease including pneumonia (<1 month)	• Central venous access
• Acute myocardial infarction	• Major surgery (>45 min)
• Congestive heart failure (<1 month)	
• Medical patient currently at bed rest	**Each Risk Factor Represents 3 Points**
• History of inflammatory bowel disease	
• History of major surgery (<1 month)	• Age 75 years or older
• Abnormal pulmonary function (COPD)	• History of DVT/PE
• Pregnancy or postpartum (<1 month)	• Positive Factor V Leiden
• Oral contraceptive or hormone replacement therapy	• Elevated serum homocysteine
• History of unexplained stillborn infant or recurrent spontaneous abortion (>3), premature birth with toxemia or growth restricted infant	• Heparin-induced thrombocytopenia
	• Elevated anticardiolipin antibodies
	• Other congenital or acquired thrombophilia
	• Family history of thrombosis
	• Positive prothrombin 20210A
	• Positive Lupus anticoagulant
	Each Risk Factor Represents 5 Points
	• Stroke (<1 month)
	• Multiple trauma (<1 month)
	• Elective major lower extremity arthroplasty
	• Hip, pelvis or leg fracture (<1 month)
	• Acute spinal cord injury (<1 month)

Total:

Table 3 Incidence rate of VTE without routine anticoagulation based on cumulative Caprini score [37]

Cumulative Caprini score	Incidence rate of VTE
0–1	0.00 %
2	0.70 %
3–4	0.97 %
5–6	1.33 %
7–8	2.58 %
9+	6.51 %

appropriate thromboprophylaxis (early ambulation, compression devices, chemoprophylaxis, or a combination) based on institutional standards according to their Caprini scores. In this study, the average Caprini score was 5.7 and the overall rate of VTE was 2.1 %. As expected, patients with higher Caprini scores were found to have higher rates VTE. The rates of VTE for patients with Caprini scores less than 6, between 7 and 8, and greater than 9 were 0.0, 3.0, and 13.1 % respectively. This study also found that patients with a history of prior VTE, malignancy, bedbound beyond 72 h, and

congestive heart failure had an association with increased risk of VTE.

These studies suggest that the Caprini score may be a useful tool to risk stratify head and neck surgery patients. There is a positive correlation between Caprini score and incidence of VTE, and this tool may successfully identify those patients most likely to benefit from VTE chemoprophylaxis. Although these studies were primarily limited by the small numbers of patients available with high Caprini scores, they do suggest that directing chemoprophylaxis towards the highest risk patients may be a viable strategy to decrease the VTE rate, while chemoprophylaxis of patients with low Caprini scores is likely unnecessary. Equally important in this data is the realization that while appropriate chemoprophylaxis may reduce VTE risk, it cannot entirely eliminate it; there remains a subset of high-risk patients that will develop VTE despite appropriate prophylaxis. Thus, VTE in head and neck surgery cannot be considered a "never" event despite appropriate preventative measures; clinical vigilance for this complication and timely recognition and treatment will continue to be crucial for head and neck surgeons to prevent the sequelae of VTE.

Table 4 Studies of VTE Incidence in Otolaryngology

Source	Study design	Study population	Hospital status	Routine anticoagulation	VTE incidence, %
Jain et al. [40] (n = 6788)	Retrospective	General otolaryngology	Inpatient and outpatient	No	0.1
Chen et al. [41] (n = 48,028)	Retrospective	General otolaryngology	Inpatient and outpatient	No	0.1
Lin et al. [42] (n = 330,629)	Retrospective	General otolaryngology	Inpatient and outpatient	No	0.3
Moreano et al. [31] (n = 12,805)	Retrospective	General otolaryngology	Inpatient and outpatient	No	Overall, 0.5 Head and neck surgery, 1.0
Lee et al. [10] (n = 10,176)	Retrospective	General otolaryngology	Inpatient and outpatient	No	0.15
Innis et al. [11] (n = 6122)	Retrospective	General otolaryngology	Inpatient and outpatient	No	Overall, 0.1 Cancer patients, 0.6
Garritano et al. [13] (n = 5616)	Retrospective	General otolaryngology	Inpatient and outpatient	No	0.085
Shuman et al. [12] (n = 2016)	Retrospective	General otolaryngology	Inpatient	No	Overall, 1.6 Caprini score > 8, 18.3
Yarlagadda et al. [39] (n = 704)	Retrospective	General otolaryngology	Inpatient	Yes, depending on Caprini score	Overall, 2.1 Caprini score > 8, 13.1 %
Hennessey et al. [43] (n = 93,663)	Retrospective	Head and neck cancer	Inpatient	Unknown	2
Thai et al. [35] (n = 134)	Retrospective	Head and neck cancer	Inpatient	No	Confirmed VTE, 1.4 Suspected VTE, 5.8
Chen et al. [44] (n = 1591)	Retrospective	Head and neck cancer	Inpatient	Yes	0.70
Ali et al. [34] (n = 413)	Retrospective	Head and neck cancer	Inpatient	Yes	2.9
Clayburgh et al. [24] (n = 100)	Prospective	Head and neck cancer	Inpatient	No	Overall, 13 Clinically significant, 8

Conclusions

Venous thromboembolism is a major source of perioperative morbidity and mortality that is largely preventable. It accounts for approximately 10 % of hospital deaths annually [3], and patients that survive are at risk for further complications. Although both surgery and cancer are major risk factors for VTE, compliance with chemoprophylaxis guidelines has traditionally been low in head and neck surgery. This is largely driven by the historically perceived low risk of VTE in head and neck patients and potential for significant complications with anticoagulation. Recent studies have demonstrated that even though most otolaryngology patients are considered to be at low risk for VTE, head and neck cancer patients constitute a unique group with different VTE risks (summarized in Table 4). Specifically, the rate of VTE in head and neck cancer patients is much higher than has been reported in previous retrospective studies, particularly in the highest-risk patients. Identification of patients at the highest risk of VTE is vital to appropriately direct surveillance and prevention resources. As such, risk assessment models like the Caprini RAM may be useful to identify those most likely to benefit from chemoprophylaxis. However, while chemoprophylaxis may reduce the risk of VTE in high-risk groups, the risk is not eliminated, and there is an associated increase in bleeding risk. Further large-scale prospective trials will be necessary to make definitive recommendations on risk stratification and VTE prophylaxis in head and neck cancer patients.

Abbreviations
BMI: Body mass index; COPD: Chronic obstructive pulmonary disease; DVT: Deep vein thrombosis; PE: Pulmonary embolus; RAM: Risk assessment model; SCD: Sequential compression device; VTE: Venous thromboembolism

Acknowledgements
None.

Funding
Not applicable.

Authors' contributions
Both FA and DC were involved in drafting the initial manuscript and editing/review. Both authors read and approved the final manuscript.

Competing interests
The authors declare that they have no competing interests.

References
1. Anderson Jr FA, Wheeler HB. Venous thromboembolism. Risk factors and prophylaxis. Clin Chest Med. 1995;16(2):235–51.
2. Heit JA, Silverstein MD, Mohr DN, Petterson TM, O'Fallon WM, Melton 3rd LJ. Risk factors for deep vein thrombosis and pulmonary embolism: a population-based case–control study. Arch Intern Med. 2000;160(6):809–15.
3. Geerts WH, Bergqvist D, Pineo GF, et al. Prevention of venous thromboembolism: American College of Chest Physicians Evidence-Based Clinical Practice Guidelines (8th Edition). Chest. 2008;133(6 Suppl):381s–453s.
4. Behranwala KA, Williamson RC. Cancer-associated venous thrombosis in the surgical setting. Ann Surg. 2009;249(3):366–75.
5. Blom JW, Vanderschoot JP, Oostindier MJ, Osanto S, van der Meer FJ, Rosendaal FR. Incidence of venous thrombosis in a large cohort of 66,329 cancer patients: results of a record linkage study. J Thromb Haemost. 2006; 4(3):529–35.
6. Merkow RP, Bilimoria KY, McCarter MD, et al. Post-discharge venous thromboembolism after cancer surgery: extending the case for extended prophylaxis. Ann Surg. 2011;254(1):131–7.
7. Zhan C, Miller MR. Excess length of stay, charges, and mortality attributable to medical injuries during hospitalization. JAMA. 2003;290(14):1868–74.
8. Ruppert A, Steinle T, Lees M. Economic burden of venous thromboembolism: a systematic review. J Med Econ. 2011;14(1):65–74.
9. Gould MK, Garcia DA, Wren SM, et al. Prevention of VTE in nonorthopedic surgical patients: Antithrombotic Therapy and Prevention of Thrombosis, 9th ed: American College of Chest Physicians Evidence-Based Clinical Practice Guidelines. Chest. 2012;141(2 Suppl):e227S–77S.
10. Lee J, Alexander A, Higgins K, Geerts W. The Sunnybrook experience: review of deep vein thrombosis and pulmonary embolism in otolaryngology. J Otolaryngol Head Neck Surg. 2008;37(4):547–51.
11. Innis WP, Anderson TD. Deep venous thrombosis and pulmonary embolism in otolaryngologic patients. Am J Otolaryngol. 2009;30(4):230–3.
12. Shuman AG, Hu HM, Pannucci CJ, Jackson CR, Bradford CR, Bahl V. Stratifying the risk of venous thromboembolism in otolaryngology. Otolaryngol Head Neck Surg. 2012;146(5):719–24.
13. Garritano FG, Lehman EB, Andrews GA. Incidence of venous thromboembolism in otolaryngology-head and neck surgery. JAMA Otolaryngol Head Neck Surg. 2013;139(1):21–7.
14. Ah-See KW, Kerr J, Sim DW. Prophylaxis for venous thromboembolism in head and neck surgery: the practice of otolaryngologists. J Laryngol Otol. 1997;111(9):845–9.
15. Swystun LL, Liaw PC. The role of leukocytes in thrombosis. Blood. 2016; 128(6):753–62.
16. Wolberg AS, Aleman MM, Leiderman K, Machlus KR. Procoagulant activity in hemostasis and thrombosis: Virchow's triad revisited. Anesth Analg. 2012; 114(2):275–85.
17. Versteeg HH, Heemskerk JW, Levi M, Reitsma PH. New fundamentals in hemostasis. Physiol Rev. 2013;93(1):327–58.
18. Witkowski M, Landmesser U, Rauch U. Tissue factor as a link between inflammation and coagulation. Trends Cardiovasc Med. 2016;26(4):297–303.
19. Morange PE, Suchon P, Tregouet DA. Genetics of Venous Thrombosis: update in 2015. Thromb Haemost. 2015;114(5):910–9.
20. Chiasson TC, Manns BJ, Stelfox HT. An economic evaluation of venous thromboembolism prophylaxis strategies in critically ill trauma patients at risk of bleeding. PLoS Med. 2009;6(6):e1000098.
21. Trousseau A. Phlegmasia alba dolens. Lectures on clinical medicine, delivered at the Hotel Dieu, Paris. New Sydenham Society. 1872;4:280–332.
22. Donati MB. Cancer and thrombosis. Haemostasis. 1994;24(2):128–31.
23. Ambrus JL, Ambrus CM, Mink IB, Pickren JW. Causes of death in cancer patients. J Med. 1975;6(1):61–4.
24. Clayburgh DR, Stott W, Cordiero T, et al. Prospective study of venous thromboembolism in patients with head and neck cancer after surgery. JAMA Otolaryngol Head Neck Surg. 2013;139(11):1143–50.
25. Pannucci CJ, Laird S, Dimick JB, Campbell DA, Henke PK. A validated risk model to predict 90-day VTE events in postsurgical patients. Chest. 2014; 145(3):567–73.
26. Gangireddy C, Rectenwald JR, Upchurch GR, et al. Risk factors and clinical impact of postoperative symptomatic venous thromboembolism. J Vasc Surg. 2007;45(2):335–41. discussion 341–332.

27. Agnelli G, Bolis G, Capussotti L, et al. A clinical outcome-based prospective study on venous thromboembolism after cancer surgery: the @RISTOS project. Ann Surg. 2006;243(1):89–95.

28. Zareba P, Wu C, Agzarian J, Rodriguez D, Kearon C. Meta-analysis of randomized trials comparing combined compression and anticoagulation with either modality alone for prevention of venous thromboembolism after surgery. Br J Surg. 2014;101(9):1053–62.

29. Lyman GH, Bohlke K, Khorana AA, et al. Venous thromboembolism prophylaxis and treatment in patients with cancer: american society of clinical oncology clinical practice guideline update 2014. J Clin Oncol. 2015; 33(6):654–6.

30. Bergqvist D, Agnelli G, Cohen AT, et al. Duration of prophylaxis against venous thromboembolism with enoxaparin after surgery for cancer. N Engl J Med. 2002;346(13):975–80.

31. Moreano EH, Hutchison JL, McCulloch TM, Graham SM, Funk GF, Hoffman HT. Incidence of deep venous thrombosis and pulmonary embolism in otolaryngology-head and neck surgery. Otolaryngol Head Neck Surg. 1998;118(6):777–84.

32. Garritano FG, Andrews GA. Current practices in venous thromboembolism prophylaxis in otolaryngology-head and neck surgery. Head Neck. 2016; 38(Suppl 1):E341–5.

33. Gavriel H, Thompson E, Kleid S, Chan S, Sizeland A. Safety of thromboprophylaxis after oncologic head and neck surgery. Study of 1018 patients. Head Neck. 2013;35(10):1410–4.

34. Ali NS, Nawaz A, Junaid M, Kazi M, Akhtar S. Venous thromboembolism-incidence of deep venous thrombosis and pulmonary embolism in patients with head and neck cancer: a tertiary care experience in Pakistan. International Archives of Otorhinolaryngology. 2015;19(3):200–4.

35. Thai L, McCarn K, Stott W, et al. Venous thromboembolism in patients with head and neck cancer after surgery. Head Neck. 2013;35(1):4–9.

36. Caprini JA, Arcelus JI, Reyna JJ. Effective risk stratification of surgical and nonsurgical patients for venous thromboembolic disease. Semin Hematol. 2001;38(2 Suppl 5):12–9.

37. Bahl V, Hu HM, Henke PK, Wakefield TW, Campbell Jr DA, Caprini JA. A validation study of a retrospective venous thromboembolism risk scoring method. Ann Surg. 2010;251(2):344–50.

38. Bahl V, Shuman AG, Hu HM, et al. Chemoprophylaxis for venous thromboembolism in otolaryngology. JAMA Otolaryngol Head Neck Surg. 2014;140(11):999–1005.

39. Yarlagadda BB, Brook CD, Stein DJ, Jalisi S. Venous thromboembolism in otolaryngology surgical inpatients receiving chemoprophylaxis. Head Neck. 2014;36(8):1087–93.

40. Jain U, Chandra RK, Smith SS, Pilecki M, Kim JY. Predictors of readmission after outpatient otolaryngologic surgery. Laryngoscope. 2014;124(8):1783–8.

41. Chen MM, Roman SA, Sosa JA, Judson BL. Postdischarge complications predict reoperation and mortality after otolaryngologic surgery. Otolaryngol Head Neck Surg. 2013;149(6):865–72.

42. Lin HW, Bhattacharyya N. Contemporary assessment of medical morbidity and mortality in head and neck surgery. Otolaryngol Head Neck Surg. 2012;146(3):385–9.

43. Hennessey P, Semenov YR, Gourin CG. The effect of deep venous thrombosis on short-term outcomes and cost of care after head and neck cancer surgery. Laryngoscope. 2012;122(10):2199–204.

44. Chen CM, Disa JJ, Cordeiro PG, Pusic AL, McCarthy CM, Mehrara BJ. The incidence of venous thromboembolism after oncologic head and neck reconstruction. Ann Plast Surg. 2008;60(5):476–9.

14

The rationale for including immune checkpoint inhibition into multimodal primary treatment concepts of head and neck cancer

Ingeborg Tinhofer[1,2*], Volker Budach[1,2], Korinna Jöhrens[3] and Ulrich Keilholz[4]

Abstract

Background: Treatment of locally advanced squamous cell carcinomas of the head and neck (SCCHN) remains unsatisfactory. Although the addition of concurrent radiochemotherapy (RCT) or the combination of radiotherapy with blockade of the epidermal growth factor receptor (EGFR) have improved outcomes over radiotherapy alone, further optimization is urgently needed. The introduction of immune checkpoint inhibitors is currently revolutionizing cancer treatment. Clinical evidence has recently been provided in melanoma that immune checkpoint blockade may cooperate with radiation. Therefore, we searched in the literature for the evidence of combining immune checkpoint inhibitors with radiotherapy in primary treatment of SCCHN.

Discussion: A substantial amount of previous studies has dissected the molecular mechanisms of immune evasion in SCCHN. The biological effects of radio- and chemotherapy in tumor cells and the immune cell microenvironment were characterized in detail, revealing significant interference of both types of treatment with anti-tumor immunity. This extensive review of the literature revealed considerable amount of evidence that addition of immune checkpoint inhibitors might boost the immunomodulatory potential of radiotherapy and RCT regimens in SCCHN.

Summary: Promising activity of immune checkpoint inhibitors has already been reported for metastatic/recurrent SCCHN. Given the immunogenic effect of radiotherapy and its enhancement by chemotherapy, combination of radiotherapy or RCT with this new type of immunotherapy might represent a valuable option for improvement of curative treatment modalities in SCCHN.

Keywords: Radiotherapy, Immune modulation, Combination therapy, Checkpoint inhibitor, Adaptive immunity

Background

Medical need for improvement of definitive treatment in locally advanced SCCHN

Patients with SCCHN completing radiotherapy-based treatment remain at considerable risk for local relapse within the radiation field, regional recurrence in the neck and hematogenous spread of tumor cells with the potential to form distant metastases. Primary radiochemotherapy (RCT) applied concurrently with cisplatin still cures less than 40 % of patients [1], and in case of disease recurrence after RCT, the 2-years survival rate is below 20 %. Furthermore, the addition of chemotherapy to radiation improves locoregional control at the cost of severe acute and late morbidity [2] but does not reduce the risk of distant metastases [1, 3].

During the last decade, there has been increasing interest in combining RCT with molecularly targeted agents. Most targeted approaches for radiosensitization tested so far have been directed against molecular pathways within cancer cells in order to increase the magnitude of DNA damage or to inhibit cellular mechanisms which interfere

---

* Correspondence: ingeborg.tinhofer@charite.de
[1]Department of Radiooncology and Radiotherapy, Translational Radiation Oncology Research Laboratory, Charite University Hospital Berlin, Charitéplatz 1, 10117 Berlin, Germany
[2]2German Cancer Research Center (DKFZ), Heidelberg, and German Cancer Consortium (DKTK) partner site Berlin, Berlin, Germany
Full list of author information is available at the end of the article

with tumor cell DNA repair, thereby increasing the efficacy of RCT. Based on the overexpression of EGFR in the majority of SCCHN cases and its causative role in radioresistance [4, 5] the EGFR signaling pathway was established as the first molecular target for radiosensitization in SCCHN [6, 7]. Consequently, the combination of cetuximab, a blocking antibody to EGFR with radiotherapy was shown to significantly improve outcome of locally advanced SCCHN when compared to radiotherapy alone [8]. However, despite improvement of locoregional control over radiotherapy alone, the cumulative rate of distant metastasis at 1 or 2 years remained unchanged by this combination [8]. Disappointingly, the RTOG study 0522 evaluating further treatment intensification by combining cetuximab with concurrent RCT failed to meet its endpoints to improve progression-free and overall survival [9]. Further trials which evaluated the combination of RCT with drugs directed against EGFR family members, a broader spectrum of receptor tyrosine kinases or the mTOR signaling pathway have not yet been completed or were stopped early due to the lack of significant activity (Table 1) which underlines the urgent need for novel concepts in this treatment setting. In view of the recent promising results of immune checkpoint inhibitors in the treatment of metastatic/recurrent SCCHN, combination of radiotherapy or RCT with this new type of immunotherapy might represent a valuable option. The aim of this review is to collect evidence from the literature which supports the notion that immune checkpoint blockade may cooperate with radiation in SCCHN.

Basic components of host immunity to cancer

In principle, the defense by the immune system against pathogenic microbes and toxins from the environment is divided into two general types of processes: the innate immunity and the adaptive immunity. Innate immunity recognizes and fights microbial invaders at the site of

Table 1 Clinical trials evaluating the combination of platinum-based RCT with targeted drugs in locally advanced SCCHN

Pathway/Target	Drug	Clinical trial	Results/Status
Tumor-specific targets (terminated trials)			
EGFR	Cetuximab	NCT00265941 (definitive, phase III, RTOG0522)	Negative
	Panitumumab	NCT00547157 (definitive, phase II, CONCERT-1)	Negative
	Cetuximab	NCT00791141 (adjuvant, phase II, ACCRA-HN)	Not yet reported
	Erlotinib	NCT00410826 (definitive, phase II)	Failed to significantly increase CRR or PFS
RTK (VEGFR2, EGFR, MET)	Vandetanib	NCT00720083 (adjuvant, phase II, RTOG0619)	Terminated early after 34 pts, no analysis
mTOR	Everolimus	NCT00858663 (definitive, phase I)	Terminated early, only assessment of outcome at 6 months - no responses seen
Tumor-specific targets (ongoing trials)			
DNA repair			
PARP	Olaparib	NCT02308072, (phase I, ORCA-2)	Recruiting
Cell cycle			
WEE-1	AZD1775	NCT02585973 (phase Ib)	Not yet recruiting
CHK-1	LY2606368	NCT02555644 (phase I)	Not yet recruiting
EGFR family			
EGFR/Her2	Lapatinib	NCT01711658 (phase II, TRYHARD)	Recruiting
AKT/PI3K			
PI3K alpha	BYL719	NCT02537223 (phase I)	Recruiting
Phospho-AKT	Nelfinavir	NCT02207439 (phase II)	Recruiting
Environmental targets (ongoing trials)			
Hypoxia	Nimorazole	NCT01880359 (phase III)	Recruiting
Immune checkpoints (ongoing trials)			
PD-1	Pembrolizumab	NCT02586207, (definitive RCT, phase I)	Recruiting
		NCT02641093 (adjuvant RT or RCT, phase II)	Recruiting
		NCT02296684 (adjuvant RCT, phase II)	Recruiting
CTLA-4	Ipilimumab	NCT01935921[a] (definitive, phase I)	Recruiting
		NCT01860430[a] (definitive, phase Ib)	Recruiting

[a]Ipilimumab combined with cetuximab-based bioradiation, not with platinum-based RCT

infection. In contrast, adaptive immunity is serving to eliminate host cells infected with viruses by recognizing peptides from intracellular viral proteins loaded onto major histocompatibility complex (MHC) molecules and displayed on the host cell surface. The adaptive immune system is also able to recognize mutated proteins in tumor cells via the same mechanism.

There are multiple mechanisms by which a tumor cell harboring immunogenic mutations can elicit adaptive immune responses, as schematically summarized in Fig. 1. Tumor cells may spontaneously undergo apoptosis or necrosis, or may be driven to do so by radiotherapy and chemotherapy. The resulting apoptotic bodies can be processed by dendritic cells (DCs). The protein repertoire of dying cells is subsequently presented on the surface to T cells (the afferent arm of adaptive immune activation). T cells recognizing peptides derived from 'foreign' mutated proteins are activated by their and, after clonal expansion, these T cells search throughout the body for tumor cells displaying exactly this mutation on their surface. The cells which are recognized as carrying this mutation are killed through the lytic machinery of T cells (the execution of the efferent arm of adaptive immunity). However, in a patient with a growing tumor, this system has obviously failed as a consequence of one or many mechanisms which tumor cells have adopted to escape immune destruction.

Immune evasion in SCCHN: hideout, defense, camouflage and balanced immune destruction

There are several ways for SCCHN to evade recognition by the adaptive immune system, as schematically

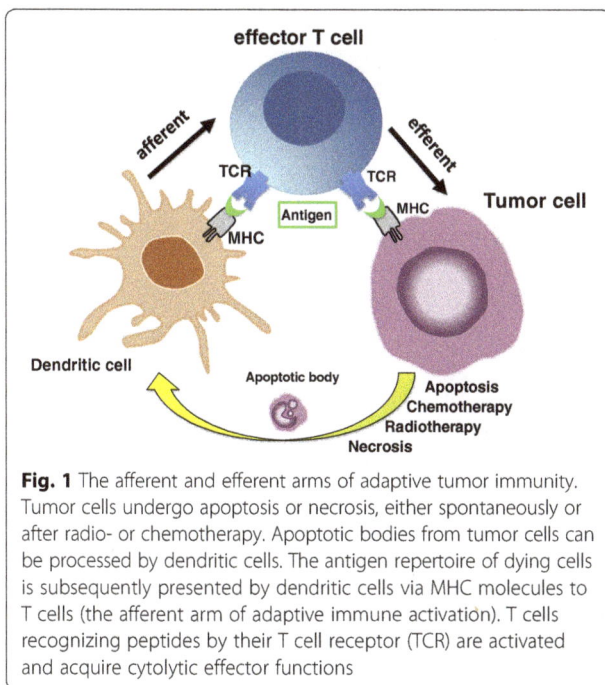

Fig. 1 The afferent and efferent arms of adaptive tumor immunity. Tumor cells undergo apoptosis or necrosis, either spontaneously or after radio- or chemotherapy. Apoptotic bodies from tumor cells can be processed by dendritic cells. The antigen repertoire of dying cells is subsequently presented by dendritic cells via MHC molecules to T cells (the afferent arm of adaptive immune activation). T cells recognizing peptides by their T cell receptor (TCR) are activated and acquire cytolytic effector functions

illustrated in Fig. 2. Early tumors may grow in a hideout, because they display neither a significant level of apoptosis or necrosis nor inflammatory signals and thus do not elicit any danger signal in the tissue (Fig. 2a). Although danger signals might subsequently be produced during the progression of the disease, the lymphocytic infiltrate may be confined to the rim of the tumor tissue with no infiltration into the tumor itself (Fig. 2b). Secretion of indoleamine 2, 3-dioxygenase (IDO) is among the major defense mechanisms used by tumors to prevent lymphocytic infiltration [10]. Tumors frequently also counterbalance infiltration by lymphocytes by down-regulation of their MHC molecules, thereby avoiding the presentation of peptides from intracellular proteins to T cells which results in an effective camouflage (Fig. 2c). As schematically depicted in Fig. 2d, in tumors with extensive inflammatory cell infiltration a delicate balance between immune destruction and immune evasion may exist which is based on immunosuppressive mechanisms including high expression of IDO and PD-L1 as well as recruitment of FoxP3+ regulatory T cells (Treg) [11]. Representative histological images from SCCHN tumor sections exemplifying the above-mentioned types of immune evasion are presented in Fig. 3.

A number of both genetic and environmental mechanisms allow such immune escape and have been described in SCCHN (for a recent detailed review see [12]), including selection of poorly antigenic cancer cell subsets, disturbances in MHC class I- and class II-mediated antigen presentation [13–15], expression and secretion of immunosuppressive cytokines [16], expression of the pro-apoptotic Fas ligand to induce activation-induced cell death in T cells [17], and recruitment of immunosuppressive immune cell subsets into the tumor [18]. More recently, evidence is increasing that expression of immune checkpoint components that may limit T cell responses also occurs frequently in these tumors [18–20].

Immunomodulatory effects of ionizing radiation

Ionizing radiation has been used for more than a century to treat cancer [21], on the basis that rapidly proliferating cancer cells are more sensitive to DNA damage induced by radiation than normal tissue. Radiotherapy has traditionally been viewed as immunosuppressive due to the inherent sensitivity of lymphocytes to radiation-induced damage but it became evident that radiotherapy can also enhance tumor-specific immune responses. Strong support of an active role of the immune system for the success of radiotherapy came from studies in which the extent of tumor control by radiotherapy was compared in immunocompetent and -deficient xenograft models. Studies in the model of melanoma revealed that the ablative effects of radiotherapy were strongly dependent on radiation-induced cytokine responses [22]

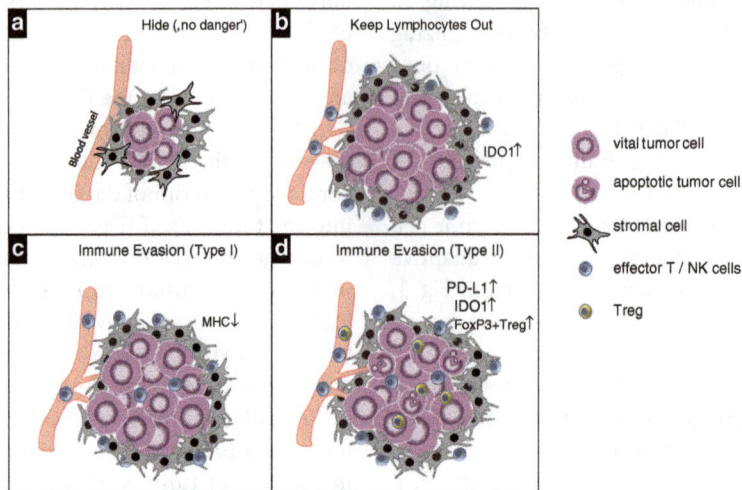

Fig. 2 Mechanisms of immune evasion by tumors. **a** In the early phase of tumor development tumors remain undetected by the immune system because of the lack of danger signals such as significant levels of apoptotic or necrotic cells or pro-inflammatory cytokines. **b** By secretion of soluble factors such as indoleamine 2,3-dioxygenase (IDO) by tumor cells the infiltration of lymphocytes is inhibited. **c** If moderate immune cell infiltration eventually occurs tumor cells downregulate the expression of components of the antigen presentation machinery including MHC class I and II which results in their impaired recognition by antigen-specific T cells. **d** In tumors with a larger extent of immune cell infiltration, tumor cell destruction by cytotoxic T cells is inhibited by high expression of immunosuppressive mechanisms such as IDO, PD-L1 and FoxP3+ Treg

and cytotoxic CD8+ T cells [23]. In a preclinical model of SCCHN, pretreatment of tumor cell lines with chemotherapeutic drugs and radiation significantly increased the extent of their cytolysis by antigen-specific CD8+ T cells [24]. All these observations suggest that not only genetic and phenotypic traits of tumor cells but also immunity

of the host are implicated into the clinical success of radiotherapy [22, 23, 25–27].

Mechanistically, radiotherapy has been shown to augment the afferent as well as efferent arms of cancer immunity. The induction of a specific T cell response to tumor cells (afferent immunity) has been observed in

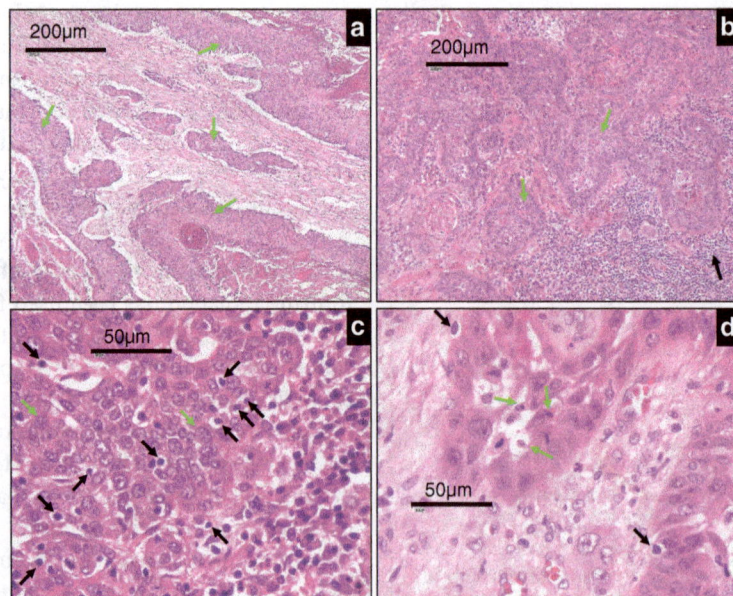

Fig. 3 Representative histological images of SCCHN tumor sections displaying different levels of immune evasion. **a** Tumor areas (*green arrows*) show the absence of any lymphocyte filtration at the rim or within the tumor cell nests. **b** Lymphocyte infiltrates are seen at the tumor border (*black arrows*) but are absent within the tumor nests (*green arrows*). **c** Despite a high extent of lymphocyte infiltration no signs of tumor cell lysis or apoptosis are visible. **d** Tumor areas with infiltrating lymphocytes are composed of vital and apoptotic tumor cells (*black arrows*), indicative of a balance between immune destruction and evasion

multiple studies. Almost 20 years ago molecular pathways were first described that were activated by treatment-induced cell stress (in particular after treatment with anthracyclins and ionizing radiation) and which induced a modality of cell death that was highly efficient in eliciting immune responses [28]. The immunogenic effects of radiation (reviewed in [29]) are thought to result from 'autovaccination' by antigens released from dying tumor cells. Translocation of a protein called calreticulin which is normally residing in the endoplasmatic reticulum to the cell surface promotes the uptake of dying cancer cells by DCs and the release of antigens that can be efficiently presented [30]. Release of ATP, heat shock proteins and high-mobility group box 1 (HMGB1) by dying cancer cells help in recruiting and activating DCs through toll-like receptor signaling pathways [31]. By integration of these danger signals DCs undergo an important maturation process. They up-regulate the expression of co-stimulatory proteins and pro-inflammatory cytokines, and acquire the ability of cross-presenting antigens to cytotoxic CD8+ T cells by which they initiate adaptive immunity [32].

Radiotherapy can also influence the efficacy of tumor cell destruction (efferent immunity) within the radiation field by altering tumor cell characteristics or the tissue microenvironment. Tumor cells in which the damage from radiation has not been sufficient to induce cell death show increased expression of MHC class-I antigen-presenting molecules [33] and adhesion molecules [34], stabilizing the binding of T cells to tumor cells and alleviating TCR activation. As a result, tumor cells that survive radiation may be eliminated through CD8+ T cell-mediated lysis [33].

It has been known for some time that irradiated tissues often show very strong changes in the local cytokine milieu. As a result of their action, a cascade of pro-inflammatory processes are triggered. Secretion of interferon-γ enhances expression of MHC class-I by cancer cells, sustaining and extending the initial effects of radiation to allow efficient recognition and killing by T cells [26, 34]. In addition, immune cell trafficking is enhanced through induction of chemokines, such as CXCL16 that attract effector T cells to the irradiated tumor site [29].

Immune effects within the radiation field, however, are not sufficient for cure, as effective treatment of a high-risk primary cancer has to secure not only local but also systemic control of the disease. In principle, the nature of the adaptive immune system should be mechanistically well suited for systemic tumor surveillance. There is emerging evidence that radiotherapy can also be associated with immune destruction of distant metastases, pointing towards efferent immunity outside of the radiotherapy field. This phenomenon termed abscopal anti-tumor effect was already described in 1953 [35]. Clinical reports of an abscopal effect after radiotherapy are few, but cover several different tumor types, including melanoma and a variety of carcinomas [36]. Growth suppression of distant non-irradiated tumors by a combination therapy of DC infusion and radiotherapy was also reported in a murine model of squamous cell carcinoma in the head and neck, indicating that indeed systemic antitumor activity can be induced by approaches which augment the immune-activating effects of radiotherapy.

The knowledge gained from mechanistic studies on the immunomodulatory effects of radiation mentioned above has changed the way the response to radiotherapy with/without chemotherapy in patients with cancer is now interpreted, by acknowledging the essential role of the host immune system for the success of radiotherapy. Importantly, these indirect effects of radiation – within and outside the field of treatment – also suggest new treatment possibilities, including combinations with established or novel forms of immunotherapy.

Immune checkpoint blockade as novel immunotherapeutic strategy in cancer

The introduction of immune checkpoint inhibitors is currently revolutionizing treatment of metastatic cancers. Previously, cancer immunology had concentrated either on afferent immune stimulation, i.e. induction of T cell immunity, most frequently by vaccination, or on stimulation of efferent T cell activity, e.g. by interleukin-2 treatment. An important limitation of these approaches was the tight regulation of the immune system by mechanisms termed immune checkpoints which are physiologically crucial to prevent autoimmune diseases (Fig. 4). At the afferent side of immunity the molecule cytotoxic T-lymphocyte protein 4 (CTLA-4) is expressed on antigen-activated T cells to dampen the magnitude of T cell activation. At the efferent side, the expression of the cell surface receptor PD-1 (programmed cell death protein 1) on activated T cells block their effector function, if bound to the ligand PD-L1 or PD-L2 on the target cell. Tumor cells frequently use the expression of PD-L1 and PD-L2 to escape immune destruction. Blocking antibodies directed to the immuno-regulatory proteins CTLA-4, PD-1 and PD-L1 have been shown to release these immune checkpoints in different ways. Antibodies to CTLA-4 (namely ipilimumab and tremelimumab) allow induction of autoimmunity, including immunity to cancer. However, there is a tight window of opportunity, as autoimmune phenomena can be quite serious after application of these agents [37]. Antibodies to PD-1 or PD-L1 do not promote induction of de-novo immunity but release the effector phase of immunity (Fig. 4), hereby allowing the execution of tumor cell destruction by T cells. Thus, the presence of tumor-specific T cells is required for efficacy of agents interfering with the PD-1/PD-L1 interaction.

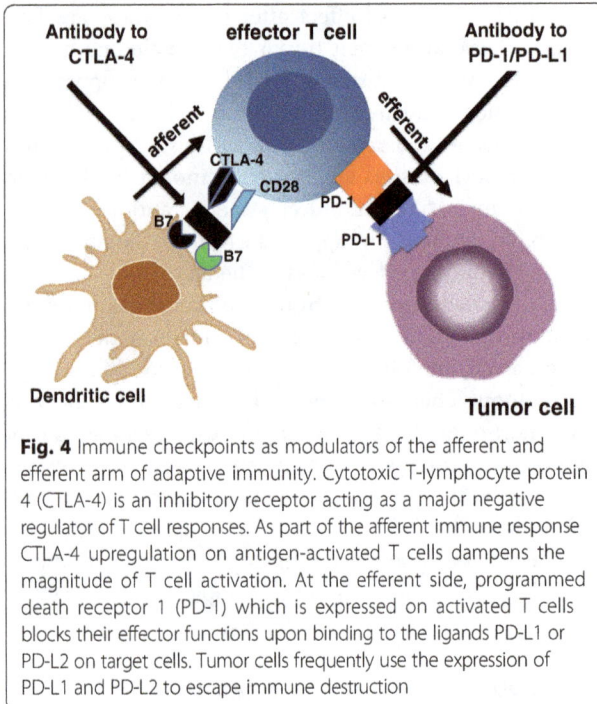

Fig. 4 Immune checkpoints as modulators of the afferent and efferent arm of adaptive immunity. Cytotoxic T-lymphocyte protein 4 (CTLA-4) is an inhibitory receptor acting as a major negative regulator of T cell responses. As part of the afferent immune response CTLA-4 upregulation on antigen-activated T cells dampens the magnitude of T cell activation. At the efferent side, programmed death receptor 1 (PD-1) which is expressed on activated T cells blocks their effector functions upon binding to the ligands PD-L1 or PD-L2 on target cells. Tumor cells frequently use the expression of PD-L1 and PD-L2 to escape immune destruction

The application of immune checkpoint inhibitors has recently been evaluated in a number of clinical trials and demonstrated remarkable activity in a broad spectrum of cancer types. Ipilimumab, nivolumab and pembrolizumab (the latter two agents both anti-PD-1 antibodies) were the first three immune checkpoint inhibitors which received FDA approval for the treatment of metastatic melanoma. A three-arm phase III trial in melanoma [38] answered the fundamental question in cancer immunology as to whether the de-novo induction of T cell responses by ipilimumab or the augmentation of a pre-existing T cell response by nivolumab may be more efficacious. Response rates and progression-free survival clearly favored nivolumab over ipilimumab, with the combination of both even more effective but at the cost of considerable immune-related toxicities [38].

There are at least eight anti-PD-1/PD-L1 antibodies currently in clinical development, covering phases I to III. In addition, the preclinical and early clinical development of inhibitors against other immune checkpoints, such as T cell immunoglobulin mucin receptor 3 (TIM3) and lymphocyte activation gene 3 protein (LAG3), and against co-stimulatory molecules, such as OX40 and CD137, are underway. Final results from several successful phase III trials with ipilimumab, nivolumab and pembrolizumab improving overall survival of metastatic cancer have been reported in melanoma and lung cancer, and it can be expected from the data available for a broad range of other histologies that this novel class of agents will be firmly established in modern treatment of many cancers.

In recurrent/metastatic SCCHN, several PD-1/PD-L1 blocking agents are currently being investigated, with most mature information on nivolumab and pembrolizumab. The phase 1b multicohort trial Keynote-012 tested the efficacy of the anti-PD-1 antibody pembrolizumab for treatment of PD-L1+ in recurrent/metastatic SCCHN [39]. A best overall response rate of 18 % was reported, with no obvious difference being observed between HPV+ (25 %) and HPV- tumors (14 %). Duration of responses was approximately 12 months [39]. Comparable results (overall response rate: 18 %; HPV+, 22 %; HPV-, 16 %) were reported for the Keynote-055 study in patients with R/M SCCHN resistant to platinum and cetuximab have been included [40]. Moreover, the randomized global phase III trial Checkmate-141, evaluating the efficacy and safety of nivolumab versus investigator's choice in patients with R/M SCCHN demonstrated an increase in 1-year overall survival (OS) rate from 16 to 36 % by nivolumab [41, 42]. Again, a survival benefit was observed in the HPV+ and HPV- subgroup [41, 42].

Early evidence of clinical activity in SCCHN were also reported from multi-arm expansion studies of anti-PD-L1 antibodies (atezolizumab, MPDL3280A [43]; durvalumab, MEDI4736 [44]). Based on these promising data, several further randomized phase III trials (NCT02358031, Keynote-048; NCT02252042, Keynote-040) have been initiated. In general, the successful clinical trials of PD-1 blocking agents are a proof of the existence of adaptive immunity towards SCCHN cells which can be very effective in a proportion of patients when unleashed by blockade of the PD-1/PD-L1 interaction.

Interference of immune checkpoints with resistance to RCT

Deregulated expression of immune checkpoint proteins has already been linked to poor efficacy of RCT in several tumor models. High expression of PD-L1 in tumor cells and stromal lymphocytes accompanied by low CD8+ T cell infiltration has recently been identified as a poor prognostic biomarker in patients with stage III non-small cell lung cancer (NSCLC) receiving cisplatin-based RCT [45]. In addition, tumor control by neoadjuvant or concurrent RCT was observed to be inefficient in patients with esophageal squamous cell carcinomas displaying elevated immunostaining for PD-L1 in neoplastic and adjacent non-malignant esophageal epithelium [46]. Preclinical studies in a variety of syngeneic mouse models of cancer [47] have also demonstrated that expression of PD-L1 can be induced by radiation itself and that such upregulation impairs both local tumor control and protection against tumor re-challenge [47]. It is therefore not surprising that blocking antibodies directed to these immune checkpoints were able to significantly enhance the immunogenic effects of radiotherapy [27, 48, 49].

In locally advanced SCCHN the magnitude of immune suppression could also be linked to the efficacy of RCT, however, a direct role of immune checkpoint proteins remains to be established. Low numbers of tumor-infiltrating cytotoxic CD8+ T cells before treatment were significantly correlated with poor outcome after RCT in several studies [50–53] but the role of CTLA-4 or PD-1/PD-L1 as negative regulators of CD8+ T cell activation has not been addressed. By inducing a change in the composition and functions of the immune cell compartment RCT was shown to relieve the extent of immune suppression: while the numbers of CD8+ and granzyme B+ cytotoxic cells only slightly decreased after RCT, a more pronounced decrease of FoxP3+ Treg was observed, resulting in an 2- to 3-fold increase in the cytotoxic T cell/FoxP3+ Treg ratio [50]. These data strongly support the idea that application of immune checkpoint inhibitors together with radio(chemo)therapy could also lead to a significant improvement of local as well as distant tumor control in SCCHN. Consequently, the first phase I/II trials evaluating the combination of pembrolizumab with standard definitive or adjuvant RCT as well as ipilimumab with cetuximab-based bioradiation (Table 2) have already been started, and several further trials with other inhibitors of PD-1 or PD-L1 are in preparation.

Potential biomarkers for patient selection for immune checkpoint blockade

Precise biomarkers to identify patients who benefit from immune checkpoint inhibition alone or in combination with RCT still have to be established. Current data in multiple cancers reveal that verification of PD-L1 overexpression by immunohistochemistry is associated with improved clinical outcome of anti-PD-1 therapy. However, the presence of robust responses in some patients with low or undetectable expression of PD-L1 complicates the issue of PD-L1 as an exclusive predictive biomarker [54].

In the Keynote-012 trial of SCCHN, an elevated expression of PD-L1 and the presence of an interferon-γ expression signature were associated with improved progression-free survival [39, 55]. The same signature had previously been established as predictive signature for outcome after pembrolizumab in metastatic melanoma [56] and its predictive value was also demonstrated in advanced gastric cancer [57]. In addition, patients with large immune cell infiltration in tumor tissue and high mutational load were more likely to benefit from immune checkpoint blockade in bladder [58] and colorectal cancer [59]. Taken together, patients with PD-L1+ tumors displaying immune-related gene expression signatures, including genes regulating T cell functions, the antigen presentation machinery and IFN-γ signaling, are most likely to benefit from immune checkpoint inhibition.

Rational development of combination regimens

While there is much excitement around the phenomenon of a radiation-induced anticancer immune response and combining radio(chemo)therapy with immunotherapy, numerous questions remain to be addressed in clinical trials. A major challenge is to identify not only the optimal immune checkpoint inhibitor as partner for a given radiotherapy schedule but also the best chronological sequence for their combined application. Preclinical evidence can serve as guidance in treatment schedule and clinical trial development. As outlined above, danger signals induced by radiation lead to the recruitment of immune cells into the tumor. However, cells of the immune system are also vulnerable to radiation, as their exposure to ionizing radiation induces apoptosis in mature natural killer (NK) cells as well as T and B cells. Since radiotherapy is generally delivered in daily fractions, re-irradiation of the tumor might therefore damage infiltrating immune cells that display cytolytic activity themselves or might significantly reduce the capacity of DCs to activate effector T cells. In addition,

Table 2 Current clinical trials (at clinicaltrials.gov) evaluating the combination of RT with immune checkpoint inhibitors

Clinical setting	Clinical trial	Drug	Combination
Resectable locally advanced SCCHN	NCT02641093 phase II	Pembrolizumab	Adjuvant RT/RCT
	NCT02296684 phase II	Pembrolizumab	Adjuvant RT/RCT
Locally advanced SCCHN	NCT01935921 phase I	Ipilimumab	Definitive RT + cetuximab
Intermediate/High risk locally advanced SCCHN	NCT01860430 phase Ib	Ipilimumab	Definitive RT + cetuximab
Locally advanced SCCHN	NCT02586207 phase I	Pembrolizumab	Definitive RT + CDDP
locally advanced laryngeal carcinoma	NCT02759575 phase I/II	Pembrolizumab	Definitive RT + CDDP
Intermediate/High risk locally advanced SCCHN	NCT02764593 phase I	Nivolumab	Definitive RT, RT+ CDDP, RT + cetuximab
	Phase III	Nivolumab	Definitive RT + CDDP
locoregional inoperable recurrence or second primary SCCHN	NCT02289209 phase II	Pembrolizumab	Reirradiation
Advanced metastatic disease (multicohort)	NCT02303990 phase I	Pembrolizumab	RT
Brain metastasis (multicohort)	NCT02669914 phase II	Durvalumab	Stereotactic radiosurgery

RT radiotherapy, *CDDP* cisplatin

DCs may find a hostile environment for T cell activation in draining lymph nodes, which represent their natural surrounding for interaction with T cells, as draining lymph nodes are systematically included into the radiation field in SCCHN. Conversely, however, the induction of immunogenic cell death (ICD) by each daily radiotherapy fraction might transiently generate a favorable milieu for immune activation within the tumor tissue, which may vanish again after termination of radiotherapy. In support of the latter, concurrent application of an anti-PD-L1 antibody together with fractionated radiotherapy significantly improved tumor control in a xenograft model [47]. In contrast, fractionated radiotherapy followed by delayed application of anti-PD-L1 was completely ineffective in enhancing the local efficacy of radiotherapy [47]. Certainly, more studies will be needed to address this important issue.

Besides the optimal time schedule also the optimal type and dosing of chemotherapy has to be established, if desired to be included into the treatment regimen. Significant differences in the ability of chemotherapeutic drugs to induce ICD have been reported previously [32]. Cisplatin which is an essential component of current state-of-the-art RCT regimens in SCCHN does not induce ICD [60] despite its presumed identical mechanism of action to that of oxaliplatin, a potent inducer of ICD. This has been attributed to the lack of calreticulin exposure after cisplatin treatment [60]. However, radiotherapy is a potent inducer of calreticulin exposure [30], and recent studies have shown that combining cisplatin with compounds that induce calreticulin exposure leads to full-scale ICD [60]. Thus, potentiation of ICD by cisplatin could still represent one of its major mechanism of action when cisplatin is administered concurrently with radiotherapy.

Taxanes including docetaxel and paclitaxel which are also common combination partners of radiotherapy in locally advanced SCCHN are known to modulate antitumor immune responses as well [61]. Similar to cisplatin, paclitaxel does not induce ICD. However, concurrent paclitaxel treatment was shown to significantly enhance radiation-induced ICD in breast cancer cell lines [62]. Similarly, docetaxel treatment itself did not induce ATP or HMGB1 secretion by tumor cells. However, calreticulin exposure of tumor cells after docetaxel treatment was observed which significantly enhanced tumor cell killing by antigen-specific CD8+ cytotoxic T cells [61].

Intriguingly, investigations on the immunogenic effects of chemotherapeutic drugs revealed also their direct interference with immune checkpoint expression. Treatment of DCs in vitro with platinum-based compounds strongly enhanced their potential to activate T cells which was caused by downregulation of PD-L2 in DCs [63]. This effect was mediated by inactivation of STAT6, the transcriptional regulator of PD-L2, and occurred also in tumor cells resulting in their enhanced recognition by T cells [63].

Overall, these preclinical observations provide a sound rationale for investigating immune checkpoint inhibitors with radiotherapy alone as well as in combination with standard cisplatin-based as well as taxane-based RCT. In addition, there is accumulating data that the efficacy of cetuximab-based regimens in treatment of recurrent/metastatic SCCHN is not only based on the inhibition of EGFR signaling pathways but also on the activation of Fcγ receptor-positive NK cells leading to DC maturation and activation of cytotoxic T cells [64]. A combination of immune checkpoint inhibitors with cetuximab-based bioradiation protocols might therefore also represent a very attractive chemotherapy-free concept for improvement of primary treatment of locally advanced SCCHN.

Toxicity of combination regimens

The toxicity of radiotherapy is mostly occurring directly at the irradiation site. Mucositis, xerostomia and swallowing dysfunctions are common side effects in radiotherapy of head and neck cancers. Clearly, the extent of early and late toxicity is dependent on the radiation technique and the applied dose: Intensity-modulated radiotherapy, which conforms closely to the tumor volume, avoids or minimizes exposure to unaffected tissue and thereby significantly reduces local side effects of irradiation [65]. On the other hand, addition of concurrent chemotherapy to radiotherapy not only improved efficacy of the treatment in locally advanced SCCHN but also increased both the toxicity and the spectrum of adverse events as compared to radiotherapy alone [66]. The toxicity of immunotherapy is dependent on the administered agent and dosage. In previous clinical trials, immune checkpoint blockade immunotherapy presented acceptable toxicity. Even occasional severe toxicity was manageable through treatment interruption or involvement of immunosuppressive drugs. During ipilimumab treatment approximately 60 % patients showed immune-related adverse events, of them 10–15 % being grade 3–4 [67]. The blockade of PD-1/-L1 showed less severe ir-AEs in previous phase I studies [68]. Diarrhea and skin rash were the most common immune-related adverse events after ipilimumab, other adverse effects included enterocolitis, hypothyroidism, hypophysitis and neuropathies [68]. The most common adverse events reported for both nivolumab and pembrolizumab were mild fatigue, rash, pruritus and diarrhea, which could be usually managed without dose interruption or discontinuation [68]. First toxicity data from a phase I study of the combined application of ipilimumab with radiotherapy for treatment of metastatic melanoma (NCT01497808, [48]) argue against an exacerbating toxicity profile of the combined regimen. No dose-limiting toxicities, defined by the study protocol as any treatment-related grade ≥4 immune-related toxicity or grade ≥3 non-immune related toxicity experienced during study treatment or within 30 days after the last injection of ipilimumab were observed [48]. Considering the different kinds and acceptable adverse events, the combinatorial treatment of radiotherapy and immune checkpoint inhibitors seems feasible for SCCHN patients.

Conclusions

The introduction of immune checkpoint inhibitors into cancer treatment has been celebrated as the breakthrough of the year 2013. Impressive activity was proven in metastatic melanoma and lung cancer, and promising results were presented for recurrent/metastatic SCCHN. Given the immunogenic effect of radiotherapy and its enhancement by chemotherapy or cetuximab, it remains to be determined whether immune checkpoint inhibitors could further increase the activation of adaptive immunity and ultimately improve overall current cure rates of locally advanced SCCHN.

Abbreviations

CTLA-4, cytotoxic T-lymphocyte protein 4; DCs: dendritic cells; DNA, deoxyribonucleic acid; EGFR, epidermal growth factor receptor; HMGB1, high-mobility group box 1; ICD, immunogenic cell death; IDO, indoleamine 2:3-dioxygenase; LAG3, lymphocyte activation gene 3 protein; MHC, major histocompatibility complex; NK, natural killer; NSCLC, non-small cell lung cancer; PD-1, programmed cell death receptor 1; PD-L1, programmed cell death 1 ligand 1; RCT, radiochemotherapy; SCCHN, squamous cell carcinoma of the head and neck; TCR, T cell receptor; TIM3, T cell immunoglobulin mucin receptor 3; Treg, regulatory T cells

Authors' contributions

IT, VB, KJ, UK conception and design. IT and UK literature search and review. IT, VB, KJ, UK interpretation of data. IT and UK manuscript drafting and writing. IT, VB, KJ, UK revision of manuscript and approval of final version.

Competing interest

The authors declare that they have no competing interests.

Author details

[1]Department of Radiooncology and Radiotherapy, Translational Radiation Oncology Research Laboratory, Charite University Hospital Berlin, Charitéplatz 1, 10117 Berlin, Germany. [2]German Cancer Research Center (DKFZ), Heidelberg, and German Cancer Consortium (DKTK) partner site Berlin, Berlin, Germany. [3]Institute of Pathology, Charite University Hospital, Berlin, Germany. [4]Comprehensive Cancer Center, Charité University Hospital, Berlin, Germany.

References

1. Pignon JP, le Maitre A, Maillard E, Bourhis J, Group M-NC. Meta-analysis of chemotherapy in head and neck cancer (MACH-NC): an update on 93 randomised trials and 17,346 patients. Radiother Oncol. 2009;92(1):4–14.

2. Machtay M, Moughan J, Trotti A, Garden AS, Weber RS, Cooper JS, Forastiere A, Ang KK. Factors associated with severe late toxicity after concurrent chemoradiation for locally advanced head and neck cancer: an RTOG analysis. J Clin Oncol. 2008;26(21):3582–9.

3. Budach V, Stuschke M, Budach W, Baumann M, Geismar D, Grabenbauer G, Lammert I, Jahnke K, Stueben G, Herrmann T, et al. Hyperfractionated accelerated chemoradiation with concurrent fluorouracil-mitomycin is more effective than dose-escalated hyperfractionated accelerated radiation therapy alone in locally advanced head and neck cancer: final results of the radiotherapy cooperative clinical trials group of the German Cancer Society 95–06 Prospective Randomized Trial. J Clin Oncol. 2005;23(6):1125–35.

4. Sartor Cl. Biological modifiers as potential radiosensitizers: targeting the epidermal growth factor receptor family. Semin Oncol. 2000;27(6 Suppl 11):15–20. discussion 92–100.

5. Ang KK, Berkey BA, Tu X, Zhang HZ, Katz R, Hammond EH, Fu KK, Milas L. Impact of epidermal growth factor receptor expression on survival and pattern of relapse in patients with advanced head and neck carcinoma. Cancer Res. 2002;62(24):7350–6.

6. Huang SM, Bock JM, Harari PM. Epidermal growth factor receptor blockade with C225 modulates proliferation, apoptosis, and radiosensitivity in squamous cell carcinomas of the head and neck. Cancer Res. 1999;59(8):1935–40.

7. Milas L, Fan Z, Andratschke NH, Ang KK. Epidermal growth factor receptor and tumor response to radiation: in vivo preclinical studies. Int J Radiat Oncol Biol Phys. 2004;58(3):966–71.

8. Bonner JA, Harari PM, Giralt J, Azarnia N, Shin DM, Cohen RB, Jones CU, Sur R, Raben D, Jassem J, et al. Radiotherapy plus cetuximab for squamous-cell carcinoma of the head and neck. N Engl J Med. 2006;354(6):567–78.

9. Ang KK, Zhang Q, Rosenthal DI, Nguyen-Tan PF, Sherman EJ, Weber RS, Galvin JM, Bonner JA, Harris J, El-Naggar AK, et al. Randomized phase III trial of concurrent accelerated radiation plus cisplatin with or without cetuximab for stage III to IV head and neck carcinoma: RTOG 0522. J Clin Oncol. 2014;32(27):2940–50.

10. Brandacher G, Perathoner A, Ladurner R, Schneeberger S, Obrist P, Winkler C, Werner ER, Werner-Felmayer G, Weiss HG, Gobel G, et al. Prognostic value of indoleamine 2,3-dioxygenase expression in colorectal cancer: effect on tumor-infiltrating T cells. Clin Cancer Res. 2006;12(4):1144–51.

11. Spranger S, Spaapen RM, Zha Y, Williams J, Meng Y, Ha TT, Gajewski TF. Up-regulation of PD-L1, IDO, and T(regs) in the melanoma tumor microenvironment is driven by CD8(+) T cells. Sci Transl Med. 2013;5(200):200ra116.

12. Ferris RL. Immunology and Immunotherapy of Head and Neck Cancer. J Clin Oncol. 2015;33(29):3293–304.

13. Grandis JR, Falkner DM, Melhem MF, Gooding WE, Drenning SD, Morel PA. Human leukocyte antigen class I allelic and haplotype loss in squamous cell carcinoma of the head and neck: clinical and immunogenetic consequences. Clin Cancer Res. 2000;6(7):2794–802.

14. Meissner M, Whiteside TL, van Kuik-Romein P, Valesky EM, van den Elsen PJ, Kaufmann R, Seliger B. Loss of interferon-gamma inducibility of the MHC class II antigen processing pathway in head and neck cancer: evidence for post-transcriptional as well as epigenetic regulation. Br J Dermatol. 2008;158(5):930–40.

15. Ferris RL, Whiteside TL, Ferrone S. Immune escape associated with functional defects in antigen-processing machinery in head and neck cancer. Clin Cancer Res. 2006;12(13):3890–5.

16. Jebreel A, Mistry D, Loke D, Dunn G, Hough V, Oliver K, Stafford N, Greenman J. Investigation of interleukin 10, 12 and 18 levels in patients with head and neck cancer. J Laryngol Otol. 2007;121(3):246–52.

17. Gastman BR, Johnson DE, Whiteside TL, Rabinowich H. Tumor-induced apoptosis of T lymphocytes: elucidation of intracellular apoptotic events. Blood. 2000;95(6):2015–23.

18. Jie HB, Gildener-Leapman N, Li J, Srivastava RM, Gibson SP, Whiteside TL, Ferris RL. Intratumoral regulatory T cells upregulate immunosuppressive molecules in head and neck cancer patients. Br J Cancer. 2013;109(10):2629–35.

19. Zandberg DP, Strome SE. The role of the PD-L1:PD-1 pathway in squamous cell carcinoma of the head and neck. Oral Oncol. 2014;50(7):627–32.

20. Yu GT, Bu LL, Huang CF, Zhang WF, Chen WJ, Gutkind JS, Kulkarni AB, Sun ZJ. PD-1 blockade attenuates immunosuppressive myeloid cells due to inhibition of CD47/SIRPalpha axis in HPV negative head and neck squamous cell carcinoma. Oncotarget. 2015;6(39):42067–80.

21. Grubbe EH. The origin and birth of x-ray therapy. Urol Cutaneous Rev. 1947;51(7):375–9.

22. Burnette BC, Liang H, Lee Y, Chlewicki L, Khodarev NN, Weichselbaum RR, Fu YX, Auh SL. The efficacy of radiotherapy relies upon induction of type i interferon-dependent innate and adaptive immunity. Cancer Res. 2011;71(7):2488–96.

23. Lee Y, Auh SL, Wang Y, Burnette B, Wang Y, Meng Y, Beckett M, Sharma R, Chin R, Tu T, et al. Therapeutic effects of ablative radiation on local tumor require CD8+ T cells: changing strategies for cancer treatment. Blood. 2009;114(3):589–95.

24. Gelbard A, Garnett CT, Abrams SI, Patel V, Gutkind JS, Palena C, Tsang KY, Schlom J, Hodge JW. Combination chemotherapy and radiation of human squamous cell carcinoma of the head and neck augments CTL-mediated lysis. Clin Cancer Res. 2006;12(6):1897–905.

25. Stone HB, Peters LJ, Milas L. Effect of host immune capability on radiocurability and subsequent transplantability of a murine fibrosarcoma. J Natl Cancer Inst. 1979;63(5):1229–35.

26. Lugade AA, Moran JP, Gerber SA, Rose RC, Frelinger JG, Lord EM. Local radiation therapy of B16 melanoma tumors increases the generation of tumor antigen-specific effector cells that traffic to the tumor. J Immunol. 2005;174(12):7516–23.

27. Deng L, Liang H, Burnette B, Beckett M, Darga T, Weichselbaum RR, Fu YX. Irradiation and anti-PD-L1 treatment synergistically promote antitumor immunity in mice. J Clin Invest. 2014;124(2):687–95.

28. Galluzzi L, Maiuri MC, Vitale I, Zischka H, Castedo M, Zitvogel L, Kroemer G. Cell death modalities: classification and pathophysiological implications. Cell Death Differ. 2007;14(7):1237–43.

29. Golden EB, Apetoh L. Radiotherapy and immunogenic cell death. Semin Radiat Oncol. 2015;25(1):11–7.

30. Obeid M, Panaretakis T, Joza N, Tufi R, Tesniere A, van Endert P, Zitvogel L, Kroemer G. Calreticulin exposure is required for the immunogenicity of gamma-irradiation and UVC light-induced apoptosis. Cell Death Differ. 2007;14(10):1848–50.

31. Yamazaki T, Hannani D, Poirier-Colame V, Ladoire S, Locher C, Sistigu A, Prada N, Adjemian S, Catani JP, Freudenberg M, et al. Defective immunogenic cell death of HMGB1-deficient tumors: compensatory therapy with TLR4 agonists. Cell Death Differ. 2014;21(1):69–78.

32. Kroemer G, Galluzzi L, Kepp O, Zitvogel L. Immunogenic cell death in cancer therapy. Annu Rev Immunol. 2013;31:51–72.

33. Garnett CT, Palena C, Chakraborty M, Tsang KY, Schlom J, Hodge JW. Sublethal irradiation of human tumor cells modulates phenotype resulting in enhanced killing by cytotoxic T lymphocytes. Cancer Res. 2004;64(21):7985–94.

34. Lugade AA, Sorensen EW, Gerber SA, Moran JP, Frelinger JG, Lord EM. Radiation-induced IFN-gamma production within the tumor microenvironment influences antitumor immunity. J Immunol. 2008;180(5):3132–9.

35. Mole RH. Whole body irradiation; radiobiology or medicine? Br J Radiol. 1953;26(305):234–41.

36. Reynders K, Illidge T, Siva S, Chang JY, De Ruysscher D. The abscopal effect of local radiotherapy: using immunotherapy to make a rare event clinically relevant. Cancer Treat Rev. 2015;41(6):503–10.

37. Michot JM, Bigenwald C, Champiat S, Collins M, Carbonnel F, Postel-Vinay S, Berdelou A, Varga A, Bahleda R, Hollebecque A, et al. Immune-related adverse events with immune checkpoint blockade: a comprehensive review. Eur J Cancer. 2016;54:139–48.

38. Larkin J, Chiarion-Sileni V, Gonzalez R, Grob JJ, Cowey CL, Lao CD, Schadendorf D, Dummer R, Smylie M, Rutkowski P, et al. Combined Nivolumab and Ipilimumab or Monotherapy in Untreated Melanoma. N Engl J Med. 2015;373(1):23–34.

39. Seiwert TY, Burtness B, Mehra R, Weiss J, Berger R, Eder JP, Heath K, McClanahan T, Lunceford J, Gause C, et al. Safety and clinical activity of pembrolizumab for treatment of recurrent or metastatic squamous cell carcinoma of the head and neck (KEYNOTE-012): an open-label, multicentre, phase 1b trial. Lancet Oncol. 2016;17:956–65.

40. Bauml J, Seiwert TY, Pfister DG, Worden FP, Liu SV, Gilbert J, Saba NF, Weiss J, Wirth LJ, Sukari A, et al. Preliminary results from KEYNOTE-055: Pembrolizumab after platinum and cetuximab failure in head and neck squamous cell carcinoma (HNSCC). J Clin Oncol. 2016;34(suppl):abstr 6011.

41. Gillison ML, Blumenschein G, Fayette J, Guigay J, Colevas AD, Licitra L, Harrington K, Kasper S, Vokes E, Even C et al. Nivolumab (nivo) vs investigator's choice (IC) for recurrent or metastatic (R/M) head and neck squamous cell carcinoma (HNSCC): CheckMate-141 [abstract]. In: Proceedings of the 107th Annual Meeting of the American Association for Cancer Research. New Orleans: AACR; 2016.

42. Ferris RL, Blumenschein G, Fayette J, Guigay J, Colevas AD, Licitra L, Harrington K, Kasper S, Vokes E, Even C, et al. Further evaluations of nivolumab (nivo) versus investigator's choice (IC) chemotherapy for recurrent or metastatic (R/M) squamous cell carcinoma of the head and neck (SCCHN): CheckMate 141. J Clin Oncol. 2016;34(suppl):abstr 6009.

43. Herbst RS, Gordon MS, Fine GD, Sosman JA, Soria J-C, Hamid O, Powderly JD, Burris HA, Mokatrin A, Kowanetz M, et al. A study of MPDL3280A, an engineered PD-L1 antibody in patients with locally advanced or metastatic tumors. J Clin Oncol. 2013;31(Suppl):abstr 3000.

44. Segal NH, Antonia SJ, Brahmer JR, Maio M, Blake-Haskins A, Li X, Vasselli J, Ibrahim RA, Lutzky J, Khleif S. Preliminary data from a multi-arm expansion study of MEDI4736, an anti-PD-L1 antibody. J Clin Oncol. 2014;32(Suppl):abstr 3002.

45. Tokito T, Azuma K, Kawahara A, Ishii H, Yamada K, Matsuo N, Kinoshita T, Mizukami N, Ono H, Kage M, et al. Predictive relevance of PD-L1 expression combined with CD8+ TIL density in stage III non-small cell lung cancer patients receiving concurrent chemoradiation. Eur J Cancer. 2016;55:7–14.

46. Chen MF, Chen PT, Chen WC, Lu MS, Lin PY, Lee KD. The role of PD-L1 in the radiation response and prognosis for esophageal squamous cell carcinoma related to IL-6 and T-cell immunosuppression. Oncotarget. 2016;7(7):7913–24.

47. Dovedi SJ, Adlard AL, Lipowska-Bhalla G, McKenna C, Jones S, Cheadle EJ, Stratford IJ, Poon E, Morrow M, Stewart R, et al. Acquired resistance to fractionated radiotherapy can be overcome by concurrent PD-L1 blockade. Cancer Res. 2014;74(19):5458–68.

48. Twyman-Saint Victor C, Rech AJ, Maity A, Rengan R, Pauken KE, Stelekati E, Benci JL, Xu B, Dada H, Odorizzi PM, et al. Radiation and dual checkpoint blockade activate non-redundant immune mechanisms in cancer. Nature. 2015;520(7547):373–7.

49. Chandra RA, Wilhite TJ, Balboni TA, Alexander BM, Spektor A, Ott PA, Ng AK, Hodi FS, Schoenfeld JD. A systematic evaluation of abscopal responses following radiotherapy in patients with metastatic melanoma treated with ipilimumab. Oncoimmunology. 2015;4(11):e1046028.

50. Distel LV, Fickenscher R, Dietel K, Hung A, Iro H, Zenk J, Nkenke E, Buttner M, Niedobitek G, Grabenbauer GG. Tumour infiltrating lymphocytes in squamous cell carcinoma of the oro- and hypopharynx: prognostic impact may depend on type of treatment and stage of disease. Oral Oncol. 2009;45(10):e167–74.

51. Balermpas P, Michel Y, Wagenblast J, Seitz O, Weiss C, Rodel F, Rodel C, Fokas E. Tumour-infiltrating lymphocytes predict response to definitive chemoradiotherapy in head and neck cancer. Br J Cancer. 2014;110(2):501–9.

52. Oguejiofor K, Hall J, Slater C, Betts G, Hall G, Slevin N, Dovedi S, Stern PL, West CM. Stromal infiltration of CD8 T cells is associated with improved clinical outcome in HPV-positive oropharyngeal squamous carcinoma. Br J Cancer. 2015;113(6):886–93.

53. Balermpas P, Rodel F, Rodel C, Krause M, Linge A, Lohaus F, Baumann M, Tinhofer I, Budach V, Gkika E, et al. CD8+ tumour-infiltrating lymphocytes in relation to HPV status and clinical outcome in patients with head and neck cancer after postoperative chemoradiotherapy: A multicentre study of the German cancer consortium radiation oncology group (DKTK-ROG). Int J Cancer. 2016;138(1):171–81.

54. Patel SP, Kurzrock R. PD-L1 Expression as a Predictive Biomarker in Cancer Immunotherapy. Mol Cancer Ther. 2015;14(4):847–56.

55. Seiwert TY, Haddad RI, Gupta S, Mehra R, Tahara M, Berger R, Lee S-H, Burtness B, Le DT, Heath K, et al. Antitumor activity and safety of pembrolizumab in patients (pts) with advanced squamous cell carcinoma of the head and neck (SCCHN): Preliminary results from KEYNOTE-012 expansion cohort. J Clin Oncol. 2015;33(Suppl):abstr LBA6008.

56. Ribas R, Robert C, Hodi FS, Wolchok JD, Joshua AM, Hwu WJ, Weber JS, Zarour HM, Kefford R, Loboda A, et al. Association of response to programmed death receptor 1 (PD-1) blockade with pembrolizumab (MK-3475) with an interferon-inflammatory immune gene signature. J Clin Oncol. 2015;33(Suppl):abstr 3001.

57. Shankaran V, Muro K, Bang Y-J, Geva R, Catenacci DVT, Gupta S, Eder JP, Berger R, Loboda A, Albright A, et al. Correlation of gene expression signatures and clinical outcomes in patients with advanced gastric cancer treated with pembrolizumab (MK-3475). J Clin Oncol. 2015;33(suppl):abstr 3026.

58. Rosenberg JE, Hoffman-Censits J, Powles T, van der Heijden MS, Balar AV, Necchi A, Dawson N, O'Donnell PH, Balmanoukian A, Loriot Y, et al.

Atezolizumab in patients with locally advanced and metastatic urothelial carcinoma who have progressed following treatment with platinum-based chemotherapy: a single-arm, multicentre, phase 2 trial. Lancet. 2016;387(10031):1909–20.

59. Le DT, Uram JN, Wang H, Bartlett BR, Kemberling H, Eyring AD, Skora AD, Luber BS, Azad NS, Laheru D, et al. PD-1 Blockade in Tumors with Mismatch-Repair Deficiency. N Engl J Med. 2015;372(26):2509–20.

60. Martins I, Kepp O, Schlemmer F, Adjemian S, Tailler M, Shen S, Michaud M, Menger L, Gdoura A, Tajeddine N, et al. Restoration of the immunogenicity of cisplatin-induced cancer cell death by endoplasmic reticulum stress. Oncogene. 2011;30(10):1147–58.

61. Hodge JW, Garnett CT, Farsaci B, Palena C, Tsang KY, Ferrone S, Gameiro SR. Chemotherapy-induced immunogenic modulation of tumor cells enhances killing by cytotoxic T lymphocytes and is distinct from immunogenic cell death. Int J Cancer. 2013;133(3):624–36.

62. Golden EB, Frances D, Pellicciotta I, Demaria S, Helen Barcellos-Hoff M, Formenti SC. Radiation fosters dose-dependent and chemotherapy-induced immunogenic cell death. Oncoimmunology. 2014;3:e28518.

63. Lesterhuis WJ, Punt CJ, Hato SV, Eleveld-Trancikova D, Jansen BJ, Nierkens S, Schreibelt G, de Boer A, Van Herpen CM, Kaanders JH, et al. Platinum-based drugs disrupt STAT6-mediated suppression of immune responses against cancer in humans and mice. J Clin Invest. 2011;121(8):3100–8.

64. Srivastava RM, Lee SC, Andrade Filho PA, Lord CA, Jie HB, Davidson HC, Lopez-Albaitero A, Gibson SP, Gooding WE, Ferrone S, et al. Cetuximab-activated natural killer and dendritic cells collaborate to trigger tumor antigen-specific T-cell immunity in head and neck cancer patients. Clin Cancer Res. 2013;19(7):1858–72.

65. Mendenhall WM, Amdur RJ, Palta JR. Intensity-modulated radiotherapy in the standard management of head and neck cancer: promises and pitfalls. J Clin Oncol. 2006;24(17):2618–23.

66. Seiwert TY, Salama JK, Vokes EE. The chemoradiation paradigm in head and neck cancer. Nat Clin Pract Oncol. 2007;4(3):156–71.

67. Hodi FS, O'Day SJ, McDermott DF, Weber RW, Sosman JA, Haanen JB, Gonzalez R, Robert C, Schadendorf D, Hassel JC, et al. Improved survival with ipilimumab in patients with metastatic melanoma. N Engl J Med. 2010;363(8):711–23.

68. Gangadhar TC, Vonderheide RH. Mitigating the toxic effects of anticancer immunotherapy. Nat Rev Clin Oncol. 2014;11(2):91–9.

15

Does concurrent chemoradiotherapy preceded by chemotherapy improve survival in locally advanced nasopharyngeal cancer patients?

Joel Yarney[1,2]*, Naa A. Aryeetey[1], Alice Mensah[4], Emmanuel D. Kitcher[2,5], Verna Vanderpuye[1,3], Charles Aidoo[1] and Kenneth Baidoo[2,5]

Abstract

Background: To find out how chemotherapy given prior to concurrent chemoradiotherapy compares with concurrent chemoradiation alone in the treatment of locally advanced nasopharyngeal cancer.

Methods: Patient charts were examined and found to have submitted to one of two regimes as follows: Neoadjuvant chemotherapy consisting of Cisplatin and 5-fluorouracil followed by concurrent chemoradiotherapy with cisplatin (group1), or concurrent cisplatin based chemoradiotherapy only (group 2). Radiation treatment dose of 70Gy in 35 fractions was given in each group.

Results: Forty-seven patients were evaluated with 68% male. Stage 4 disease comprised 83%, WHO type 3 was the commonest histologic type (53.2%). Median follow up period was 20 months (4–129). The 3-year overall survival for group 1 was 52.1%, and for group 2:65.7% ($p = 0.47$). The 3-year disease free survival for group 1 was 61.4, and 81.4% for group 2 ($p = 0.03$).

Conclusion: The study revealed that concurrent chemoradiation alone yields better disease free survival compared to chemotherapy given prior to it. There is however no difference in overall survival between the two regimes.

Keywords: Neoadjuvant chemotherapy, Radiation, Nasopharyngeal cancer, Survival, Locally advanced disease

Background

Nasopharyngeal cancer is relatively uncommon worldwide, but shows distinct geographical and ethnic distribution [1]. It is endemic in Southeast Asia, where cured fish is a staple, the incidence is rising in North Africa [2]. It is the commonest head and neck malignancy at the Korle-Bu Teaching Hospital in Accra, Ghana, West Africa. The epidemiology of the disease has previously been described by the authors [3].

Infection with Epstein Barr virus (EBV) increases the risk of developing nasopharyngeal cancer in addition to genetic predisposition. EBV DNA and other nuclear components including nuclear antigens and viral encoded RNA(EBER) have been identified in tumor cells and plasma, providing opportunity for early detection and novel therapeutic approaches [4, 5].

The landmark paper published by Al- Saraf et al., that compared Cisplatin based concurrent chemoradiation with radiotherapy alone, established the former as the standard of care [6]. This finding has been validated by several studies and meta-analyses. In a meta-analysis of 8 randomized trials comparing radiotherapy to concurrent chemo-radiotherapy, concurrent chemo-radiotherapy resulted in overall survival benefit [7]. A previous meta-analysis had also confirmed concurrent chemo-radiotherapy as the most effective way of improving survival with a 20% improvement in overall survival at 5 years [8]. This finding was again replicated in a recent update to meta-analysis of chemotherapy in

* Correspondence: kodwoahen@gmail.com
[1]National Center for Radiotherapy and NuclearMedicine Korle bu Teaching, Hospital P.O. Box KB 369, Accra, Ghana
[2]School of Medicine and Dentistry, Accra, Ghana
Full list of author information is available at the end of the article

nasopharyngeal carcinoma collaborative group study (MAC-NPC) which showed no added benefit of adjuvant chemotherapy when concomitant chemoradiotherapy is used [9]. Induction chemotherapy followed by radiotherapy alone on the other hand has failed to demonstrate significant benefit [10]. Recent randomized studies have yielded conflicting outcomes when chemotherapy is given prior to concomitant chemoradiotherapy [11, 12].

The pattern of recurrence after concurrent chemoradiation alone for locally advanced disease which represents the norm in our setting [3], includes local, regional as well as distant failure, suggesting the need for novel therapeutic approaches to enable better disease control.

The authors previously reported 73.1% of patients presenting with stage IVB disease in Accra [3], this proportion of disease is much higher than in most series, and therefore presents unique challenges to treatment, indeed two thirds of all failures occurred loco-regionally. For these patients, rapid downsizing of disease which can be achieved with neoadjuvant chemotherapy is desirable.

The objectives of this study therefore were:

1. To describe the demography of nasopharyngeal cancer with respect to age, sex, and histological type.
2. To compare, the 3-year disease free and overall survival in patients treated with concurrent chemoradiotherapy only to those treated with neoadjuvant chemotherapy followed by concurrent chemoradiotherapy in locally advanced nasopharyngeal cancer patients.

Methods
Design
This is a single institution observational retrospective chart review.

Inclusion criteria
All patients with histologically confirmed nasopharyngeal cancer referred for treatment were considered for chart review with the intention to select patient charts that meet the eligibility criteria for study. To be eligible for inclusion in the study, patients ought to have been treated with curative intent from January, 2000 to June, 2012, the end point for analysis was 31 December 2013. Eligible patients were required to have Eastern Cooperative Oncology Group (ECOG) performance status of at most 2. Patients ought to have adequate renal, liver and hematopoietic function.

Exclusion criteria
Patients treated with palliative intent or for metastatic disease were excluded. Patients were not excluded from the study on the basis of toxicity.

Staging
Patients were staged by physical and radiological examination using the 6th edition of American Joint Cancer Committee on staging. Physical examination included fibre-optic endoscopy and biopsy under anesthesia with a description of the extent of disease. Staging work-up comprised Computed Tomography (CT) scan of the head and neck region, Chest X ray (CXR) and ultrasound of the abdomen and pelvis, and bone scintigraphy where indicated. CT scan: chest, abdomen and pelvis was performed only when CXR and ultrasound of the abdomen were equivocal.

Treatment
Chemotherapy
Neoadjuvant chemotherapy consisted of 3 weekly Cisplatin at 80 mg/m^2 on day 1 with 5-fluorouracil at 1000 mg/m^{2}on day 1–4 or Capecitabine at 1000 mg/m^2 twice a day for fourteen days (only two patients), 3 weekly for 2–3 cycles followed by chemo- radiation. Patients received only Cisplatin at a dose of 100 mg/m^2 during radiotherapy on days 1,22 and 43 of radiotherapy.

Radiation
All patients were immobilized in a Med Tec mask, and simulated with a conventional simulator after submitting to dental assessment. Some patients underwent hearing test as well. Patients received external beam radiation using 2-D planning as follows: Treatment fields consisted of two lateral opposed fields matched with a supraclavicular field, with appropriate shielding and using shrinking field technique. A posterior neck field was placed with a central block to shield the spinal cord whilst treating the involved nodes to the prescribed dose.

Patients were prescribed to receive:70Gy in 35 fractions at 2 Gy per fraction per day to the mid plane over seven weeks to the primary and involved nodes. Uninvolved neck was treated to 50Gy using similar fractionation schedule.

Megavoltage verification or port films were obtained of all fields prior to, and mid-way through treatment, and localization adjusted accordingly. The institution participates in the International Atomic Energy Agency postal audits on a yearly basis and records figures within 5% accuracy level.

Toxicity
Patients were reviewed once a week during treatment to determine toxicity with weekly complete blood count, urea, electrolytes and creatinine. Acute and late toxicities were gleaned from the patient chart as recorded by treating Physician. Only grade 3 and 4 toxicities in eligible patients were assessed. A feeding tube was placed when required.

Follow up

Following completion of treatment, patients were reviewed by Oncologists and Otolaryngologists three monthly for the first 2 years, and at most 6 monthly thereafter with clinical examination including fibre-optic examination.

Re-staging CT scan was ordered based on clinical suspicion of recurrence with biopsy where indicated. The date of death was ascertained by making telephone calls to next of kin or from death certificates.

Statistics

Patient age, sex, histology, primary tumor stage T, and nodal stage N, were extracted from the charts and analyzed for summary statistics using Statistical Package for Social Science version 16 software, with description of mean, frequency, range and standard deviation where appropriate. Log-rank test was performed to determine differences in overall and disease free survival on the Kaplan Meier curve. Probability of < 0.05 was chosen as the level of significance.

Limitations

The study is limited by the small number of patients and its retrospective nature.

Results

Ninety-nine patients were identified to have been referred with a histologically confirmed diagnosis of nasopharyngeal cancer between January 2000 and June 2012, to the Radiotherapy Department, Korle-Bu Teaching Hospital in Accra, Ghana. Out of this number, only forty-seven met the inclusion criteria, the rest were excluded on the following basis: twenty-eight were excluded because they were treated with palliative intent, nine received radiation only, four were non-Ghanaian, left the country after treatment, and therefore had no follow- up data, and eleven were excluded because they absconded treatment before two weeks into it.

The mean age was 34.1 years with a range of 10–83 years. Only one patient was in the pediatric age bracket of twelve years or less. The commonest histological type going by WHO classification was type 3 (53.2%), followed by type 1 (25.5%), the least common was type 2(14. 9%), unknown comprised 6.4%. Male to female ratio was 2.1: 1.

Patients with Stage 4 disease comprised 83% (38.3% in group 1 and 44.7% in group 2). Staging characteristics is shown in Table 1.

Patients who fulfilled the inclusion criteria were identified to have been treated with either of two regimes. Group 1 received neoadjuvant chemotherapy followed by concurrent chemoradiation, they were 22 in number; Group 2 patients received chemoradiation only and

Table 1 Staging characteristics

Stage						
T-Stage	N-Stage					Total
	0	1	2	3	X	
1	0	0	1	2	0	3
2	0	1	1	7	0	9
3	0	5	2	8	0	15
4	4	2	6	7	1	20
Total	4	8	10	24	1	47

comprised 25 patients. Characteristics of patients in each group is shown in Table 2, other than age, there was no statistical difference between the two groups in the parameters examined.

Two patients in group 2 had persistent neck disease at the end of treatment, 2 more in this group failed in the neck during the follow up period. Four patients had persistent disease in the neck in group 1. There were five distant events including one in the liver and lung, and three in bone for group one. Group 2 patients had two failures in bone. Six and three patients suffered recurrence in the nasopharynx in groups 1 and 2 respectively. Some of the recurrences were concurrent events.

The median follow-up period was 20 months (4–129). The three-year disease free survival rates for groups one and two were 61.4 and 81.4% respectively yielding a p value

Table 2 Group characteristics

	Group 1	Group 2	P – Value @ 95% CI
Toxicity			
Neutropenia	8	5	
Trismus	5	9	
Age (years)			
< 20	15	8	0.013
> 20	7	17	
Sex			
Male	17	15	0.205
Female	5	10	
Stage			
I	–	1	0.422
III	3	3	
IV	18	21	
Unknown	1	–	
Who type			
1	5	7	0.214
2	4	3	
3	13	12	
Not stated	–	3	

of 0.03 on log rank test. The three-year overall survival for groups one and two were 52.1 and 65.7% respectively, yielding a p value of 0.47. Kaplan Meier curves for disease free and overall survival are shown in Figs. 1 and 2 respectively. More patients in Group 1, 8 in all, developed neutropenia, compared to 5 in Group 2. Nine patients in Group 2 developed trismus compared to 5 in Group 1. Average number of chemotherapy cycles received during concurrent chemoradiotherapy was not significantly different between the two groups.

Discussion

Head and Neck cancer is the third commonest malignancy seen at the Radiotherapy Centre in Accra, and nasopharyngeal cancer is the commonest amongst them. This observation probably reflects low incidence of smoking in Ghana relative to the developed world where laryngeal cancer is more common.

The observed incidence of nasopharyngeal cancer is probably due to consumption of salt cured fish which is a delicacy, EBV infection, as well as genetic predisposition. Epstein Bar viral antigen was not tested in this chart review.

Concurrent chemoradiation has been established as the standard of care in the management of nasopharyngeal cancer, all patients therefore submitted to concurrent chemoradiation, it was however left to the discretion of the treating Physician to determine whether this would be preceded by neoadjuvant chemotherapy as it holds the promise of down-sizing tumors especially with extracted evidence from management of other head and neck cancer. The safety and efficacy of induction chemotherapy followed by concomitant chemoradiation was reported by Al-Amro et al. in 2005 [13], in addition,

adjuvant chemotherapy has not been shown to impact on overall survival [7, 8, 14].

The observed male to female ratio is similar to previous reports. World Health Organization (WHO) type 3 is the commonest variety, consistent with the picture in endemic regions, followed by type 1.

Following the study by Al Saraf et al. that included patients with predominantly non-endemic variety, concerns were expressed regarding the applicability of the findings of that study to endemic regions. Subsequent studies have however validated the conclusion of that study in different geographical settings with varying distribution of WHO type, thus establishing concurrent chemoradiotherapy as the standard of care in all geographical regions [7–9].

The ten-year-old patient was treated with the Al Saraf protocol because of the presence of extensive disease at presentation. This was based on the recommended dose range of 50–72 Gy in patients 10 years and older, this dose is reduced by 5–10% in children under 10 years [15–17]. The other patients were twelve years or older.

Owing to the limited number of patients studied, the number of failures were also small. From the results on recurrence pattern: the number of regional failures were the same for both groups. There were more failures in the nasopharynx and distantly for group 1 relative to group 2, we are however unable to comment on the statistical significance of this observation owing to the small numbers.

Chen YP et al. reported that neoadjuvant chemotherapy followed by concurrent chemoradiotherapy is associated with reduced distant failures, as compared with concurrent chemoradiotherapy alone and whether the addition of neoadjuvant chemotherapy can improve

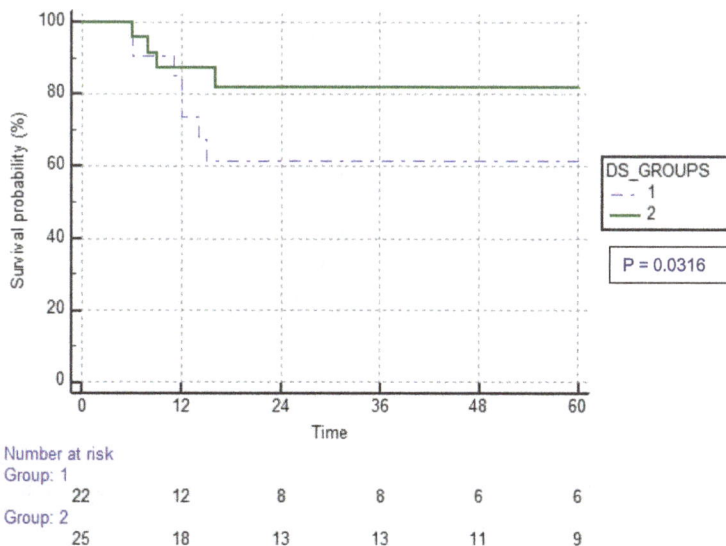

Fig. 1 Kaplan Meier curve of disease free survival in months

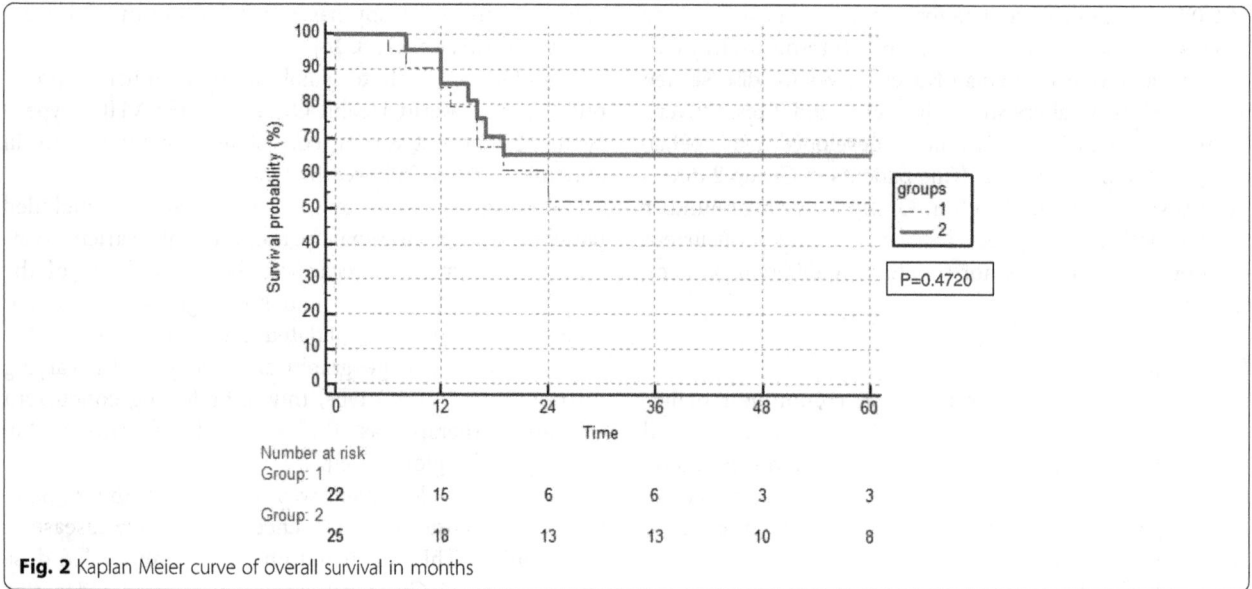

Fig. 2 Kaplan Meier curve of overall survival in months

survival for locoregionally advanced nasopharyngeal cancer should be further explored. Optimizing regimes and identifying patients at high-risk of metastases may enhance the efficacy of neoadjuvant chemotherapy followed by concurrent chemoradiotherapy [18].

In a study from South Korea, 300 patients were selected after matching for analysis. Higher 5-year locoregional failure free survival was observed in the chemoradiotherapy only arm (85% vs 72%, $p = 0.014$). No significant difference in distant failure-free survival (DFFS), disease- free survival (DFS), and overall survival were observed between the groups. In subgroup analysis, the neoadjuvant chemotherapy arm showed superior DFFS and DFS in stage IV patients younger than 60 years. No significant difference in compliance and toxicity was observed between groups, except the radiation therapy duration was slightly shorter in the concurrent chemoradiotherapy only arm. The authors concluded that the study did not show superiority of neoadjuvant chemotherapy followed by concurrent chemoradiotherapy over concurrent chemoradiotherapy alone. Because neoadjuvant chemotherapy could increase the risk of locoregional recurrence, it can only be considered in selected young patients with advanced stage IV disease. The role of neoadjuvant chemotherapy remains to be defined and should not be viewed as the standard of care [19]. Even though small, our study seems to support findings from other studies that neoadjuvant chemotherapy patients appear to have more local failures.

Our 3-year overall survival of 65.7%, and disease free survival of 81.4% in the concurrent chemoradiation only group is modest considering the high proportion of Stage 4 disease.

Comparing the overall survival between the two groups on log-rank test, we were unable to detect a statistically significant difference between the two groups, $p = 0.47$. There was however a statistically significant difference between the two groups in relation to disease free survival in favor of chemoradiation only, with a 3-year value of 81.4% in the chemoradiation only group, versus 61.4% in the neoadjuvant followed by chemoradiation group, $p = 0.03$ on log-rank test.

It is evident from other studies that even though neoadjuvant chemotherapy can achieve substantial tumor downsizing, it does not translate into improved disease free or overall survival [14]. In this study, neoadjuvant chemotherapy was found to be inferior to chemoradiation only, in terms of disease free survival.

Fountzilas G et al. [11] demonstrated that induction chemotherapy with three cycles of cisplatin, epirubicin and taxol followed by concomitant chemoradiation did not significantly improve response rates, progression free or overall survival relative to concomitant chemoradiation alone; 3- year overall survival was quoted as 66.6 and 71.8% respectively ($p = 0.652$). Contrary to the afore mentioned trial, Hui EP et al. [12] in a phase II trial, reported 3- year overall survival of 94.1 and 67.7% with a p value of 0.012 in favor of neoadjuvant chemotherapy. A recent trial by Sun Y and colleagues demonstrated a 3- year failure free survival of 80% in the group that received neoadjuvant chemotherapy using cisplatin, docetaxel and 5- fluorouracil followed by concurrent chemoradiation, relative to 72% in the group that received concurrent chemoradiation alone, $p = 0.034$, but with more toxicity [20].

There are similar studies that seem to suggest that upfront chemotherapy followed by concomitant chemoradiotherapy has high efficacy, demonstrated by progression free and overall survival, but these outcomes were not compared to concomitant chemoradiation alone [18, 21].

Neoadjuvant chemotherapy followed by radiotherapy may significantly reduce the risk of locoregional recurrence and distant metastases and may improve disease specific survival in locally advanced nasopharyngeal cancer as demonstrated by Chua et al. [10], and therefore has a theoretical potential to confer improvement in overall survival, it must however be noted that in that study it was compared to radiotherapy alone. In a phase 2 study involving neoadjuvant chemotherapy followed by concurrent chemoradiation by Kong L et al., docetaxel was given in addition to cisplatin and 5-fluorouracil prior to concurrent cisplatin based chemoradiation and a 3-year overall survival of 90.2% was reported in patients with stage IVA/IVB disease, thus demonstrating the potential high efficacy of this maneuver [22].

Despite the above, an interim analysis of a phase 3 study in which patients received three cycles of a 3-weekly regimen that employed relatively newer agents viz gemcitabine, carboplatin and paclitaxel prior to cisplatin based concurrent chemoradiation compared to concurrent chemoradiation alone was reported early because it had crossed the statistical boundary for futility in the use of neoadjuvant chemotherapy. There was no statistically significant difference between the two arms for overall survival, disease free survival and distant metastases free survival [23]. There was however considerably higher hematological toxicity and fatigue in the neoadjuvant chemotherapy group even though global quality of life scores were identical.

A recent study from Taiwan comparing concurrent chemoradiotherapy to neoadjuvant chemotherapy followed by radiation alone also failed to show superiority of neoadjuvant chemotherapy, reporting similar 5-year overall survival, indeed among patients who were recurrence-free in the first 2 years after treatment, those treated with neoadjuvant chemotherapy experienced poorer locoregional control that reached statistical significance [24]. It is believed that neoadjuvant chemotherapy leads to selection of resistant cell, accelerated repopulation and reduced compliance to chemoradiation, perhaps this deficiency is offset by concurrent chemoradiation more efficiently than radiation alone.

Toxicity reporting in our study was inadequate.

Modern radiotherapy is performed using Intensity Modulated Radiation Therapy (IMRT) or Volume Modulated Arc Therapy (VMAT). We also acknowledge that there could be stage migration if the patients had been staged with Magnetic Resonance Imaging (MRI); this imaging modality can also improve tumor localization during target volume delineation and therefore afford better tumor control. Despite these deficiencies, we believe that both groups were subjected to the same staging procedures, and treatment, and therefore any difference in outcomes is attributable to the treatment they received and not the sophistication of the treatment received.

Conclusion
The epidemiology of nasopharyngeal cancer in our setting is similar to endemic regions with a predominance of the type 3 variety. Neoadjuvant chemotherapy followed by concurrent chemoradiation did not improve disease free or overall survival compared to concurrent chemoradiation alone in this group of patients. Neoadjuvant chemotherapy appears to be associated with more hematological toxicity, and may be responsible for more failures in the nasopharynx.

Abbreviations
CT scan: Computed tomography scan; CXR: Chest X Ray; DNA: Deoxy ribonucleic acid; EBER: Epstein barr encoded RNA; EBV: Epstein barr virus; ECOG: Eastern cooperative oncology group; IMRT: Intensity modulated radiation therapy; VMAT: Volume modulated arc therapy; WHO: World health organization

Acknowledgements
Nil.

Funding
The authors did not receive any funding in executing this research.

Authors' contributions
JY: Developed the concept, managed patients, contributed to statistical analysis, did chart review and wrote sections of the paper. NAA: Wrote sections of the paper and did chart review. AM: Did the statistical analysis and wrote sections of the paper. CA: Contributed to the statistical analysis. VV: Managed patients and wrote sections of the paper. KB: Contributed patients and wrote sections of the paper. EDK: Contributed patients, did chart review and wrote sections of the paper. All authors read and approved the final manuscript.

Competing interests
The authors declare that they have no competing interests.

Author details
[1]National Center for Radiotherapy and NuclearMedicine Korle bu Teaching, Hospital P.O. Box KB 369, Accra, Ghana. [2]School of Medicine and Dentistry, Accra, Ghana. [3]School of Biomedical and Allied Health Science University of Ghana, Accra, Ghana. [4]Department of Mathematics and Statistics, Accra Technical University, Accra, Ghana. [5]Ear Nose and Throat Unit, Department of Surgery, Accra, Ghana.

References

1. Torre LA, Bray F, Siegel RL, Ferlay J, Lortet- Tieulent J, Jemal A. Global Cancer Statistics 2012 CA. Cancer J Clin. 2015;65:87–108.

2. Wee J, Tan EH, Tai BC, Wong HB, Leong SS, Tan T, et al. Randomized trial of radiotherapy versus concurrent chemoradiotherapy followed by adjuvant chemotherapy in patients with American Joint Committee on Cancer/ International Union against cancer stage III and IV nasopharyngeal cancer of the endemic variety. J Clin Oncol. 2005;23:6730–8.

3. Yarney J, Vanderpuye V, Kitcher ED. Treatment outcome of locally advanced nasopharyngeal cancer with concurrent chemoradiotherapy. West Afr J Med. 2008;27(2):65–8.

4. Chan KC, Hung EC, Woo JK, Chan PK, Leung SF, Lai FP, et al. Early detection of nasopharyngeal carcinoma by plasma Epstein Barr virus DNA analysis in a surveillance programme. Cancer. 2013;119(10):1839–44.

5. Taylor GS, Jia H, Harrington K, Lee LW, Turner J, Ladell K, et al. A recombinant modified vaccinia Ankara vaccine encoding Epstein- Barr virus targeted antigens: a phase 1 trial in UK patients with EBV-positive cancer. Clin Cancer Res. 2014;20:5009–22.

6. Al-Sarraf M, LeBlanc M, Giri PG, Fu KK, Cooper J, Vuong T, et al. Chemoradiotherapy versus radiotherapy in patients with advanced nasopharyngeal cancer: phase III randomized Intergroup study 0099. J Clin Oncol. 1998;16:1310–7.

7. Baujat B, Audry H, Bourhis J, Chan AT, Onat H, Chua DT, et al. Chemotherapy in locally advanced nasopharyngeal carcinoma: an individual patient data meta-analysis of eight randomized trials and 1753 patients. Int J Radiat Oncol Biol Phys. 2006;4:47–56.

8. Langendijk JA, Leemans CR, Buter J, Berkhof J, Slotman BJ. The additional value of chemotherapy to radiotherapy in locally advanced nasopharyngeal carcinoma: a meta-analysis of the published literature. J Clin Oncol. 2004;22:4604–12.

9. Blanchard P, Lee A, Marguet S, Leclercq J, Ng WT, Ma J, et al. Chemotherapy and radiotherapy in nasopharyngeal carcinoma: an update of the MAC-NPC meta-analysis. Lancet Oncol. 2015;16(6):645–55.

10. Chua DT, Ma J, Sham JS, Mai HQ, Choy DT, Hong MH, et al. Long- term survival after cisplatin-based induction chemotherapy and radiotherapy for nasopharyngeal carcinoma: a pooled data analysis of two phase III trials. J Clin Oncol. 2005;23:1118–24.

11. Fountzilas G, Ciuleanu E, Bobos M, Kalogera-Fountzila A, Eleftheraki AG, Karayannopoulou G, et al. Induction chemotherapy followed by concomitant radiotherapy and weekly cisplatin versus the same concomitant chemoradiotherapy in patients with nasopharyngeal carcinoma: a randomized phase II study conducted by the Hellenic Cooperative Oncology Group (HeCOG) with biomarker evaluation. Ann Oncol. 2012;23:427–35.

12. Hui EP, Ma BB, Leung SF, King AD, Mo F, Kam MK, et al. Randomized phase II trial of concurrent cisplatin-radiotherapy with or without neoadjuvant docetaxel and cisplatin in advanced nasopharyngeal carcinoma. J Clin Oncol. 2009;27:242–9.

13. Al- Amro A, Al Rajhi N, Khfaga Y, Memon M, Al Hebshi A, El-Enbabi A, et al. Neoadjuvant chemotherapy followed by concurrent chemo-radiation in locally advanced nasopharyngeal cancer. Int J Rad Oncol. 2005;62(2):508–13.

14. Chen L, Hu CS, Chen XZ, Hu GQ, Cheng ZB, Sun Y. Concurrent chemoradiotherapy plus adjuvant chemotherapy versus concurrent chemotherapy alone in patients with locoregionally advanced nasopharyngeal carcinoma: a phase 3 multi-centre randomized controlled trial. Lancet Oncol. 2012;13(2):163–71.

15. Kao WC, Chen J-S, Yen C-J. Advanced nasopharyngeal carcinoma in children. J Cancer Res Pract. 2016;3(3):84–8.

16. Liu W, Tang Y, Gao L, Huang X, Luo J, Zhang S, et al. Nasopharyngeal carcinoma in children and adolescents-a single institution experience of 158 patients Radiation. Oncology. 2014;9:274.

17. Ayan I, Kaytan E, Ayan N. Childhood nasopharyngeal carcinoma: from biology to treatment. Lancet Oncol. 2003;4(1):13–21.

18. Chen YP, Guo R, Liu N, Liu X, Mao YP, Tang L-L, et al. Efficacy of the additional neoadjuvant chemotherapy to concurrent chemoradiotherapy for patients with locoregionally advanced nasopharyngeal carcinoma: a Bayesian network meta- analysis of randomized controlled trials. J Cancer. 2015;6(9):883–92.

19. Song JH, Wu H-G, Keam BS, Han JH, Ahn YC, Oh D, et al. The role of neoadjuvant chemotherapy in the treatment of nasopharyngeal carcinoma: a multi-institutional retrospective study (KROG 11–06) using propensity score matching analysis. Cancer Res Treat. 2016;48(3):917–27.

20. Sun Y, Li W-F, Chen N-Y, Zhang N, Hu G-Q, Xie F-Y, et al. Induction chemotherapy plus concurrent chemotherapy versus concurrent chemotherapy alone in locoregionally advanced nasopharyngeal carcinoma: a phase 3, multicenter randomized controlled trial. Lancet Oncol. 2016;17(11):1509–20.

21. Golden DW, Rudra S, Witt ME, Nwizu T, Cohen EEW, Blair E. Outcomes of induction chemotherapy followed by concurrent chemoradiation for nasopharyngeal cancer. Oral Oncol. 2013;49(3):277–82.

22. Kong L, Hu C, Niu X, Zhang Y, Guo Y, Tham IW. Neoadjuvant chemotherapy followed by concurrent chemoradiation for locally advanced nasopharyngeal carcinoma: Interim results from two prospective phase 2 clinical trials. Cancer. 2013;119(23):4111–8.

23. Tan T, Lim WT, Fong KW, Cheah SL, Soong YL, Ang MK et al. Randomized phase III trial of concurrent chemoradiation with or without neoadjuvant gemcitabine, carboplatin, and paclitaxel in locally advanced nasopharyngeal cancer. J ClinOncol 32:5 s, 2014(suppl; abstr 6003).

24. Wu SY, Wu YH, Yang MW, Hsueh WT, Hsiao JR, Tsai ST, et al. Comparison of concurrent chemoradiotherapy versus neoadjuvant chemotherapy followed by radiation in patients with advanced nasopharyngeal carcinoma in endemic area: experience of 128 consecutive cases with 5-year follow-up. BMC Cancer. 2014;14:787.

16

A review of weight loss and sarcopenia in patients with head and neck cancer treated with chemoradiation

Shrujal S. Baxi[1]* (iD), Emily Schwitzer[2] and Lee W. Jones[2]

Abstract

Background: Concurrent chemotherapy and radiation (CTRT) improves disease-free survival in locally advanced head and neck cancer but is associated with numerous acute and chronic toxicities resulting in substantial alterations in body mass and composition. We aim to summarize the current evidence on body composition changes experienced by patients undergoing CTRT, examine the impact of these changes on clinical outcomes and address potential interventions aimed at mitigating the loss.

Main Body: Loss of 20 % of pre-CTRT weight predicts poorer treatment tolerance and 30-day mortality. While clinical practice focuses on body weight, emerging data indicates that CTRT causes profound adverse changes in lean body mass (sarcopenia). Higher prevalence of sarcopenia predicts poorer disease-free survival as well as overall survival, lower quality of life and functional performance. The magnitude of CTRT-induced sarcopenia is the equivalent to that observed in a decade of aging in a healthy adult. Alterations in body composition are only explained, in part, by decreased caloric intake; other significant predictors include body mass index, stage, and dysphagia. Lifestyle interventions aimed at preventing loss of whole-body and especially lean mass include nutritional counseling, nutritional supplements, dietary supplements and exercise training. Personalized nutritional counseling has been associated with improvement in quality of life, while the benefits of feeding tube placement are inconsistent. There are inconsistently reported benefits of resistance training in this population.

Conclusion: Patients with head and neck cancer undergoing CTRT therapy experience dramatic shifts in body composition, including sarcopenia, which can negatively impact clinical outcomes. Efforts to understand the magnitude, clinical importance and mechanisms of sarcopenia are needed to inform a more personalized approach to mitigating the body composition changes associated with CTRT.

Keywords: Head and neck cancer, Sarcopenia, Chemoradiation, Quality of life, Cardiopulmonary fitness, Nutrition

Background

Head and neck squamous cell carcinoma (HNSCC) is a group of diseases arising from the upper aerodigestive tract including the oral cavity, pharynx and larynx. There are an estimated 59,000 cases of HNSCC diagnosed annually in the US, representing 3 % of all newly identified cancers [1, 2]. Despite remaining relatively consistent in overall incidence, the epidemiology of HNSCC has changed over the last three decades, most notably in Western countries [3]. Once considered a disease resulting mostly from chronic exposure to tobacco and alcohol, it is now recognized that there are other causative factors for HNSCC. One of the fastest growing subsets of patients are those diagnosed with HNSCC tumors arising from the oropharynx secondary to human papilloma-virus (HPV) [4]. Patients with HPV-positive tumors have a striking improvement in survival compared with patients with historical, HPV-negative tumors with 3-year survival of 82 % versus 57 %, respectively $(p < 0.001)$ [5]. Patients with HPV-associated tumors also appear to have a lower risk of

* Correspondence: baxis@mskcc.org
[1]Head and Neck Oncology Service, Department of Medicine, Memorial Sloan Kettering Cancer Center, 300 East 66th Street, Rm 1459, New York, NY 10065, USA
Full list of author information is available at the end of the article

developing second primary malignancies, resulting in longer long-term survival [5, 6]. Changing epidemiology along with treatment advances have resulted in a rise in the number of survivors of HNSCC who are expected to live well beyond their cancer diagnosis and treatment. Efforts are underway to better understand the toxicities associated with treatment and implement strategies aimed at improving the long-term quality of life and survival in this emerging cohort of cancer survivors [7].

Main text

Approximately 70 % of patients with HNSCC will present with locally advanced disease and many will be treated with concurrent chemotherapy and radiation (CTRT). Concurrent chemotherapy and radiation is associated with significant in-field and systemic toxicities including mucositis, dysphagia, odynophagia, nausea, vomiting, anorexia, fatigue and dysgeusia resulting in difficulty eating [8–10]. Furthermore, many patients present with symptomatic tumors that lead to difficulty eating prior to the initiation of treatment, with most patients experiencing a loss of more than 5 % of pretreatment body weight in the 6 months around CTRT [11–14]. In part, this has been exacerbated by a change in resting energy expenditure, which furthers the loss of lean body mass seen during and immediately after treatment [11, 15]. Predictors of excessive weight loss during treatment include higher weight at baseline, dysphagia at diagnosis, and higher stage tumors [16]. More specifically, a recent study from Denmark reported that patients with a body mass index (BMI) ≥ 25 are three times more likely to lose more than 5 % of baseline weight than patients with BMI < 25 ($p < 0.0001$) [12].

Weight loss has been negatively associated with tumor control and survival outcomes in HNSCC [13]. For example, patients with early significant weight loss (defined as >20 % loss from baseline) are more likely to die from a treatment-related complication within 30 days of completing CTRT compared to those who do not ($p = 0.029$). In a secondary analysis from the phase III SAKK 10/94 trial of hyperfractionated radiation versus cisplatin and standard fraction radiation, Ghadjar and colleagues found that weight loss during treatment on either arm was common, but only weight loss experienced before treatment was associated with decreased time to treatment failure, disease free survival (DFS), and overall survival (OS) ($p < 0.05$ for all); weight loss occurring during treatment was not associated with survival outcomes [14]. The results from this study highlight two important aspects of weight loss and HNSCC. First, patients who are already losing weight at diagnosis are at a disadvantage and may be presenting with more aggressive disease at baseline. Second, while weight loss during treatment

is common, it is not universally prognostic. One explanation for this discrepancy is that in some patients the weight loss is caused of decreased caloric intake, while in others weight loss is a manifestation of cachexia, or a syndrome of dysregulated catabolism and anabolism [17]. Historically, high-risk patients would have a percutaneous endoscopic gastrostomy (PEG) placed prior to starting treatment in order to prevent decreased caloric intake, but more recently there has been movement away from using feeding tubes due to concerns about delayed recovery of swallowing post-CTRT [18–20]. Interestingly, the placement of a PEG, or increased caloric intake alone, does not alleviate all the weight loss experienced during CTRT [12, 19, 21].

The weight loss experienced by patients with HNSCC undergoing CTRT is more specifically a change in body composition. Body weight or body mass is composed of fat, bone, water and lean body mass and the loss of lean body mass accounts for more than 70 % of weight lost during CTRT [15, 22]. Loss of lean body mass in cancer is mostly explained by sarcopenia, or loss of skeletal muscle [23]. Patients with HNSCC undergoing CTRT are often losing more than 5 % of their total muscle mass in less than 6 months time which is equivalent to the amount of muscle mass lost in the average, inactive adult over the course of a decade [24–26]. Skeletal muscle is the largest organ in the body and makes up approximately 50 % of total body weight and is essential for movement, strength, balance, body temperature regulation and respiration. Maintaining muscle mass involves a balance of protein breakdown (catabolism) and muscle synthesis (anabolism) and is tightly regulated through a network of external signaling pathways leading to intracellular gene transcription [22]. Lean body mass, mostly composed of muscle, can be measured using both validated direct and indirect methods. Examples of possible techniques include bioelectrical impedance (BIA), measurement of air displacement plethysmography, dual energy x-ray (DXA, and cross-sectional imaging on computed tomography (CT) or magnetic resonance imaging (MRI) [27].

Importantly, loss of lean body mass is associated with poorer treatment tolerance and worse cancer outcomes [28–30]. For example, in patients receiving systemic chemotherapy for colorectal cancer, loss of ≥ 9 % muscle mass during a 3 month period was independently predictive of lower survival at 6 months compared to patients who had < 9 % loss, 33 % versus 69 %, respectively, despite no difference in treatment modifications [31]. Similar associations have been described in patients with HNSCC. Grossberg and colleagues recently reported that in a cohort of 190 patients with HNSCC treated with definitive radiation, decreased overall survival was associated with baseline sarcopenia (Hazard

Ratio (HR) 1.92, 95 % confidence interval [CI] 1.19–3.11) and post-radiation sarcopenia (HR 2.03, 95 % CI 1.02–4.24). However, in this analysis, weight loss alone, without associated loss of skeletal muscle, was not associated with worse clinical outcomes [32]. Further, when they evaluated by subsites, skeletal muscle depletion was associated with decreased survival in patients with non-oropharyngeal cancer ($n = 51$) but not in patients with oropharyngeal cancer ($n = 139$). This is a retrospective study and while causation cannot be gleaned, the results highlight that patients with more significant loss of skeletal muscle are experiencing poorer clinical outcomes. Further, it also highlights that patients with HNSCC are a heterogenous group and more research is necessary to understand what, and if any, relationship exists between change in body composition and oncologic outcomes. Emerging data suggests that patients with HPV-related oropharyngeal cancer, generally a healthier and younger population at diagnosis, are also experiencing significant alterations in body composition as a result of CTRT, but that this may not negatively impact the expected excellent clinical outcomes, at least not at early follow-up [33].

Sarcopenia is not only relevant for oncologic outcomes, but is predictive of worse survival in the general, non-cancer, and population as well. It is associated with numerous negative outcomes, including an impaired stress response, frailty, functional impairment, lower quality of life and decreased overall survival [34–37]. As such, acute sarcopenia, could then explain, at least in part, the dramatic drop in quality of life experienced by even the most functional patients at baseline who undergo CTRT for HNSCC [38]. In a large cross-sectional study in people over the age of 65, sarcopenia predicted for three times more functional impairment in females and two times more functional impairment in males compared to age- and sex-matched participants with normal lean body mass [39]. Further, a large portion of age-associated decline in cardiopulmonary fitness, measured by VO_{2peak}, is also explained by sarcopenia [40]. Low cardiorespiratory fitness is an important precursor for premature mortality regardless of underlying cardiovascular risk factors [41]. Altogether, this highlights the need for studies to better understand the impact of sarcopenia sustained during CTRT and its impact on cardiorespiratory fitness and subsequent non-oncologic mortality in patients with HNSCC.

The current strategies employed to combat metabolic derangements experienced by patients during CTRT generally focus on weight maintenance. Patients are encouraged to eat "as many calories as they can" and when food gets harder to swallow, supplementing it with either oral or parenteral nutrition via a PEG [42]. However, decreased caloric intake is probably only partially responsible for sarcopenia and simply increasing calories may not address loss of muscle mass. In a review of sarcopenia and cachexia in patients with all stages of HNSCC, Couch and colleagues describe the dysregulated metabolism and the resulting sarcopenia seen in patients with HNSCC, suggesting that nutrition alone is not enough to counteract the impact of body composition [21]. In spite of this, numerous studies have tried to optimize nutritional support in patients undergoing CTRT. Clinical trials have evaluated the benefit of individualized nutrition counseling, oral supplementation, and the right type and route of supplemental nutrition. In a systematic review on the effect of nutritional interventions on weight, quality of life and mortality in HNSCC patients treated with RT or CTRT, individualized dietary counseling was beneficial on quality of life, but the impact of tube feedings was not conclusive [43]. For example, in a prospective study of patients with HNSCC undergoing RT, Ravasco and colleagues found that nutritional counseling with regular foods was superior to only adding nutritional supplements in maintaining quality of life during and at 3 months post-RT, but the impact of these interventions on weight was not reported [44]. In a large retrospective review of patients on RTOG 90-03, investigators performed a secondary analysis of patients with HNSCC treated with four different radiation strategies, Rabinovitch and colleagues found that beginning nutritional supplementation before starting RT was a negative prognostic indicator for locoregional failure and death, HR 1.47, 95 % CI 1.21–1.79, $p < .0001$ and HR 1.41, 95 % CI 1.19–1.67, $p < .0001$, respectively [45]. Given the retrospective nature of this analysis, nutritional supplement was likely initiated pre-RT in patients who presented with weight loss at diagnosis. This suggests that patients with baseline weight loss have a worse clinical outcomes and not that nutritional supplement itself is having a negative impact on outcomes.

Integration of optimal nutritional support into clinical practice for HNSCC patients has been impeded due to the inconsistent methodology across studies, measuring various time points and outcomes. In response, a group of investigators published a review of the current state of the science on nutrition and malnutrition in HNSCC and provided a set of consensus criteria for implementation and definitions in studies on nutrition in this population [46].

There is growing interest in using pharmacologic supplements to combat cancer-related sarcopenia and cachexia, including amino acids, anabolic steroids, anti-inflammatory agents, and ghrelin-analogues, to counteract the deranged metabolism experienced by cancer patients. Most research in this space has been completed in patients with metastatic disease, often non-small cell lung cancer [44]. One agent of interest in HNSCC patients is eicosapentaenoic acid (EPA), which is an alpha-3-omega fatty acid found in fish oil. In vitro, EPA has been shown to mitigate the lipolysis and inflammatory underpinnings of cachexia [47, 48]. Patients with HNSCC undergoing primary surgical approach did show short-term benefit in loss of muscle mass with EPA, but longer-term follow is needed [49]. A Cochrane review on the use of EPA in cancer cachexia was completed in 2007 and recommended against regular use of EPA [50]. An alternative approach recently explored is anamorelin, an oral ghrelin mimetic. Ghrelin is a ligand for the growth hormone secretagogue receptor and leads to

release of growth hormone. There have been two large phase III, double blind placebo-controlled trials of anamorelin in patients with cachexia resulting from unresectable lung cancer. The two studies included a combination of more 900 patients and reported improvement in body weight and anorexia with anamorelin but no improvement in overall survival or strength [51]. Hopefully, pharmacologic interventions will follow a better understanding of the exact mechanism of sarcopenia in patients with HNSCC undergoing CTRT.

Another intervention with the potential to counteract the negative effects of CTRT on body composition is exercise. Exercise has emerged as a promising

Table 1 Prospective Studies on resistance training in patients with head and neck cancer

Author	Subjects	Exercise Intervention	Major Findings
McNeely et al. 2008	52 HNSCC patients after neck dissection	12 week supervised PRT (2-3x/week) versus standard of care.	Adherence: 95 % for PRT group and 87 % for control group.
			Outcomes: PRT was superior to standard of care for improving shoulder pain and disability ($p < 0.001$), upper extremity strength ($p < 0.001$), and upper extremity endurance ($p < 0.039$)
Lonbro, DAHANCA 25A 2013	30 HNSCC patients after curative radiotherapy +/- chemotherapy	12 week partially supervised PRT (2-3x/week) with or without a seven day creatinine load	Adherence: 97 % in those that completed the study with a completion rate of 70 %
			Outcomes: Addition of creatinine to PRT did not improve lean body mass ($p = 0.07$). Regardless of nutritional intervention, improvement noted after PRT in lean body mass and maximal isometric and isokinetic muscle strength.
Lonbro, DAHANCA 25B 2013	41 HNSCC patients after curative radiotherapy +/- chemotherapy	24 week study of early versus delayed 12 week supervised PRT (2-3x/week).	Adherence: Not reported
			Outcomes: Increase in lean body mass by 4.3 % and 4.2 % in early versus delayed PRT. Improvement larger than change after self-chosen physical activity ($p < 0.005$). Regardless of PRT start-up time, the odds ratio of increasing LBM by more than 4 % after PRT was 6.26 ($p < 0.05$).
Rogers et al. 2013	15 HNSCC patients during radiation therapy	12 week supervised PRT (2x/week) for 6 weeks then at home PRT (2x/week) versus standard of care.	Adherence: 83 % for supervised exercise and 62 % for exercise telephone counseling.
			Outcomes: PRT improved in fatigue and quality of life at 6 weeks versus control. Chair rise time (seconds) improved at 6 and 12 weeks in PRT arm versus standard of care (-1.6 vs 0.4 respectively, $p < 0.05$).
Samuel et al. 2013	48 HNSCC patients during CRT	6 week supervised general exercise program (5-6x/week) versus routine physical activity encouragement.	Adherence: not recorded
			Outcomes: Increased 6MWD in the intervention arm, decreased in the control arm with a 138 m difference between groups ($p < 0.001$).
Capozzi et al. 2016	60 newly diagnosed HNSCC patients during RT or CRT	24 week study of immediate versus delayed with a 12 week supervised PRT (2x/week) and nutrition intervention.	Adherence: 45.2 % in immediate group and 61.5 % in delayed group.
			Outcomes: No difference in lean body mass or percentage body fat at 24 weeks.

AE adverse event, *CRT* concurrent chemoradiotherapy, *HNSCC* head and neck squamous cell cancer, *PRT* progressive resistance training, *RT* radiation therapy, *6MWD* six minute walk distance

component of cancer care and has been shown to improve clinical and survival outcomes [52–54]. In a large systematic review and meta-analysis, Speck and colleagues reported favorable changes of exercise on body composition, cardiopulmonary fitness, muscular fitness, psychological well-being, flexibility and quality of life for cancer patients both during and after treatment. While this study included 82 trials, few of the included studies focused on patients with HNSCC [55]. Of those that did, the majority used a progressive resistance training program to improve muscle quantity, quality and function. As sarcopenia and impaired physical functioning remain primary concerns for these patients, this becomes clinically important. Indeed, randomized studies from both breast and prostate cancer patients have shown that resistance training can increase lean muscle mass compared to the control (i.e., sedentary) group [52, 54, 56, 57]. This contrasts to aerobic (or endurance) exercise training, which primarily focuses on improving one's peak oxygen consumption (VO_{2peak}) – another independent predictor of survival in both oncologic and non-oncologic populations alike. Together, aerobic and resistance exercise training, are complementary to both the cardiovascular and musculoskeletal system.

Against this background, exercise is increasingly being explored as a potential method to combat the negative impact of HNSCC and its treatment on patients. A prior cross-sectional study demonstrated that HNSCC patients get less than the recommended level of activity at all time points; specifically, only 30.5 % are active at baseline, falling to only 8.5 % of patients at the end of treatment [58]. This demonstrates the great potential for exercise to improve outcomes in this currently inactive group. There is good data available on the benefit of therapeutic exercises for shoulder dysfunction or trismus resulting from fibrosis following treatment, but the systemic impacts of exercise in HNSCC are less well understood. We performed a review and summarized the data from studies on progressive resistance training in patients treated for locally advanced HNSCC (Table 1). There was considerable heterogeneity in the study methodology, differing in the type and timing of exercise intervention, as well as the outcomes measured. Regardless, it is clear from the control arms, when available, that there is a negative impact of no intervention [59, 60]. Much like the limitations of current literature in nutritional interventions for HNSCC, there is a need to standardize research in exercise interventions including the type, timing, frequency and duration of studied regimens. Only then can the results from one study be compared to the next and provide measurable, reproducible and generalizable interventions that are relevant to clinical practice.

Conclusions

HNSCC survivors remain at a substantial risk for long-term disability and early mortality despite achieving initial tumor control [58, 61]. Younger patients are now presenting with HNSCC due to the epidemic of HPV-related oropharyngeal cancer and have an expected better overall prognosis. As these patients live longer past diagnosis, maintaining quality of life and long-term survival is paramount. Longitudinal studies are required to measure the rates of recovery of weight and lean body mass and then in turn, discover new strategies to assist patients as they try to return to baseline functional capacity after aggressive CTRT therapy. Patients with HNSCC are unique in the challenges they face, and the applicability of studies performed in other cancer populations may not be directly relevant to these patients; standardized nutritional and exercise interventions are needed for HNSCC.

Abbreviations
CI, confidence interval; CTRT, concurrent chemotherapy and radiation; DFS, disease free survival; HNSCC, head and neck squamous cell carcinoma; HPV, human papillomavirus; HR, hazards ratio; OS, Overall survival; PEG, percutaneous endoscopic gastrostomy; RT, radiation

Acknowledgements
We have no acknowledgements to report.

Funding
This work was also supported by a Cancer Center Support Grant from the National Cancer Institute to Memorial Sloan Kettering Cancer Center (award number P30 CA008748).

Authors' contributions
SB made substantial contributions to conception and design, drafted the manuscript and ensures the integrity of the work. ES made substantial contributions to conception and design, drafted parts of the manuscript and ensures the integrity of the work. LJ contributed to the conception and design and ensures the integrity of the work. All authors read and approved the final manuscript.

Competing interests
The authors declare that they have no competing interests however SSB does serve on an advisory board for AstraZeneca and Lilly Oncology and serves as a consultant for Bristol Myers Squibb.

Author details
[1]Head and Neck Oncology Service, Department of Medicine, Memorial Sloan Kettering Cancer Center, 300 East 66th Street, Rm 1459, New York, NY 10065, USA. [2]Department of Medicine, Memorial Sloan Kettering Cancer Center, 1275 York Ave, New York, NY 10065, USA.

References
1. Siegel R, Miller K, Jemal A. Cancer statistics, 2015. CA Cancer J Clin. 2015; 64(1):5–29. doi:10.3322/caac.21254.
2. Jemal A, Bray F, Center MM, Ferlay J, Ward E, Forman D. Global cancer statistics. CA Cancer J Clin. 2011;61(2):69–90. doi:10.3322/caac.20107.

3. Chaturvedi A, Anderson W, Lortet-Tieulent J, Curado M, Ferlay J, Franceschi S, et al. Worldwide trends in incidence rates for oral cavity and oropharyngeal cancers. J Clin Oncol. 2013;31(36):4550–9. doi:10.1200/JCO.2013.50.3870.

4. Simard EP, Torre LA, Jemal A. International trends in head and neck cancer incidence rates: differences by country, sex and anatomic site. Oral Oncol. 2014;50(5):387–403. doi:10.1016/j.oraloncology.2014.01.016.

5. Ang K, Harris J, Wheeler R, Weber R, Rosenthal D, Nguyen-Tan P, et al. Human papillomavirus and survival of patients with oropharyngeal cancer. N Engl J Med. 2010;363(1):24–35. doi:10.1056/NEJMoa0912217.

6. Licitra L, Perrone F, Bossi P, Suardi S, Mariani L, Artusi R, et al. High-risk human papillomavirus affects prognosis in patients with surgically treated oropharyngeal squamous cell carcinoma. J Clin Oncol. 2006;24(36):5630–6. doi:10.1200/JCO.2005.04.6136.

7. Ringash J. Survivorship and quality of life in head and neck cancer. J Clin Oncol. 2015;33(29):3322–7. doi:10.1200/jco.2015.61.4115.

8. Adelstein D, Li Y, Adams G, Wagner H, Kish J, Ensley J, et al. An intergroup phase III comparison of standard radiation therapy and two schedules of concurrent chemoradiotherapy in patients with unresectable squamous cell head and neck cancer. J Clin Oncol. 2003;21(1):92–8.

9. Forastiere A, Goepfert H, Maor M, Pajak T, Weber R, Morrison W, et al. Concurrent chemotherapy and radiotherapy for organ preservation in advanced laryngeal cancer. N Engl J Med. 2003;349(22):2091–8. doi:10.1056/NEJMoa031317.

10. List MA, Siston A, Haraf D, Schumm P, Kies M, Stenson K, et al. Quality of life and performance in advanced head and neck cancer patients on concomitant chemoradiotherapy: a prospective examination. J Clin Oncol. 1999;17(3):1020.

11. García-Peris P, Lozano MA, Velasco C, de La Cuerda C, Iriondo T, Bretón I, et al. Prospective study of resting energy expenditure changes in head and neck cancer patients treated with chemoradiotherapy measured by indirect calorimetry. Nutrition. 2005;21(11–12):1107–12. http://dx.doi.org/10.1016/j.nut.2005.03.006.

12. Lonbro S, Petersen GB, Andersen JR, Johansen J. Prediction of critical weight loss during radiation treatment in head and neck cancer patients is dependent on BMI. Support Care Cancer. 2016;24(5):2101–9. doi:10.1007/s00520-015-2999-8.

13. Mick R, Vokes EE, Weichselbaum RR, Panje WR. Prognostic factors in advanced head and neck cancer patients undergoing multimodality therapy. Otolaryngol Head Neck Surg. 1991;105(1):62–73.

14. Ghadjar P, Hayoz S, Zimmermann F, Bodis S, Kaul D, Badakhshi H, et al. Impact of weight loss on survival after chemoradiation for locally advanced head and neck Cancer: secondary results of a randomized phase III trial (SAKK 10/94). Radiat Oncol. 2015;10(1):21.

15. Silver HJ, Dietrich MS, Murphy BA. Changes in body mass, energy balance, physical function, and inflammatory state in patients with locally advanced head and neck cancer treated with concurrent chemoradiation after low-dose induction chemotherapy. Head Neck. 2007;29(10):893–900. doi:10.1002/hed.20607.

16. Nourissat A, Bairati I, Samson E, Fortin A, Gelinas M, Nabid A, et al. Predictors of weight loss during radiotherapy in patients with stage I or II head and neck cancer. Cancer. 2010;116(9):2275–83. doi:10.1002/cncr.25041.

17. Couch ME, Dittus K, Toth MJ, Willis MS, Guttridge DC, George JR, et al. Cancer cachexia update in head and neck cancer: pathophysiology and treatment. Head Neck. 2015;37(7):1057–72. doi:10.1002/hed.23696.

18. Caudell JJ, Schaner PE, Meredith RF, Locher JL, Nabell LM, Carroll WR, et al. Factors associated with long-term dysphagia after definitive radiotherapy for locally advanced head-and-neck cancer. Int J Radiat Oncol Biol Phys. 2009;73(2):410–5. http://dx.doi.org/10.1016/j.ijrobp.2008.04.048.

19. Langmore S, Krisciunas GP, Miloro KV, Evans SR, Cheng DM. Does PEG use cause dysphagia in head and neck cancer patients? Dysphagia. 2011;27(2):251–9. doi:10.1007/s00455-011-9360-2.

20. Mekhail TM, Adelstein DJ, Rybicki LA, Larto MA, Saxton JP, Lavertu P. Enteral nutrition during the treatment of head and neck carcinoma. Cancer. 2001;91(9):1785–90. doi:10.1002/1097-0142(20010501)91:9<1785::AID-CNCR1197>3.0.CO;2-1.

21. Couch M, Lai V, Cannon T, Guttridge D, Zanation A, George J et al. Cancer cachexia syndrome in head and neck cancer patients: part I. Diagnosis, impact on quality of life and survival, and treatment. Head Neck. 2007;29. doi:10.1002/hed.20447.

22. Lenk K, Schuler G, Adams V. Skeletal muscle wasting in cachexia and sarcopenia: molecular pathophysiology and impact of exercise training. J Cachexia Sarcopenia Muscle. 2010;1. doi:10.1007/s13539-010-0007-1.

23. Carmeli E, Coleman R, Reznick AZ. The biochemistry of aging muscle. Exp Gerontol. 2002;37(4):477–89. http://dx.doi.org/10.1016/S0531-5565(01)00220-0.

24. Doherty TJ. Invited Review: aging and sarcopenia. J Appl Physiol. 2003;95(4):1717–27. doi:10.1152/japplphysiol.00347.2003.

25. Tzankoff SP, Norris AH. Effect of muscle mass decrease on age-related BMR changes. J Appl Physiol. 1977;43(6):1001–6.

26. Forbes GB, Reina JC. Adult lean body mass declines with age: some longitudinal observations. Metabolism. 1970;19(9):653–63.

27. Mijnarends DM, Meijers JM, Halfens RJ, ter Borg S, Luiking YC, Verlaan S, et al. Validity and reliability of tools to measure muscle mass, strength, and physical performance in community-dwelling older people: a systematic review. J Am Med Dir Assoc. 2013;14(3):170–8. doi:10.1016/j.jamda.2012.10.009.

28. Prado CMM, Baracos VE, McCargar LJ, Reiman T, Mourtzakis M, Tonkin K, et al. Sarcopenia as a determinant of chemotherapy toxicity and time to tumor progression in metastatic breast cancer patients receiving capecitabine treatment. Clin Cancer Res. 2009;15(8):2920–6. doi:10.1158/1078-0432.ccr-08-2242.

29. McMillan DC, Watson WS, Preston T, McArdle CS. Lean body mass changes in cancer patients with weight loss. Clin Nutr. 2000;19(6):403–6. http://dx.doi.org/10.1054/clnu.2000.0136.

30. Kadar L, Albertsson M, Areberg J, Landberg T, Mattsson S. The prognostic value of body protein in patients with lung cancer. Ann N Y Acad Sci. 2000;904:584–91.

31. Blauwhoff-Buskermolen S, Versteeg KS, de van der Schueren MA, den Braver NR, Berkhof J, Langius JA, et al. Loss of muscle mass during chemotherapy is predictive for poor survival of patients with metastatic colorectal cancer. J Clin Oncol. 2016;34(12):1339–44.

32. Grossberg AJ, Chamchod S, Fuller CD, Mohamed AS, Heukelom J, Eichelberger H, et al. Association of body composition with survival and locoregional control of radiotherapy-treated head and neck squamous cell carcinoma. JAMA Oncol. 2016;2(6):782–9. doi:10.1001/jamaoncol.2015.6339.

33. Baxi SS Jones L, Eaton A, Gandelman S, Halpenny D, Jackson J, et al. Changes in body composition and prognostic importance of sarcopenia in patients receiving CTRT for oropharyngeal cancer. J Clin Oncol. 2016;34(supplement):abstr 6077.

34. Collins J, Noble S, Chester J, Coles B, Byrne A. The assessment and impact of sarcopenia in lung cancer: a systematic review. BMJ Open. 2014;46. doi:10.1136/bmjopen-2013-003697.

35. Pereira CT, Barrow RE, Sterns AM, Hawkins HK, Kimbrough CW, Jeschke MG, et al. Age-dependent differences in survival after severe burns: a unicentric review of 1,674 patients and 179 autopsies over 15 years. J Am Coll Surg. 2006;202(3):536–48. doi:10.1016/j.jamcollsurg.2005.11.002.

36. Evans WJ. What is sarcopenia? J Gerontol A Biol Sci Med Sci. 1995;50(Spec No):5–8.

37. Fulster S, Tacke M, Sandek A, Ebner N, Tschope C, Doehner W, et al. Muscle wasting in patients with chronic heart failure: results from the studies investigating co-morbidities aggravating heart failure (SICA-HF). Eur Heart J. 2013;34(7):512–9. doi:10.1093/eurheartj/ehs381.

38. Sharma A, Méndez E, Yueh B, Lohavanichbutr P, Houck J, Doody DR, et al. Human papillomavirus–positive oral cavity and oropharyngeal cancer patients do not have better quality-of-life trajectories. Otolaryngol Head Neck Surg. 2012;146(5):739–45.

39. Janssen I, Heymsfield SB, Ross R. Low relative skeletal muscle mass (sarcopenia) in older persons is associated with functional impairment and physical disability. J Am Geriatr Soc. 2002;50(5):889–96.

40. Fleg JL, Lakatta EG. Role of muscle loss in the age-associated reduction in VO2 max. J Appl Physiol. 1988;65(3):1147–51.

41. Blair SN, Kampert JB, Kohl HW, Barlow CE, Macera CA, Paffenbarger RS, et al. Influences of cardiorespiratory fitness and other precursors on cardiovascular disease and all-cause mortality in men and women. JAMA. 1996;276(3):205–10.

42. Ravasco P, Monteiro-Grillo I, Vidal PM, Camilo ME. Nutritional deterioration in cancer: the role of disease and diet. Clin Oncol. 2003;15(8):443–50. doi:10.1016/S0936-6555(03)00155-9.

43. Langius JA, Zandbergen MC, Eerenstein SE, van Tulder MW, Leemans CR, Kramer MH, et al. Effect of nutritional interventions on nutritional status,

quality of life and mortality in patients with head and neck cancer receiving (chemo)radiotherapy: a systematic review. Clin Nutr. 2013;32(5):671–8. doi:10.1016/j.clnu.2013.06.012.

44. Ravasco P, Monteiro-Grillo I, Marques Vidal P, Camilo ME. Impact of nutrition on outcome: a prospective randomized controlled trial in patients with head and neck cancer undergoing radiotherapy. Head Neck. 2005;27(8): 659–68. doi:10.1002/hed.20221.

45. Rabinovitch R, Grant B, Berkey BA, Raben D, Ang KK, Fu KK, et al. Impact of nutrition support on treatment outcome in patients with locally advanced head and neck squamous cell cancer treated with definitive radiotherapy: a secondary analysis of RTOG trial 90-03. Head Neck. 2006;28(4):287–96. doi:10.1002/hed.20335.

46. Dechaphunkul T, Martin L, Alberda C, Olson K, Baracos V, Gramlich L. Malnutrition assessment in patients with cancers of the head and neck: A call to action and consensus. Crit Rev Oncol Hematol. 2013;88(2):459–76. doi:10.1016/j.critrevonc.2013.06.003.

47. Wigmore SJ, Fearon KC, Maingay JP, Ross JA. Down-regulation of the acute-phase response in patients with pancreatic cancer cachexia receiving oral eicosapentaenoic acid is mediated via suppression of interleukin-6. Clin Sci. 1997;92(2):215–21.

48. Price SA, Tisdale MJ. Mechanism of inhibition of a tumor lipid-mobilizing factor by eicosapentaenoic acid. Cancer Res. 1998;58(21):4827–31.

49. Weed HG, Ferguson ML, Gaff RL, Hustead DS, Nelson JL, Voss AC. Lean body mass gain in patients with head and neck squamous cell cancer treated perioperatively with a protein-and energy-dense nutritional supplement containing eicosapentaenoic acid. Head Neck. 2011;33(7):1027–33.

50. Dewey A, Baughan C, Dean T, Higgins B, Johnson I. Eicosapentaenoic acid (EPA, an omega-3 fatty acid from fish oils) for the treatment of cancer cachexia. Cochrane Database Syst Rev. 2007(1):CD004597. doi:10.1002/14651858.CD004597.pub2.

51. Temel JS, Abernethy AP, Currow DC, Friend J, Duus EM, Yan Y, et al. Anamorelin in patients with non-small-cell lung cancer and cachexia (ROMANA 1 and ROMANA 2): results from two randomised, double-blind, phase 3 trials. Lancet Oncol. 2016;17(4):519–31. http://dx.doi.org/10.1016/S1470-2045(15)00558-6.

52. Schmitz KH, Ahmed RL, Hannan PJ, Yee D. Safety and efficacy of weight training in recent breast cancer survivors to alter body composition, insulin, and insulin-like growth factor axis proteins. Cancer Epidemiol Biomark Prev. 2005;14. doi:10.1158/1055-9965.epi-04-0736.

53. Mock V, Pickett M, Ropka ME, Muscari Lin E, Stewart KJ, Rhodes VA et al. Fatigue and quality of life outcomes of exercise during cancer treatment. Cancer Pract. 2001;9. doi:10.1046/j.1523-5394.2001.009003119.x.

54. Courneya KS, Mackey JR, Bell GJ, Jones LW, Field CJ, Fairey AS. Randomized controlled trial of exercise training in postmenopausal breast cancer survivors: cardiopulmonary and quality of life outcomes. J Clin Oncol. 2003; 21(9):1660–8.

55. Speck RM, Courneya KS, Masse LC, Duval S, Schmitz KH. An update of controlled physical activity trials in cancer survivors: a systematic review and meta-analysis. J Cancer Surviv. 2010;4. doi:10.1007/s11764-009-0110-5.

56. Segal RJ, Reid RD, Courneya KS, Malone SC, Parliament MB, Scott CG, et al. Resistance exercise in men receiving androgen deprivation therapy for prostate cancer. J Clin Oncol. 2003;21(9):1653–9. doi:10.1200/JCO.2003.09.534.

57. Galvão DA, Taaffe DR, Spry N, Joseph D, Newton RU. Combined resistance and aerobic exercise program reverses muscle loss in men undergoing androgen suppression therapy for prostate cancer without bone metastases: a randomized controlled trial. J Clin Oncol. 2010;28(2):340–7.

58. Rogers L, Courneya K, Robbins KT, Malone J, Seiz A, Koch L, et al. Physical activity and quality of life in head and neck cancer survivors. Support Care Cancer. 2006;14(10):1012–9. doi:10.1007/s00520-006-0044-7.

59. Samuel SR, Maiya GA, Babu AS, Vidyasagar MS. Effect of exercise training on functional capacity & quality of life in head & neck cancer patients receiving chemoradiotherapy. Indian J Med Res. 2013;137(3):515–20.

60. Rogers LQ, Anton PM, Fogleman A, Hopkins-Price P, Verhulst S, Rao K, et al. Pilot, randomized trial of resistance exercise during radiation therapy for head and neck cancer. Head Neck. 2013;35(8):1178–88. doi:10.1002/hed.23118.

61. Baxi SS, Pinheiro LC, Patil SM, Pfister DG, Oeffinger KC, Elkin EB. Causes of death in long-term survivors of head and neck cancer. Cancer. 2014;120(10):1507–13. doi:10.1002/cncr.28588.

17

Targeting phosphoinositide 3-kinase (PI3K) in head and neck squamous cell carcinoma (HNSCC)

Kyungsuk Jung[1]* ⓘ, Hyunseok Kang[2] and Ranee Mehra[2]

Abstract: The landscape of head and neck squamous cell carcinoma (HNSCC) has been changing rapidly due to growing proportion of HPV-related disease and development of new therapeutic agents. At the same time, there has been a constant need for individually tailored treatment based on genetic biomarkers in order to optimize patient survival and alleviate treatment-related toxicities. In this regard, aberrations of PI3K pathway have important clinical implications in the treatment of HNSCC. They frequently constitute 'gain of function' mutations which trigger oncogenesis, and PI3K mutations can also lead to emergence of drug resistance after treatment with EGFR inhibitors. In this article, we review PI3K pathway as a target of treatment for HNSCC and summarize PI3K/mTOR inhibitors that are currently under clinical trials. In light of recent advancement of immune checkpoint inhibitors, consideration of PI3K inhibitors as potential immune modulators is also suggested.

Keywords: HNSCC, PI3K, mTOR, Akt, EGFR, *PIK3CA*, HPV, Drug resistance, Precision medicine

Background

Head and neck squamous cell carcinoma (HNSCC) arises from mucosal epithelium of oral cavity, pharynx and larynx. An estimate of 61,000 new cases of HNSCC were diagnosed in the US in 2016, with 13,190 deaths attributable to the disease [1]. Traditional risk factors include tobacco smoking, alcohol consumption, betel nut chewing and genetic predisposition such as Fanconi anemia [2–4]. Human papillomavirus (HPV) has recently emerged as a major and distinct risk factor for HNSCC. HPV-related HNSCC most commonly arises in oropharynx and has been associated with younger age of disease onset, less smoking history, better performance status and favorable prognosis [5]. The proportion of HPV-positive oropharyngeal squamous cell cancer has significantly increased for the past decade regardless of sex and race [6], raising the need for a separate therapeutic strategy.

Comprehensive genomic analysis of HNSCC revealed frequent alterations in genes encoding molecules in phosphoinositide 3-kinase (PI3K) pathway including *PIK3CA*, *PTEN* and *PIK3R1* [7, 8]. In particular, HPV-

related HNSCC frequently harbors mutations in the helical domain of *PIK3CA*, yet its biological significance has not been fully elucidated. In the era of precision medicine, it is becoming more important to understand key genomic alterations and their therapeutic implications [9]. This review will focus on the role of PI3K-Akt-mTOR pathway in relation to epidermal growth factor receptor (EGFR) and their clinical applications in HNSCC.

Phosphoinositide 3-kinase (PI3K) and PI3K-Akt-mTOR pathway

PI3K is a family of phospholipid kinase that is divided into three classes based on structure, function and substrate specificity. Class I PI3K is a heterodimer that consists of a regulatory and a catalytic subunit. It is further divided into class IA and IB. For class IA PI3K, there are three variants of catalytic subunit, p110α, p110β and p110δ (encoded by *PIK3CA*, *PIK3CB* and *PIK3CD*), and five variants of regulatory subunit, p85α, p55α, p50α (encoded by *PIK3R1* and splice variants), p85β and p55δ (encoded by *PIK3R2* and *PIK3R3*). p85 regulatory subunit contains Src homology 2 (SH2) domain which binds to phosphorylated Y-X-X-M motif in receptor tyrosine kinase [10]. It was found that five isoforms of regulatory subunit express different affinities to tyrosine kinases

* Correspondence: kyungsukjung@fccc.edu
[1]Department of Medicine, Fox Chase Cancer Center, 333 Cottman Ave, Philadelphia, PA, USA
Full list of author information is available at the end of the article

[11], and each p110 subunit is selectively recruited to receptor activation [12, 13]. These findings are consistent with selective mutation of p110 in various types of cancer and provides important prospect for targeted therapy. *PIK3CA* is one of the most commonly mutated and extensively studied oncogenes in various types of human cancer. An analysis of The Cancer Genome Atlas (TCGA) data showed that *PIK3CA* was the most frequently mutated gene in breast cancer samples, second most frequently mutated gene in uterine corpus endometrial cancer and third most commonly mutated gene in HNSCC [14]. *PIK3CA* is also heavily mutated in lung squamous cell carcinoma, urothelial carcinoma of bladder and colorectal adenocarcinoma [14]. Molecular composition of p110α, the product of *PIK3CA*, and p85α are illustrated in Fig. 1.

Class IB PI3K consists of p110γ catalytic subunit (encoded by *PIK3CG*) and p101 or p87 regulatory subunit (encoded by *PIK3R5*, *PIK3R6*). Class IA and IB PI3K phosphorylate 3-hydroxyl group of phosphatidylinositol (PI), phosphatidylinositol 4-phosphate (PIP) and phosphatidylinositol 4,5-bisphosphate (PIP2), producing phosphatidylinositol 3-phosphate (PI-3-P), phosphatidylinositol 3,4-bisphosphate (PI-3,4-P2) and phosphatidylinositol 3,4,5-triphosphate (PIP3), respectively [15]. Expressions of p110δ and p110γ are found exclusively in lymphocytic immune system whereas p110α and p110β are expressed ubiquitously [16]. Idelalisib, a drug used for treatment of lymphoma, is a selective inhibitor of p110δ which is abundantly expressed in malignant B cells [17].

Class II PI3K is a monomer of catalytic isoforms, C2α, C2β and C2γ (encoded by *PIK3C2A*, *PIK3C2B* and *PIK3C2G*), and lacks regulatory subunit. Class II lipid kinase produces PI-3,4-P2 from PIP and PI-3-P from PI. C2α isoform found in endosomes was suggested to play a role in angiogenesis and vascular barrier formation [18]. Class III PI3K is a heterodimer of a regulatory (Vps15, encoded by *PIK3R4*) subunit and a catalytic subunit (Vps34, encoded by *PIK3C3*), which converts PI to PI-3-P. Little is known about physiologic role of class III PI3K, but it was implicated in induction of autophagy in the state of nutrient deficiency [19].

The family of PI3K proteins mainly regulates cellular growth and cycle. Its activation is triggered by upstream receptor tyrosine kinase such as ErbB family receptor (including EGFR), platelet-derived growth factor receptor (PDGFR), insulin-like growth factor 1 receptor (IGF-1R) or G protein-coupled receptor (GPCR). PI3K attaches a phosphate group to the 3′ hydroxyl of the inositol head of PIP2, converting it to PIP3 [20]. Inositol phospholipids constitute a minor part of the cellular membrane and phosphorylation of inositol head has little effect on membrane structure. However, phosphorylated inositol head protruding from the membrane provides an anchoring site for secondary signaling molecules that are floating in the cytosol. Once PIP3 is formed by PI3K, cytosolic molecules such as Akt/Protein kinase B localize to plasma membrane and become tethered to the head of PIP3 via Pleckstrin homology (PH) domain in N terminal [21]. Activated Akt, in turn, phosphorylates a series of molecules including mechanistic target of rapamycin

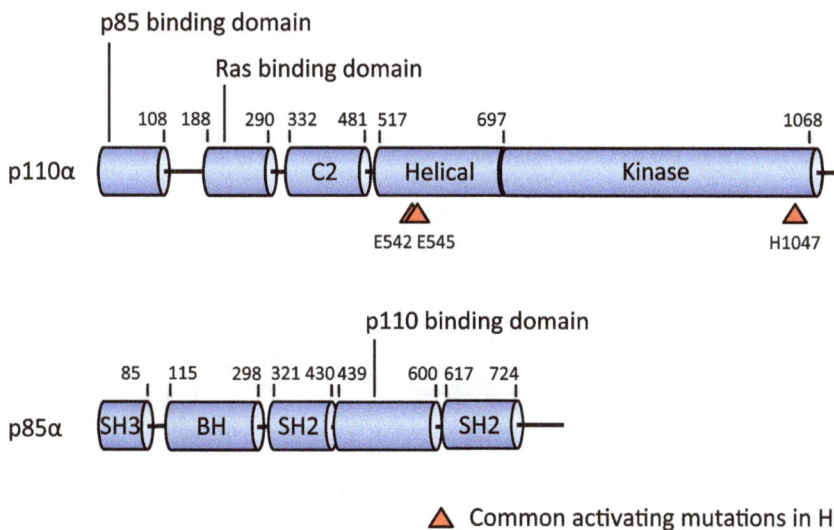

Fig. 1 Linear composition of p110α and p85α molecules. Red arrowheads in p110α indicate 'hotspot' mutations. C2 in p110α is a putative membrane-binding domain. Breakpoint cluster region-homology (BH) domain in p85α has shown GTPase activating protein (GAP) activity toward Rab family. Rab GTPase induces degradation and deregulation of activated growth factor receptors, and mutated Rab GAP induces cell transformation [148]. However, it is unclear if this function is still active in complex with p110α [149]. BH domain in p85α is flanked by proline-rich domain, implying an auto-regulatory mechanism in interaction with its SH3 domain [150]

(mTOR) that promotes cell survival, proliferation and motility. The action of PI3K, conversion of PIP2 to PIP3, is negatively regulated by reverse phosphatases, such as phosphatase and tensin homolog (PTEN). Other cytoplasmic molecules that contain PH domain and interact with PIP3 include Rho-guanine nucleotide exchange factor (GEF). Rho family proteins, when activated by GEF, remodel cytoskeleton, decrease contact inhibition and increase cell motility, all of which elevate invasiveness in cancer cells [22].

Implications of PI3K pathway alteration for EGFR pathway in HNSCC

EGFR is a cell surface receptor tyrosine kinase in ErbB family and has been an attractive therapeutic target for various human cancers including HNSCC. The receptor becomes activated by ligand binding which transitions EGFR monomers to the allosteric homodimer. Receptor dimerization stimulates tyrosine kinase activity in C terminal domain and initiates downstream phosphorylation cascade through PI3K-Akt-mTOR, Raf-MEK-MAP kinase or JAK/STAT pathways (Fig. 2).

It has been well known that EGFR overexpression is involved in carcinogenesis of HNSCC [23, 24], and associated with poor prognosis [25, 26]. EGFR-targeting strategy with a monoclonal antibody, cetuximab, has prolonged survival of patients with locally advanced HNSCC in

combination with radiotherapy [27]. Cetuximab is currently used with platinum-based chemotherapy as the first line treatment for HNSCC or for recurrent or metastatic (R/M) disease [28, 29]. However, efforts to develop a predictive biomarker for EGFR-targeting treatment have not been successful. In particular, overexpression of EGFR assessed by immunohistochemistry (IHC) could not be correlated with the level of treatment response to cetuximab [30–32]. Additionally, resistance to cetuximab has been widely observed in various types of cancer including HNSCC. Several evasive mechanisms may serve to restore original oncogene dependence, circumventing the initial targeting treatment. Receptors can potentially abrogate inhibitory action of therapeutic agents as they obtain second mutations that result in pharmacokinetic changes [33]. A well-known mutation of EGFR, T790M, enhances affinity of the kinase pocket for ATP, which competitively blocks binding of tyrosine kinase inhibitors [34]. Copy number gains of target genes also reactivate dependent pathway and counteract the treatment effect. For example, amplification of *BRAF* via copy number gains was found in 8% of the tumor samples from metastatic melanoma treated with BRAF inhibitors [35]. Studies with HNSCC demonstrated as well that copy number alteration by amplification of 7p11.2 accounts for a number of cases of EGFR activation [36–38]. It was also hypothesized that ligand overexpression or receptor cross phosphorylation triggers

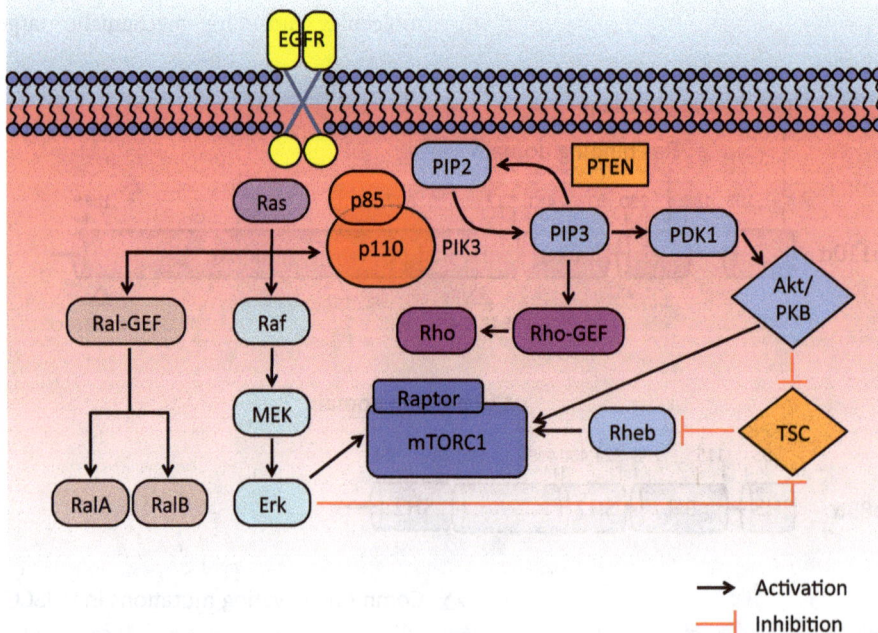

Fig. 2 Interactive signaling pathway of EGFR-PI3K-mTOR. PI3K binds to cytoplasmic tail of receptor tyrosine kinase via SH domains within p85 regulatory subunit. Activation signal can also be transferred through Ras-binding domain in p110 catalytic subunit which tethers PI3K molecule to Ras protein in growth receptors. p110 activation by Ras binding is inhibited by p85 subunit which can be released by co-stimulation of SH domain by tyrosine kinase [151]

uncontrolled EGFR hyperactivity. A genetic profiling of HNSCC samples with EGFR activation revealed that EGFR ligands (including TGFα) were highly expressed in a subset, suggesting an establishment of an autocrine loop [39].

Alternatively, the function of target gene can be bypassed by activating downstream molecules of the signaling cascade or switching dependence to an alternative pathway for cell growth and proliferation [40]. As the tumor progresses and develops genomic heterogeneity, cells with genetic survival benefit outgrow through evolutionary selection pressure. In consistent with this theory, whole-exome sequencing of melanoma cells that are resistant to BRAF inhibitor revealed diverse genetic alterations in the downstream MAPK pathway [41]. Similarly, KRAS amplification or mutation was found in tumor samples from colorectal cancer patients who developed resistance to EGFR inhibitors [42]. Relevant to our review, compensatory activation of downstream pathway, mainly PI3K, has been proposed as one of the major resistance mechanisms to EGFR inhibitors in HNSCC. Gene expression of the molecules in PI3K pathway was elevated in cetuximab-resistant strains compared to cetuximab-susceptible cells [43], and addition of mTOR/PI3K inhibitor effectively achieved control of cell growth in HNSCC that acquired resistance to EGFR inhibitors [44, 45].

PI3K-mTOR alteration in HNSCC

66% of HNSCC harbor genomic alterations in one of the major components of PI3K pathway [46]. An analysis of whole-exome sequencing of 151 HNSCC tumors revealed that PI3K is the most commonly mutated mitogenic pathway among PI3K, JAK/STAT and MAPK and that presence of multiple mutations in PI3K signaling pathway is correlated with more advanced disease [8]. Physiologic data confirms that an aberrant PI3K-mTOR pathway is associated with cell motility, invasion and metastasis. PI3K-PTEN balance has a direct effect on chemotaxis and cell motility as it controls actin cytoskeleton via Rho family proteins, such as Rho, Rac and CDC42 [22, 47]. PIP3 and PIP2 determine epithelial polarity in individual cells, thus dysfunctional PI3K results in epithelial-mesenchymal transition, a critical event in tumor invasion [48].

PI3KCA is among the most frequently mutated genes in HNSCC, affected both in HPV-positive and negative diseases (56 and 34%, respectively) [7]. PIK3CA mutations in HPV-positive HNSCCs are concentrated in helical domain, whereas mutations are more spread out in HPV-negative diseases [9, 49]. TCGA data presents that 73% of PIK3CA mutations are located at E542, E545 in the helical domain and in H1047 in the kinase domain

[7]. Frequency of these 'hotspot' mutations is also higher in HPV-positive oropharyngeal cancers [50].

Targeting PIK3CA alteration in human squamous cell xenografts has demonstrated susceptibility to treatment in vitro and in vivo, leading a path for its clinical implication. Inhibition of PI3K by competitive blockage of ATP binding site led to decreased phosphorylation of Akt in several studies [51–54]. In a number of the patient-derived xenografts harboring E545K and H1047R mutations, PI3K inhibitors were effective in achieving control of tumor growth [43, 55, 56]. Additionally, activation of PI3K/mTOR pathway from either mutation or gene amplification was positively correlated with tumor susceptibility to PI3K inhibitors in xenograft models [52, 57–59]. However, preclinical data also suggested that additional molecular change should interact with PIK3CA alteration for tumorigenesis. Cell lines engineered to harbor PIK3CA mutations in the 'hotspots' responded more favorably to PI3K/mTOR dual inhibition than PI3K inhibition only, indicating that tumor survival is not strictly dependent on the activated PI3K [60]. In a similar sense, PI3K inhibition demonstrated markedly synergistic effect when combined with EGFR or MEK inhibition [61]. Interestingly, PIK3CA activation in HPV-positive HNSCC did not necessarily lead to increased Akt target phosphorylation, but instead, led to increased mTOR activity and showed more sensitivity to PI3K/mTOR dual inhibition than Akt inhibition [62]. This finding can be extended to more favorable efficacy of PI3K/mTOR inhibitors over Akt inhibitors in clinical settings [63].

Locations of mutations affect PI3K structure and function, resulting in different responsiveness to inhibition and clinical outcome. Regulatory subunit p85 normally suppresses catalytic function of p110 at resting stage. Consequently, C terminal truncation or internal deletion of p85 releases p110 from negative regulation and constitutively activates the PI3K pathway [64, 65]. Additionally, as frequently mutated E542 and E545 in p110 are located at a distance from the kinase domain, it is plausible that mutations at these spots alter regulatory control of p85. Indeed, E545K mutation in the helical domain of p110 changes acid-base charge and disrupts inhibitory interaction between p85 and p110 [66]. H1047R mutation in the kinase domain, on the other hand, shifts orientation of the residue and changes conformation of the two loops of kinase that contact cell membrane. This allows for kinase access to phospholipid that is less regulated by p85 [67].

Independently from p110, p85 as a monomer also down-regulates PI3K activation: p85 is naturally more abundant than p110 and excess p85 monomers can sequestrate insulin receptor substrate 1 (IRS-1), an adaptor molecule that mediates signal transduction between IGF-1R and downstream PI3K [68]. Thus, in wild-type cells, the p85 monomer competes with the p85-p110 dimer for IRS binding and signal transduction. In heterozygous knock out cells, the amount of p85 monomers decreases more than p85-p110 dimers which up-regulates the PI3K pathway [69]. However, in null cells, complete absence of regulatory subunit to stabilize p110 leads to significantly decreased signal transduction causing cell apoptosis [69]. Although not as frequent as in PIK3CA, mutations in PIK3R1 (encoding p85α) can be found in 3% of HPV-positive HNSCC and 1% of HPV-negative HNSCC according to TCGA data [7].

Alteration of PTEN tumor suppressor gene is among the frequently found somatic mutations in human cancers as well as germline mutations causing hereditary cancer syndromes. PTEN dephosphorylates PIP3 to PIP2, inhibiting mitogenic signal transduction in the PI3K pathway. PTEN also interacts with PI3K, which plays a key role in chemotaxis and tumor metastasis [47, 48]. Clinical data has shown that loss of PTEN expression is a poor prognostic marker in oral squamous cell cancer [70]. However, PTEN loss was found in only a small number of HNSCC (8.16%), implying that it is a relatively minor component in PI3K pathway activation [8].

Targeting PI3K-Akt-mTOR pathway in clinic
PI3K inhibitor
Buparlisib (BKM120)

Buparlisib is an orally bioavailable pan-PI3K inhibitor, targeting the ATP binding site of p110 kinase domain. Its inhibitory potency is equitable on class IA isoforms of p110α, β and δ, but slightly less against class IB p110γ [51]. An in vitro study demonstrated IC_{50} values for Akt inhibition of 104 ± 18, 234 ± 47 and 463 ± 87 nmol/L for PI3Kα, β and δ, respectively [51]. Buparlisib is rapidly absorbed orally and its serum concentration increases proportionately to dosage [71]. The molecule also penetrates blood brain barrier and administration of buparlisib by gavage effectively controlled metastatic growth of human breast cancer in mouse brain [72]. Based on preclinical data, its antitumor activity was also attributed to suppression of microtubular dynamics [73], and antiangiongenic effect [51]. A combination of buparlisib, cetuximab and radiation exerted a synergistic antiproliferative effect on human head and neck cancer cell lines [74, 75]. In vivo, buparlisib inhibited PI3K activity in cell lines with wild-type PIK3CA as well as mutant form harboring any hotspot mutation of E542K, E545K or H1047R [76]. In a phase I dose-escalation study for advanced solid tumors, most common side effects included rash, abnormal hepatic function, alteration in glucose metabolism and fatigue [71]. In a recent randomized phase II trial with R/M HNSCC, adding buparlisib to paclitaxel improved progression-free survival (PFS) to

4–6 months compared to 3–5 months in the placebo plus paclitaxel group ($p = 0.011$) [77]. In this trial, comparable proportions of the patients had a mutation in PIK3CA, 11% and 13% in the buparlisib and control arm, respectively. Patients taking buparlisib also maintained stable quality of life and demonstrated good tolerance to the treatment compared to the placebo group, as similar proportions of patients discontinued the treatment due to adverse effects [77]. However, this study failed to demonstrate significant improvement in overall survival (OS) with buparlisib partly because of insufficient power. There are several ongoing clinical trials to evaluate the efficacy and safety of buparlisib with or without additional therapy (Table 1).

PX-866

PX-866 is an analog of wortmannin that irreversibly inhibits class I PI3K by binding to Lys in ATP catalytic site [78]. Potent and irreversible binding of PX-866 enables sub-nanomolar IC_{50} values of 0.1, 1.0 and 2.9 nmol/L for PI3Kα PI3Kγ and PI3Kδ, respectively, in contrast to much higher IC_{50} of > 300 nmol/L for PI3Kβ [79]. In vivo studies revealed antitumor activities of PX-866 against human colon cancer, ovarian cancer and lung cancer xenografts [80]. It enhanced antitumor activities of cisplatin and radiation treatment in colon cancer and ovarian cancer cells, respectively [80]. PX-866 also effectively overcame resistance to EGFR inhibitor in human lung cancer cells lacking expression of ErbB-3 [79]. PX-866 induced cessation of tumor growth in xenograft models of human HNSCC which included one case of PIK3CA gene amplification and another case of E545K [43]. However, clinical trials of PX-866 failed to show promising results. In phase II clinical trials, combined use of PX-866 with either cetuximab or docetaxel failed to achieve improved PFS or OS compared to each treatment alone [81, 82].

Alpelisib (BYL719)

Theoretically, a selective inhibitor of PI3Kα can achieve antitumor activity without affecting other isoforms of PI3K, allowing for a more favorable side effect profile. Alpelisib was designed as a specific inhibitor of PI3Kα, the product of frequently mutated PIK3CA [83]. The molecule inhibits wild-type PI3Kα ($IC_{50} = 4.6$ nmol/L) as well as PI3Kα with common PIK3CA mutations, such as E545K or H1047R ($IC_{50} = 4$ nmol/L), more potently than PI3Kδ ($IC_{50} = 290$ nmol/L) or PI3Kγ ($IC_{50} = 250$ nmol/L) [52]. Preclinical data also suggested that PIK3CA mutation makes cancer cells more vulnerable to PI3K inhibition by alpelisib. In vitro pharmacologic sensitivity screen among a broad panel of cancer cell lines revealed that sensitivity to alpelisib was positively associated with the presence of PIK3CA mutation, amplification or copy number gain

Table 1 Clinical trials evaluating PI3K or mTOR inhibitor in patients with HNSCC

Agent	Clinical Trial Identifier	Other Targeted Agent	Additional Therapy	Conditions	Phase	Status
PI3K inhibitor						
Alpelisib (BYL719)	NCT02145312	–	–	R/M HNSCC, failed to respond to platinum-based therapy	II	Not yet recruiting
	NCT02537223	–	Cisplatin, radiation	Locoregionally advanced HNSCC, not previously treated	I	Active, recruiting
	NCT01602315	Cetuximab	–	R/M HNSCC	I/II	Terminated (sponsor withdrawal)
	NCT02298595	Cetuximab	Cisplatin	HPV-associated oropharyngeal SCC	I/II	Not yet recruiting
Buparlisib (BKM120)	NCT01816984	Cetuximab	–	R/M HNC	I/II	Active, not recruiting
	NCT01737450	–	–	Recurrent or progressive HNC	II	Active, recruiting
	NCT02113878	–	Cisplatin, radiation	Locally advanced HNSCC	I	Active, recruiting
PX-866	NCT01252628	Cetuximab		R/M HNSCC	II	Completed
	NCT01204099	Docetaxel		Locally advanced or R/M HNSCC	II	Completed
Copanlisib	NCT02822482	Cetuximab	–	HNSCC with PI3KCA mutation/ amplification or PTEN loss	I/II	Active, recruiting
INCB050465	NCT02646748	Itacitinib	Pembrolizumab	Advanced solid tumors	I	Active, recruiting
mTOR inhibitor						
Sirolimus	NCT01195922	–	–	Advanced HNSCC, not previously treated	I/II	Completed
Temsirolimus	NCT01172769	–	–	R/M HNSCC	II	Completed
	NCT01009203	Erlotinib	–	Advanced HNSCC, refractory to platinum	II	Terminated (high patient withdrawal rate)
	NCT01016769	–	Paclitaxel, carboplatin	R/M HNSCC	I/II	Active, not recruiting
	NCT02215720	Cetuximab	–	Advanced or metastatic solid tumors	I	Active, recruiting
	NCT00703625	–	Docetaxel	Resistant solid malignancies	I	Completed
Everolimus (RAD001)	NCT01332279	Erlotinib	Radiation	Recurrent HNC, previously treated with radiation	I	Withdrawn (sponsor withdrawal)
	NCT01313390	–	Docetaxel	R/M HNSCC	I/II	Terminated (lack of recruitment)
	NCT01009346	Cetuximab	Cisplatin, carboplatin	R/M HNSCC	I/II	Terminated (toxicity)
	NCT01051791	–	–	R/M HNSCC	II	Active, not recruiting
PI3K/mTOR dual inhibitor						
SF1126	NCT02644122	–	–	R/M HNSCC	II	Active, recruiting
Gedatolisib	NCT03065062	Palbociclib	–	Advanced HNSCC	I	Active, recruiting
Dactolisib (BEZ235)	NCT00620594	–	–	Advanced solid tumors	I	Completed
PI3K/HDAC dual inhibitor						
CUDC-907	NCT02307240	–	–	Advanced or relapsed solid tumors	I	Active, recruiting

[84], which was confirmed by an in vivo study using mouse models [52]. In a HNSCC cell line (Cal-33) and a patient-derived xenograft model, both harboring H1047R mutation in *PIK3CA*, administration of alpelisib using nanoparticles induced inhibition of tumor growth and sensitization to radiation [55]. Compared to HNSCC cell lines with wild-type *PIK3CA*, cell lines with *PIK3CA* H1047R mutation were more susceptible to antiproliferative effect of alpelisib [56]. In another in vivo study, *PIK3CA* mutation, regardless of its location, was the

strongest predictive feature that correlated with favorable response to alpelisib [52]. Compensatory hyperactivation of PIK3CA is one of the major mechanisms of treatment resistance, thus PI3K inhibitors are being tested with other targeted therapies, such as EGFR inhibitors. Inhibition of PI3K with alpelisib enhanced tumor sensitivity to cetuximab in HNSCC xenograft models [85]. A phase I trial of alpelisib combined with cetuximab in R/M HNSCC resulted in one partial response (PR), three unconfirmed PRs and five stable diseases (SDs) among 32 cases with relatively good patient tolerance [86]. PI3K activation status was unknown in this trial. In a more recent phase I trial of alpelisib, any of complete response (CR), PR or SD was achieved in 13 out of 19 study participants with PIK3CA-mutant HNSCC (NCT01219699) [87].

Copanlisib

Copanlisib is a potent inhibitor of class I PI3K with sub-nanomolar IC_{50}. The molecule exhibits preferential activity against PI3Kα and PI3Kδ over PI3Kβ and PI3Kγ (IC_{50} values of 0.5 and 0.7 nmol/L over 3.7 and 6. 4 nmol/L, respectively) [57, 88]. It demonstrated superior inhibitory effect in cells with PIK3CA activating mutations over wild-type in breast cancer and non-small cell lung cancer xenografts [57]. Phase I trials in patients with advanced or refractory solid tumors presented good patient tolerance and evidence of disease control [89, 90]. Efficacy and safety of combined copanlisib and cetuximab for HNSCC is under study (NCT02822482).

mTOR inhibitor
Sirolimus (rapamycin)

Sirolimus was initially developed as an antifungal metabolite, extracted from the bacterium Streptomyces hygroscopicus [91]. However, since its immunosuppressive and antiproliferative properties were revealed, this macrolide molecule has been more widely used for oncologic treatment and for prevention of graft rejection or coronary stent blockage. Sirolimus binds with FKBP12 (12 kDa FK506-binding protein) to form a gain-of-function complex that function as an inhibitor of mTOR complex 1 (mTORC1) [92]. This compound, as a result, inhibits metabolic alteration and cell proliferation which is triggered by upstream gain-of-function mutations, such as PI3K and Akt. Sirolimus demonstrated antiproliferative activity in HNSCC cell lines inducing synergistic effect with chemotherapeutic agents or radiation [93, 94]. In HNSCC xenograft models with activated PI3K-Akt pathway, administration of sirolimus induced marked inhibition of tumor growth and cell apoptosis [58, 59]. It also suppressed lymphangiogenesis in HNSCC xenograft models and prevented spread of the cancer cells to adjacent lymph nodes [95]. In a phase I trial of sirolimus and bevacizumab for patients with advanced malignancies, no objective response was observed among the participants with HNSCC [96]. However, among the patients with stage II-IVA, untreated HNSCC, neoadjuvant trial of sirolimus followed by definitive therapy (surgery or chemoradiation) demonstrated significant clinical responses (one CR, one PR and 14 SDs among 16 patients) with good patient tolerance [97]. Sirolimus is known for poor bioavailability and low predictability of serum concentration after intestinal absorption, thus its narrow therapeutic window and a long half-life require regular drug concentration monitoring [98]. Based on these concerns, analogs of sirolimus have been developed to improve pharmacokinetic properties.

Temsirolimus

Temsirolimus is a water-soluble analog of sirolimus and can be administered parenterally [99]. It undergoes hydrolysis after administration to form sirolimus, but the medication itself is also capable of inhibiting mTOR. Temsirolimus is currently FDA approved for the treatment of advanced renal cell carcinoma [100]. Several preclinical studies proved that a combination of temsirolimus and cetuximab induces synergistic antitumor effect, as it mitigates or prevents compensatory downstream mTOR over-activation induced by EGFR inhibitor [101–105]. There have been a number of phase I/II trials using temsirolimus in patients with HNSCC. In a phase I study of temsirolimus used with carboplatin and paclitaxel in R/M HNSCC, 22% of the patients exhibited objective PRs [106]. The information regarding PI3K activation status was lacking in this study. In TEMHEAD trial, a phase II study of temsirolimus in R/M HNSCC refractory to platinum and cetuximab, tumor shrinkage occurred in 39.4% of the patients mostly within the first six weeks of the treatment. However, no objective response was achieved, nor did PI3KCA mutational status (H1048Y and G1050S) predict treatment success [107]. In another trial including a broad range of advanced malignances, the combination of bevacizumab, cetuximab and temsirolimus was effective in achieving PRs in 25% of the patients with HNSCC, but a few patients were withdrawn from the trial because of toxicities [108]. In this study, treatment-responders did not carry PIK3CA mutation in HNSCC cells. A trial combining temsirolimus with erlotinib for R/M HNSCC was closed early due to toxicity and patient death [109]. In a phase I pharmacokinetic study of temsirolimus, dose-limiting toxicities occurred such as thrombocytopenia, stomatitis or mucositis, asthenia, manic-depressive syndrome and rash [110]. Thus, the treatment effect of temsirolimus should be evaluated against potential toxicities and more clinical trials are ongoing.

Everolimus (RAD001)

Everolimus is a hydroxyethyl derivative of rapamycin, offering improved oral bioavailability. The medication has a short half-life, allowing for quick establishment of stable status and improved drug safety [111]. After intestinal absorption, everolimus is not converted to rapamycin, instead forms a complex with FKBP12 and inhibits mTOR [112]. It is currently approved by the FDA for treatment of multiple malignancies including advanced breast cancer, kidney cancer, neuroendocrine tumor (NET) of pancreas, progressive NET of GI and lung, tuberous sclerosis-associated renal angiomyolipoma and subependymal giant cell astrocytoma [113]. Although everolimus was effective in arresting tumor growth in HNSCC xenograft models [114, 115], clinical data was not as encouraging. Several phase I studies demonstrated PRs among patients with HNSCC [116–119], but the doses of everolimus used were different depending on other treatments combined, such as platinum, docetaxel, cetuximab or radiation. Phase II trials with everolimus also failed to demonstrate clinical benefit for HNSCC. Either as monotherapy or combination with erlotinib, treatment with everolimus was not successful in achieving objective response in patients with previously treated R/M HNSCC [120, 121]. There is a currently active clinical trial testing everolimus monotherapy in patients with R/M HNSCC (NCT01051791).

PI3K/mTOR dual inhibitor
SF1126

SF1126 is a peptide-conjugated prodrug of LY294002, with improved water solubility and pharmacokinetics. RGDS conjugation enables the molecule to bind to specific integrins within the tumor, enhancing drug permeability [53]. LY294002 is a pan-PI3K inhibitor, with IC_{50} values of 720 nmol/L, 306 nmol/L, 1.33 μmol/L and 1.6 μmol/L for PI3Kα, PI3Kβ, PI3Kδ and PI3Kγ respectively, and similar IC_{50} for mTOR (1.5 μmol/L) [53, 122]. In a phase I trial, SF1126 as a single agent was effective in maintaining stable diseases in patients with GIST and clear cell renal cancer, and in combination with rituximab decreased absolute lymphocyte count and lymph node/spleen size in CLL [123]. SF1126 monotherapy is now being evaluated for treatment of R/M HNSCC (NCT02644122).

Gedatolisib

Gedatolisib is a potent and reversible inhibitor of class I PI3K and mTOR. IC_{50} values for PI3Kα, PI3Kβ, PI3Kδ, PI3Kγ and mTOR are 0.4 nmol/L, 6 nmol/L, 8 nmol/L, 6 nmol/L and 10 nmol/L, respectively [124]. The inhibitory activity against PI3Kα with hotspot mutations, such as E545K and H1047R, are comparatively low (0.6 nmol/L and 0.8 nmol/L) [124]. Its antitumor activity was demonstrated in in vitro studies using mutant cells harboring E545K or H1047R in *PIK3CA* as well as wild-type [124, 125]. Gedatolisib also inhibited cell proliferation and increased radiosensitivity of human nasopharyngeal cancer cells with PI3K/mTOR hyperactivation [126]. Additionally, use of gedatolisib in EGFR inhibitor-resistant HNSCC suppressed cell survival and induced apoptosis [45]. Phase I trials with gedatolisib for patients with advanced cancer demonstrated potential antitumor activities with PRs and acceptable tolerance [127, 128]. However, no apparent relationship between *PIK3CA* alteration and treatment response was observed in these trials. There is an ongoing phase I trial of gedatolisib combined with palbociclib (CDK4/CDK6 inhibitor) for advanced solid tumors including HNSCC (NCT0306 5062).

Dactolisib (BEZ235)

Dactolisib is an ATP-competitive dual inhibitor of PI3K and mTOR, exerts more potency on PI3Kα, PI3Kδ, PI3Kγ and mTOR (IC_{50} values of 4, 7, 5 and 21 nmol/L, respectively) than PI3Kβ (IC_{50} = 75 nmol/L) [54, 129]. Dactolisib exhibited potent antiproliferative activity, halting cell cycles at G1 [54] and attenuating VEGF expression [129]. HNSCC cell lines with H1047R mutation were more susceptible to inhibition with lower IC_{50}, whereas E545K conferred only slightly increased sensitivity [60]. In clinical settings, however, there has been little evidence to support drug efficacy and safety. When dactolisib was used for patients with castration-resistant prostate cancer or everolimus-resistant pancreatic NET, the trials were discontinued due to dose-limiting toxicities, such as stomatitis, vomiting, diarrhea or hyperglycemia [130, 131]. Combination of dactolisib and everolimus tested in patients with various advanced solid tumors, including one case of HNSCC, failed to demonstrate objective response [132]. Another phase I trial of dactolisib treatment for various, advanced solid tumors is now complete and the result is being awaited (NCT00620594).

PI3K/HDAC dual inhibitor
CUDC-907

CUDC-907 is an orally administered inhibitor of class I PI3K isoforms and histone deacetylase (HDAC). IC_{50} values for PI3Kα, PI3Kβ, PI3Kδ and PI3Kγ are 19, 54, 38 and 311 nmol/L, respectively [133]. Simultaneous inhibition of PI3K and HDAC has demonstrated synergistic effect compared to the combined level of growth suppression achieved by single compound of HDAC inhibitor, vorinostat, and PI3K inhibitor, GDC-0941 [133]. CUDC907 has proved to be therapeutic against B cell lymphoma by decreasing MYC protein levels [134]. The effect of dual inhibition synergistically induced apoptosis of MYC-altered cells in diffuse large B-cell lymphoma (DLBCL) [135]. For cancer cells that developed resistance to PI3K inhibition through alternative pathway activation, concurrent inhibition of HDAC can down-regulate other signaling proteins and circumvent treatment resistance. This potential benefit of dual inhibition was supported by an in vitro finding which demonstrated that administration of HDAC inhibitor successfully overcame resistance to mTOR inhibitor in lymphoma cells [136]. An in vivo study has also revealed that dual inhibition of PI3K and HDAC can defeat cancer resistance to platinum-based treatment by suppressing multidrug resistance transporters and DNA repairs [137]. The first phase I trial of CUDC-907 for the treatment of relapsed/refractory lymphoma achieved two CRs and three PRs in patients with DLBCL [138]. There is an actively ongoing phase I trial of CUDC-907 for the patients with advanced or relapsed solid tumors (NCT02307240), and another phase I trial for the patients with metastatic or locally advanced thyroid cancer (NCT03002623).

Inhibition of PI3K pathway and immune system

It has been well known that inhibitors of mTOR, such as sirolimus, modulate immune system. Clinically, they have been used as immune suppressive agents to prevent rejection for patients who had undergone organ transplant. In fact, PI3K family controls many aspects of cell development, differentiation and function in both innate and adaptive immune system [139]. Especially, PI3Kγ and PI3Kδ are highly expressed in all subtypes of leukocyte, and inhibition of PI3Kγ suppressed progression of breast cancer in an animal model by inhibiting tumor inflammation and myeloid cell-mediated angiogenesis [140]. Furthermore, it has been revealed that PI3Kγ in macrophage has a critical role in the interplay between immune stimulation and suppression during inflammation or cancer development [141]. Class I PI3K signaling becomes activated by antigen receptors expressed by T and B cells, altering adaptive immune system. Therefore, inhibition of PI3Kδ dampens regulatory T cells, enhances activity of cytotoxic T cells and induces tumor regression as shown in animal models of melanoma, lung cancer, thymoma and breast cancer [142]. Various mutations in genes encoding PI3Kδ may as well lead to immunodeficiency syndromes [143].

Immune checkpoint inhibitors such as anti-programmed death 1 (anti-PD1) antibodies have demonstrated remarkable activities in HNSCC [144, 145]. Interestingly, the level of immune checkpoint ligands such as programmed death ligand 1 (PD-L1) appears to be regulated by the PI3K-Akt-mTOR pathway: inhibition of PI3K, Akt or mTOR decreased expression of PD-L1 in a non-small cell lung cancer model in vitro and in vivo [146]. Furthermore, combination of PI3Kγ blockade and immune checkpoint blockade with anti-PD1 therapy induced a synergistic growth inhibitory effect in animal models of both HPV-positive and negative HNSCC [141]. In this study, the authors showed that PI3Kγ

in macrophages plays a key role in inducing immune suppression by inhibiting NFκB pathway. Inhibition of PI3Kγ in macrophages, therefore, stimulated NFκB activation and promoted an immunostimulatory transcriptional program, restoring T cell activation. Another report suggests that PI3K-Akt pathway activation may mediate Tim-3 expression in HNSCC, which is associated with more exhausted phenotype of tumor infiltrating lymphocytes, and cause resistance to immune checkpoint blockade [147]. However, the role of PI3K pathway in cancer immunology needs to be clinically investigated further. There are phase I trials of combining PI3Kδ inhibitor (INCB050465) with pembrolizumab in advanced solid tumors (NCT02646748), and combining PI3Kβ inhibitor (GSK2636771) with pembrolizumab in advanced melanoma (NCT03131908). With recent approvals of immune checkpoint inhibitors for the treatment of R/M HNSCC, effects of adding PI3K inhibitors to immune checkpoint inhibitors will be further explored.

Conclusions

PI3K plays a key role in the progression of HNSCC and development of resistance against cetuximab. Genomic alterations affecting PI3K are common among both HPV-positive and HPV-negative diseases and serve as an attractive target for the treatment of HNSCC. Early clinical trials evaluating PI3K inhibitors have shown disappointing results, but further evaluation with more potent agents and careful patient selection might lead to development of effective PI3K inhibitors in HNSCC. In light of recent success of immune checkpoint inhibitors, potential impacts of PI3K inhibition on immune system should be considered in the future development of PI3K-targeted therapy.

Abbreviations

anti-PD1: anti-programmed death 1; BH: Breakpoint cluster region-homology; CR: Complete response; DLBCL: Diffuse large B-cell lymphoma; EGFR: Epidermal growth factor receptor; Erk: Extracellular signal-regulated kinase; FKBP12: 12 kDa FK506-binding protein; GAP: GTPase activating protein; GEF: Guanine nucleotide exchange factor; GPCR: G protein-coupled receptor; HDAC: Histone deacetylase; HNSCC: Head and neck squamous cell carcinoma; HPV: Human papillomavirus; IGF-1R: Insulin-like growth factor 1 receptor; IHC: Immunohistochemistry; IRS-1: Insulin receptor substrate 1; MEK: MAPK(mitogen-activated protein kinase)/Erk kinase; mTOR: mechanistic target of rapamycin; mTORC1: mTOR complex1; NET: Neuroendocrine tumor; OS: Overall survival; PDGFR: Platelet-derived growth factor receptor; PDK1: Phosphoinositide-dependent kinase 1; PD-L1: Programmed death-ligand 1; PFS: Progression-free survival; PH: Pleckstrin homology; PI: Phosphatidylinositol; PI-3,4-P2: Phosphatidylinositol 3,4-bisphosphate; PI3K: Phosphoinositide 3-kinase; PI-3-P: Phosphatidylinositol 3-phosphate; PIP: Phosphatidylinositol 4-phosphate; PIP2: Phosphatidylinositol 4,5-bisphosphate; PIP3: Phosphatidylinositol 3,4,5-triphosphate; PKB: Protein kinase B; PR: Partial response; PTEN: Phosphatase and tensin homolog; Ral: Ras-like protein; Rheb: Ras homolog enriched in brain; SD: Stable disease; SH: Src homology; TCGA: The cancer genome atlas; TSC: Tuberous sclerosis complex

Funding

There was no financial support or funding for this review article.

Authors' contributions

KJ searched literature and RM compiled current clinical trials. KJ and HK wrote the initial manuscript. RM and HK provided revisions. All authors read and approved the final manuscript.

Competing interests

The authors declare that they have no competing interest.

Author details

[1]Department of Medicine, Fox Chase Cancer Center, 333 Cottman Ave, Philadelphia, PA, USA. [2]Department of Oncology, The Sidney Kimmel Comprehensive Cancer Center at Johns Hopkins, 201 N Broadway, Baltimore, MD, USA.

References

1. American Cancer Society. Cancer Facts & Figures, vol. 2016. Atlanta: American Cancer Society; 2016.
2. Maier H, Dietz A, Gewelke U, Heller WD, Tobacco WH. Alcohol and the risk of head and neck cancer. Clin Investig. 1992;70(3–4):320–7.
3. Goldenberg D, Lee J, Koch WM, Kim MM, Trink B, Sidransky D, et al. Habitual risk factors for head and neck cancer. Otolaryngol Head Neck Surg. 2004; 131(6):986–93.
4. Kutler DI, Auerbach AD, Satagopan J, Giampietro PF, Batish SD, Huvos AG, et al. High incidence of head and neck squamous cell carcinoma in patients with Fanconi anemia. Arch Otolaryngol Head Neck Surg. 2003;129(1):106–12.
5. Ang KK, Harris J, Wheeler R, Weber R, Rosenthal DI, Nguyen-Tan PF, et al. Human papillomavirus and survival of patients with oropharyngeal cancer. N Engl J Med. 2010;363(1):24–35.
6. D'Souza G, Westra WH, Wang SJ, van Zante A, Wentz A, Kluz N, et al. Differences in the prevalence of human papillomavirus (HPV) in head and neck squamous cell cancers by sex, race, anatomic tumor site, and HPV detection method. JAMA Oncol. 2017;3(2):169–77.
7. Cancer Genome Atlas N. Comprehensive genomic characterization of head and neck squamous cell carcinomas. Nature. 2015;517(7536):576–82.
8. Lui VW, Hedberg ML, Li H, Vangara BS, Pendleton K, Zeng Y, et al. Frequent mutation of the PI3K pathway in head and neck cancer defines predictive biomarkers. Cancer Discov. 2013;3(7):761–9.
9. Kang H, Kiess A, Chung CH. Emerging biomarkers in head and neck cancer in the era of genomics. Nat Rev Clin Oncol. 2015;12(1):11–26.
10. Songyang Z, Shoelson SE, Chaudhuri M, Gish G, Pawson T, Haser WG, et al. SH2 domains recognize specific phosphopeptide sequences. Cell. 1993; 72(5):767–78.
11. Inukai K, Funaki M, Anai M, Ogihara T, Katagiri H, Fukushima Y, et al. Five isoforms of the phosphatidylinositol 3-kinase regulatory subunit exhibit different associations with receptor tyrosine kinases and their tyrosine phosphorylations. FEBS Lett. 2001;490(1–2):32–8.
12. Foukas LC, Claret M, Pearce W, Okkenhaug K, Meek S, Peskett E, et al. Critical role for the p110alpha phosphoinositide-3 OH kinase in growth and metabolic regulation. Nature. 2006;441(7091):366–70.
13. Papakonstanti EA, Zwaenepoel O, Bilancio A, Burns E, Nock GE, Houseman B, et al. Distinct roles of class IA PI3K isoforms in primary and immortalised macrophages. J Cell Sci. 2008;121(Pt 24):4124–33.
14. Kandoth C, McLellan MD, Vandin F, Ye K, Niu B, Lu C, et al. Mutational landscape and significance across 12 major cancer types. Nature. 2013; 502(7471):333–9.
15. Leevers SJ, Vanhaesebroeck B, Waterfield MD. Signalling through phosphoinositide-3-kinases: the lipids take Centre stage. Curr Opin Cell Biol. 1999;11(2):219–25.
16. Okkenhaug K, Vanhaesebroeck B. PI3K in lymphocyte development, differentiation and activation. Nat Rev Immunol. 2003;3(4):317–30.
17. Furman RR, Sharman JP, Coutre SE, Cheson BD, Pagel JM, Hillmen P, et al. Idelalisib and rituximab in relapsed chronic lymphocytic leukemia. N Engl J Med. 2014;370(11):997–1007.
18. Yoshioka K, Yoshida K, Cui H, Wakayama T, Takuwa N, Okamoto Y, et al. Endothelial PI3K-C2alpha, a class II PI3K, has an essential role in angiogenesis and vascular barrier function. Nat Med. 2012;18(10):1560–9.
19. Backer JM. The regulation and function of class III PI3Ks: novel roles for Vps 34. Biochem J. 2008;410(1):1–17.
20. Lee JY, Engelman JA, Cantley LC. Biochemistry. PI3K charges ahead. Science. 2007;317(5835):206–7.
21. Scheid MP, Woodgett JR. PKB/AKT: functional insights from genetic models. Nat Rev Mol Cell Biol. 2001;2(10):760–8.
22. Komiya Y, Onodera Y, Kuroiwa M, Nomimura S, Kubo Y, Nam JM, et al. The rho guanine nucleotide exchange factor ARHGEF5 promotes tumor malignancy via epithelial-mesenchymal transition. Oncogene. 2016;5(9):e258.
23. Ozanne B, Richards CS, Hendler F, Burns D, Gusterson B. Over-expression of the EGF receptor is a hallmark of squamous cell carcinomas. J Pathol. 1986; 149(1):9–14.
24. Grandis JR, Tweardy DJ. Elevated levels of transforming growth factor alpha and epidermal growth factor receptor messenger RNA are early markers of carcinogenesis in head and neck cancer. Cancer Res. 1993;53(15):3579–84.
25. Ang KK, Berkey BA, Tu X, Zhang HZ, Katz R, Hammond EH, et al. impact of epidermal growth factor receptor expression on survival and pattern of relapse in patients with advanced head and neck carcinoma. Cancer Res. 2002;62(24):7350–6.
26. Keren S, Shoude Z, Lu Z, Beibei Y. Role of EGFR as a prognostic factor for survival in head and neck cancer: a meta-analysis. Tumour Biol. 2014;35(3):2285–95.
27. Bonner JA, Harari PM, Giralt J, Azarnia N, Shin DM, Cohen RB, et al. Radiotherapy plus cetuximab for squamous-cell carcinoma of the head and neck. N Engl J Med. 2006;354(6):567–78.
28. Vermorken JB, Mesia R, Rivera F, Remenar E, Kawecki A, Rottey S, et al. Platinum-based chemotherapy plus cetuximab in head and neck cancer. N Engl J Med. 2008;359(11):1116–27.
29. Erbitux. http://pi.lilly.com/us/erbitux-uspi.pdf. Accessed 5 May 2017.
30. Licitra L, Storkel S, Kerr KM, Van Cutsem E, Pirker R, Hirsch FR, et al. Predictive value of epidermal growth factor receptor expression for first-line chemotherapy plus cetuximab in patients with head and neck and colorectal cancer: analysis of data from the EXTREME and CRYSTAL studies. Eur J Cancer. 2013;49(6):1161–8.
31. Tinhofer I, Klinghammer K, Weichert W, Knodler M, Stenzinger A, Gauler T, et al. Expression of amphiregulin and EGFRvIII affect outcome of patients with squamous cell carcinoma of the head and neck receiving cetuximab-docetaxel treatment. Clin Cancer Res. 2011;17(15):5197–204.
32. Ang KK, Zhang Q, Rosenthal DI, Nguyen-Tan PF, Sherman EJ, Weber RS, et al. Randomized phase III trial of concurrent accelerated radiation plus cisplatin with or without cetuximab for stage III to IV head and neck carcinoma: RTOG 0522. J Clin Oncol. 2014;32(27):2940–50.
33. Choi YL, Soda M, Yamashita Y, Ueno T, Takashima J, Nakajima T, et al. EML4-ALK mutations in lung cancer that confer resistance to ALK inhibitors. N Engl J Med. 2010;363(18):1734–9.
34. Kobayashi S, Boggon TJ, Dayaram T, Janne PA, Kocher O, Meyerson M, et al. EGFR mutation and resistance of non-small-cell lung cancer to gefitinib. N Engl J Med. 2005;352(8):786–92.
35. Rizos H, Menzies AM, Pupo GM, Carlino MS, Fung C, Hyman J, et al. BRAF inhibitor resistance mechanisms in metastatic melanoma: spectrum and clinical impact. Clin Cancer Res. 2014;20(7):1965–77.
36. Chung CH, Ely K, McGavran L, Varella-Garcia M, Parker J, Parker N, et al. Increased epidermal growth factor receptor gene copy number is associated with poor prognosis in head and neck squamous cell carcinomas. J Clin Oncol. 2006;24(25):4170–6.
37. Temam S, Kawaguchi H, El-Naggar AK, Jelinek J, Tang H, Liu DD, et al. Epidermal growth factor receptor copy number alterations correlate with poor clinical outcome in patients with head and neck squamous cancer. J Clin Oncol. 2007;25(16):2164–70.
38. Sheu JJ, Hua CH, Wan L, Lin YJ, Lai MT, Tseng HC, et al. Functional genomic analysis identified epidermal growth factor receptor activation as the most common genetic event in oral squamous cell carcinoma. Cancer Res. 2009; 69(6):2568–76.
39. Chung CH, Parker JS, Karaca G, Wu J, Funkhouser WK, Moore D, et al. Molecular classification of head and neck squamous cell carcinomas using patterns of gene expression. Cancer Cell. 2004;5(5):489–500.

40. Alifrangis CC, McDermott U. Reading between the lines; understanding drug response in the post genomic era. Mol Oncol. 2014;8(6):1112–9.

41. Van Allen EM, Wagle N, Sucker A, Treacy DJ, Johannessen CM, Goetz EM, et al. The genetic landscape of clinical resistance to RAF inhibition in metastatic melanoma. Cancer Discov. 2014;4(1):94–109.

42. Misale S, Yaeger R, Hobor S, Scala E, Janakiraman M, Liska D, et al. Emergence of KRAS mutations and acquired resistance to anti-EGFR therapy in colorectal cancer. Nature. 2012;486(7404):532–6.

43. Keysar SB, Astling DP, Anderson RT, Vogler BW, Bowles DW, Morton JJ, et al. A patient tumor transplant model of squamous cell cancer identifies PI3K inhibitors as candidate therapeutics in defined molecular bins. Mol Oncol. 2013;7(4):776–90.

44. Wang Z, Martin D, Molinolo AA, Patel V, Iglesias-Bartolome R, Degese MS, et al. mTOR co-targeting in cetuximab resistance in head and neck cancers harboring PIK3CA and RAS mutations. J Natl Cancer Inst. 2014;106(9):dju215.

45. D'Amato V, Rosa R, D'Amato C, Formisano L, Marciano R, Nappi L, et al. The dual PI3K/mTOR inhibitor PKI-587 enhances sensitivity to cetuximab in EGFR-resistant human head and neck cancer models. Br J Cancer. 2014; 110(12):2887–95.

46. Vander Broek R, Mohan S, Eytan DF, Chen Z, Van Waes C. The PI3K/Akt/ mTOR axis in head and neck cancer: functions, aberrations, cross-talk, and therapies. Oral Dis. 2015;21(7):815–25.

47. Kolsch V, Charest PG, Firtel RA. The regulation of cell motility and chemotaxis by phospholipid signaling. J Cell Sci. 2008;121(Pt 5):551–9.

48. Martin-Belmonte F, Mostov K. Regulation of cell polarity during epithelial morphogenesis. Curr Opin Cell Biol. 2008;20(2):227–34.

49. Koncar RF, Feldman R, Bahassi EM, Hashemi Sadraei N. Comparative molecular profiling of HPV-induced squamous cell carcinomas. Cancer Med. 2017;6(7):1673–85.

50. Nichols AC, Palma DA, Chow W, Tan S, Rajakumar C, Rizzo G, et al. High frequency of activating PIK3CA mutations in human papillomavirus-positive oropharyngeal cancer. JAMA Otolaryngol Head Neck Surg. 2013;139(6):617– 22.

51. Maira SM, Pecchi S, Huang A, Burger M, Knapp M, Sterker D, et al. Identification and characterization of NVP-BKM120, an orally available pan-class I PI3-kinase inhibitor. Mol Cancer Ther. 2012;11(2):317–28.

52. Fritsch C, Huang A, Chatenay-Rivauday C, Schnell C, Reddy A, Liu M, et al. Characterization of the novel and specific PI3Kalpha inhibitor NVP-BYL719 and development of the patient stratification strategy for clinical trials. Mol Cancer Ther. 2014;13(5):1117–29.

53. Garlich JR, De P, Dey N, Su JD, Peng X, Miller A, et al. A vascular targeted pan phosphoinositide 3-kinase inhibitor prodrug, SF1126, with antitumor and antiangiogenic activity. Cancer Res. 2008;68(1):206–15.

54. Maira SM, Stauffer F, Brueggen J, Furet P, Schnell C, Fritsch C, et al. Identification and characterization of NVP-BEZ235, a new orally available dual phosphatidylinositol 3-kinase/mammalian target of rapamycin inhibitor with potent in vivo antitumor activity. Mol Cancer Ther. 2008;7(7):1851–63.

55. Mizrachi A, Shamay Y, Shah J, Brook S, Soong J, Rajasekhar VK, et al. Tumour-specific PI3K inhibition via nanoparticle-targeted delivery in head and neck squamous cell carcinoma. Nat Commun. 2017;8:14292.

56. Keam B, Kim S, Ahn YO, Kim TM, Lee SH, Kim DW, et al. In vitro anticancer activity of PI3K alpha selective inhibitor BYL719 in head and neck cancer. Anticancer Res. 2015;35(1):175–82.

57. Liu N, Rowley BR, Bull CO, Schneider C, Haegebarth A, Schatz CA, et al. BAY 80-6946 is a highly selective intravenous PI3K inhibitor with potent p110alpha and p110delta activities in tumor cell lines and xenograft models. Mol Cancer Ther. 2013;12(11):2319–30.

58. Amornphimoltham P, Patel V, Sodhi A, Nikitakis NG, Sauk JJ, Sausville EA, et al. Mammalian target of rapamycin, a molecular target in squamous cell carcinomas of the head and neck. Cancer Res. 2005;65(21):9953–61.

59. Liu D, Hou P, Liu Z, Wu G, Xing M. Genetic alterations in the phosphoinositide 3-kinase/Akt signaling pathway confer sensitivity of thyroid cancer cells to therapeutic targeting of Akt and mammalian target of rapamycin. Cancer Res. 2009;69(18):7311–9.

60. Wirtz ED, Hoshino D, Maldonado AT, Tyson DR, Weaver AM. Response of head and neck squamous cell carcinoma cells carrying PIK3CA mutations to selected targeted therapies. JAMA Otolaryngol Head Neck Surg. 2015;141(6):543–9.

61. Mazumdar T, Byers LA, Ng PK, Mills GB, Peng S, Diao L, et al. A comprehensive evaluation of biomarkers predictive of response to PI3K inhibitors and of resistance mechanisms in head and neck squamous cell carcinoma. Mol Cancer Ther. 2014;13(11):2738–50.

62. Sewell A, Brown B, Biktasova A, Mills GB, Lu Y, Tyson DR, et al. Reverse-phase protein array profiling of oropharyngeal cancer and significance of PIK3CA mutations in HPV-associated head and neck cancer. Clin Cancer Res. 2014;20(9):2300–11.

63. Argiris A, Cohen E, Karrison T, Esparaz B, Mauer A, Ansari R, et al. A phase II trial of perifosine, an oral alkylphospholipid, in recurrent or metastatic head and neck cancer. Cancer Biol Ther. 2006;5(7):766–70.

64. Luo J, Cantley LC. The negative regulation of phosphoinositide 3-kinase signaling by p85 and it's implication in cancer. Cell Cycle. 2005;4(10):1309–12.

65. Philp AJ, Campbell IG, Leet C, Vincan E, Rockman SP, Whitehead RH, et al. The phosphatidylinositol 3'-kinase p85alpha gene is an oncogene in human ovarian and colon tumors. Cancer Res. 2001;61(20):7426–9.

66. Miled N, Yan Y, Hon WC, Perisic O, Zvelebil M, Inbar Y, et al. Mechanism of two classes of cancer mutations in the phosphoinositide 3-kinase catalytic subunit. Science. 2007;317(5835):239–42.

67. Mandelker D, Gabelli SB, Schmidt-Kittler O, Zhu J, Cheong I, Huang CH, et al. A frequent kinase domain mutation that changes the interaction between PI3Kalpha and the membrane. Proc Natl Acad Sci U S A. 2009;106(40): 16996–7001.

68. Luo J, Field SJ, Lee JY, Engelman JA, Cantley LC. The p85 regulatory subunit of phosphoinositide 3-kinase down-regulates IRS-1 signaling via the formation of a sequestration complex. J Cell Biol. 2005;170(3):455–64.

69. Ueki K, Fruman DA, Brachmann SM, Tseng YH, Cantley LC, Kahn CR. Molecular balance between the regulatory and catalytic subunits of phosphoinositide 3-kinase regulates cell signaling and survival. Mol Cell Biol. 2002;22(3):965–77.

70. Lee JI, Soria JC, Hassan KA, El-Naggar AK, Tang X, Liu DD, et al. Loss of PTEN expression as a prognostic marker for tongue cancer. Arch Otolaryngol Head Neck Surg. 2001;127(12):1441–5.

71. Ando Y, Inada-Inoue M, Mitsuma A, Yoshino T, Ohtsu A, Suenaga N, et al. Phase I dose-escalation study of buparlisib (BKM120), an oral pan-class I PI3K inhibitor, in Japanese patients with advanced solid tumors. Cancer Sci. 2014; 105(3):347–53.

72. Nanni P, Nicoletti G, Palladini A, Croci S, Murgo A, Ianzano ML, et al. Multiorgan metastasis of human HER-2+ breast cancer in Rag2–/–;Il2rg–/– mice and treatment with PI3K inhibitor. PLoS One. 2012;7(6):e39626.

73. Brachmann SM, Kleylein-Sohn J, Gaulis S, Kauffmann A, Blommers MJ, Kazic-Legueux M, et al. Characterization of the mechanism of action of the pan class I PI3K inhibitor NVP-BKM120 across a broad range of concentrations. Mol Cancer Ther. 2012;11(8):1747–57.

74. Lattanzio L, Tonissi F, Monteverde M, Vivenza D, Russi E, Milano G, et al. Treatment effect of buparlisib, cetuximab and irradiation in wild-type or PI3KCA-mutated head and neck cancer cell lines. Investig New Drugs. 2015; 33(2):310–20.

75. Bozec A, Ebran N, Radosevic-Robin N, Chamorey E, Yahia HB, Marcie S, et al. Combination of phosphotidylinositol-3-kinase targeting with cetuximab and irradiation: a preclinical study on an orthotopic xenograft model of head and neck cancer. Head Neck. 2017;39(1):151–9.

76. Kong D, Yamori T, Yamazaki K, Dan S. In vitro multifaceted activities of a specific group of novel phosphatidylinositol 3-kinase inhibitors on hotspot mutant PIK3CA. Investig New Drugs. 2014;32(6):1134–43.

77. Soulieres D, Faivre S, Mesia R, Remenar E, Li SH, Karpenko A, et al. Buparlisib and paclitaxel in patients with platinum-pretreated recurrent or metastatic squamous cell carcinoma of the head and neck (BERIL-1): a randomised, double-blind, placebo-controlled phase 2 trial. Lancet Oncol. 2017;18(3):323–35.

78. Zask A, Kaplan J, Toral-Barza L, Hollander I, Young M, Tischler M, et al. Synthesis and structure-activity relationships of ring-opened 17-hydroxywortmannins: potent phosphoinositide 3-kinase inhibitors with improved properties and anticancer efficacy. J Med Chem. 2008;51(5):1319–23.

79. Ihle NT, Paine-Murrieta G, Berggren MI, Baker A, Tate WR, Wipf P, et al. The phosphatidylinositol-3-kinase inhibitor PX-866 overcomes resistance to the epidermal growth factor receptor inhibitor gefitinib in A-549 human non-small cell lung cancer xenografts. Mol Cancer Ther. 2005;4(9):1349–57.

80. Ihle NT, Williams R, Chow S, Chew W, Berggren MI, Paine-Murrieta G, et al. Molecular pharmacology and antitumor activity of PX-866, a novel inhibitor of phosphoinositide-3-kinase signaling. Mol Cancer Ther. 2004;3(7):763–72.

81. Jimeno A, Bauman JE, Weissman C, Adkins D, Schnadig I, Beauregard P, et al. A randomized, phase 2 trial of docetaxel with or without PX-866, an irreversible oral phosphatidylinositol 3-kinase inhibitor, in patients with relapsed or metastatic head and neck squamous cell cancer. Oral Oncol. 2015;51(4):383–8.

82. Jimeno A, Shirai K, Choi M, Laskin J, Kochenderfer M, Spira A, et al. A randomized, phase II trial of cetuximab with or without PX-866, an irreversible oral phosphatidylinositol 3-kinase inhibitor, in patients with relapsed or metastatic head and neck squamous cell cancer. Ann Oncol. 2015;26(3):556–61.

83. Furet P, Guagnano V, Fairhurst RA, Imbach-Weese P, Bruce I, Knapp M, et al. Discovery of NVP-BYL719 a potent and selective phosphatidylinositol-3 kinase alpha inhibitor selected for clinical evaluation. Bioorg Med Chem Lett. 2013;23(13):3741–8.

84. Huang A, Fritsch C, Wilson C, Reddy A, Liu M, Lehar J, et al. Abstract 3749: single agent activity of PIK3CA inhibitor BYL719 in a broad cancer cell line panel. Cancer Res. 2012;72(8 Supplement):3749.

85. Sheng Q, Wang H, Das R, Chen Y, Liang J, Cao A, et al. Abstract 4261: targeting HER3 and PI3K in head and neck squamous cancer cells. Cancer Res. 2013;73(8 Supplement):4261.

86. Razak ARA, Ahn MJ, Yen CJ, Solomon BJ, Lee SH, Wang HM, et al. Phase Ib/II study of the PI3K alpha inhibitor BYL719 in combination with cetuximab in recurrent/metastatic squamous cell cancer of the head and neck (SCCHN). J Clin Oncol. 2014;32(15)

87. Juric D, Rodon J, Tabernero J, Janku F, Burris HA, Schellens JHM, et al. Phosphatidylinositol 3-Kinase alpha-Selective Inhibition With Alpelisib (BYL719) in PIK3CA-Altered Solid Tumors: Results From the First-in-Human Study. J Clin Oncol. 2018;36(13):1291-9.

88. Scott WJ, Hentemann MF, Rowley RB, Bull CO, Jenkins S, Bullion AM, et al. Discovery and SAR of novel 2,3-Dihydroimidazo[1,2-c]quinazoline PI3K inhibitors: identification of Copanlisib (BAY 80-6946). ChemMedChem. 2016; 11(14):1517–30.

89. Doi T, Fuse N, Yoshino T, Kojima T, Bando H, Miyamoto H, et al. A phase I study of intravenous PI3K inhibitor copanlisib in Japanese patients with advanced or refractory solid tumors. Cancer Chemother Pharmacol. 2017; 79(1):89–98.

90. Patnaik A, Appleman LJ, Tolcher AW, Papadopoulos KP, Beeram M, Rasco DW, et al. First-in-human phase I study of copanlisib (BAY 80-6946), an intravenous pan-class I phosphatidylinositol 3-kinase inhibitor, in patients with advanced solid tumors and non-Hodgkin's lymphomas. Ann Oncol. 2016;27(10):1928–40.

91. Seto B. Rapamycin and mTOR: a serendipitous discovery and implications for breast cancer. Clin Transl Med. 2012;1(1):29.

92. Li J, Kim SG, Blenis J. Rapamycin: one drug, many effects. Cell Metab. 2014; 19(3):373–9.

93. Aissat N, Le Tourneau C, Ghoul A, Serova M, Bieche I, Lokiec F, et al. Antiproliferative effects of rapamycin as a single agent and in combination with carboplatin and paclitaxel in head and neck cancer cell lines. Cancer Chemother Pharmacol. 2008;62(2):305–13.

94. Shinohara ET, Maity A, Jha N, Lustig RA. Sirolimus as a potential radiosensitizer in squamous cell cancer of the head and neck. Head Neck. 2009;31(3):406–11.

95. Patel V, Marsh CA, Dorsam RT, Mikelis CM, Masedunskas A, Amornphimoltham P, et al. Decreased lymphangiogenesis and lymph node metastasis by mTOR inhibition in head and neck cancer. Cancer Res. 2011;71(22):7103–12.

96. Cohen EE, Sharma MR, Janisch L, Llobrera M, House L, Wu K, et al. A phase I study of sirolimus and bevacizumab in patients with advanced malignancies. Eur J Cancer. 2011;47(10):1484–9.

97. Shirai K, Day TA, Szabo E, Van Waes C, O'Brien PE, Matheus MG, et al. A pilot, single arm, prospective trial using neoadjuvant rapamycin prior to definitive therapy in head and neck squamous cell carcinoma. J Clin Oncol. 2015;33(15)

98. Mukherjee S, Mukherjee U. A comprehensive review of immunosuppression used for liver transplantation. J Transp Secur 2009; 2009;701464.

99. Dancey J, Sausville EA. Issues and progress with protein kinase inhibitors for cancer treatment. Nat Rev Drug Discov. 2003;2(4):296–313.

100. Torisel. http://labeling.pfizer.com/showlabeling.aspx?id=490. Accessed 24 Apr 2017.

101. Bozec A, Etienne-Grimaldi MC, Fischel JL, Sudaka A, Toussan N, Formento P, et al. The mTOR-targeting drug temsirolimus enhances the growth-inhibiting effects of the cetuximab-bevacizumab-irradiation combination on head and neck cancer xenografts. Oral Oncol. 2011;47(5):340–4.

102. Jimeno A, Kulesza P, Wheelhouse J, Chan A, Zhang X, Kincaid E, et al. Dual EGFR and mTOR targeting in squamous cell carcinoma models, and development of early markers of efficacy. Br J Cancer. 2007;96(6):952–9.

103. Lattanzio L, Milano G, Monteverde M, Tonissi F, Vivenza D, Merlano M, et al. Schedule-dependent interaction between temsirolimus and cetuximab in head and neck cancer: a preclinical study. Anti-Cancer Drugs. 2016;27(6): 533–9.

104. Bozec A, Ebran N, Radosevic-Robin N, Sudaka A, Monteverde M, Toussan N, et al. Combination of mTOR and EGFR targeting in an orthotopic xenograft model of head and neck cancer. Laryngoscope. 2016;126(4):E156–63.

105. Nathan CO, Amirghahari N, Rong X, Giordano T, Sibley D, Nordberg M, et al. Mammalian target of rapamycin inhibitors as possible adjuvant therapy for microscopic residual disease in head and neck squamous cell cancer. Cancer Res. 2007;67(5):2160–8.

106. Fury MG, Sherman E, Ho A, Katabi N, Sima C, Kelly KW, et al. A phase I study of temsirolimus plus carboplatin plus paclitaxel for patients with recurrent or metastatic (R/M) head and neck squamous cell cancer (HNSCC). Cancer Chemother Pharmacol. 2012;70(1):121–8.

107. Grunwald V, Keilholz U, Boehm A, Guntinas-Lichius O, Hennemann B, Schmoll HJ, et al. TEMHEAD: a single-arm multicentre phase II study of temsirolimus in platin- and cetuximab refractory recurrent and/or metastatic squamous cell carcinoma of the head and neck (SCCHN) of the German SCCHN group (AIO). Ann Oncol. 2015;26(3):561–7.

108. Liu X, Kambrick S, Fu S, Naing A, Subbiah V, Blumenschein GR, et al. advanced malignancies treated with a combination of the VEGF inhibitor bevacizumab, anti-EGFR antibody cetuximab, and the mTOR inhibitor temsirolimus. Oncotarget. 2016;7(17):23227–38.

109. Bauman JE, Arias-Pulido H, Lee SJ, Fekrazad MH, Ozawa H, Fertig E, et al. A phase II study of temsirolimus and erlotinib in patients with recurrent and/ or metastatic, platinum-refractory head and neck squamous cell carcinoma. Oral Oncol. 2013;49(5):461–7.

110. Raymond E, Alexandre J, Faivre S, Vera K, Materman E, Boni J, et al. Safety and pharmacokinetics of escalated doses of weekly intravenous infusion of CCI-779, a novel mTOR inhibitor, in patients with cancer. J Clin Oncol. 2004; 22(12):2336–47.

111. Tanaka C, O'Reilly T, Kovarik JM, Shand N, Hazell K, Judson I, et al. Identifying optimal biologic doses of everolimus (RAD001) in patients with cancer based on the modeling of preclinical and clinical pharmacokinetic and pharmacodynamic data. J Clin Oncol. 2008;26(10):1596–602.

112. Nguyen SA, Walker D, Gillespie MB, Gutkind JS, Day TA. mTOR inhibitors and its role in the treatment of head and neck squamous cell carcinoma. Curr Treat Options in Oncol. 2012;13(1):71–81.

113. Afinitor. https://www.pharma.us.novartis.com/sites/www.pharma.us.novartis. com/files/afinitor.pdf. Accessed 24 Apr 2017.

114. Li SH, Lin WC, Huang TL, Chen CH, Chiu TJ, Fang FM, et al. Significance of mammalian target of rapamycin in patients with locally advanced stage IV head and neck squamous cell carcinoma receiving induction chemotherapy with docetaxel, cisplatin, and fluorouracil. Head Neck. 2016;38(Suppl 1):E844–52.

115. Klinghammer K, Raguse JD, Plath T, Albers AE, Joehrens K, Zakarneh A, et al. A comprehensively characterized large panel of head and neck cancer patient-derived xenografts identifies the mTOR inhibitor everolimus as potential new treatment option. Int J Cancer. 2015;136(12):2940–8.

116. Fury MG, Lee NY, Sherman E, Ho AL, Rao S, Heguy A, et al. A phase 1 study of everolimus + weekly cisplatin + intensity modulated radiation therapy in head-and-neck cancer. Int J Radiat Oncol Biol Phys. 2013;87(3):479–86.

117. Fury MG, Sherman E, Haque S, Korte S, Lisa D, Shen R, et al. A phase I study of daily everolimus plus low-dose weekly cisplatin for patients with advanced solid tumors. Cancer Chemother Pharmacol. 2012;69(3):591–8.

118. Fury MG, Sherman E, Ho AL, Xiao H, Tsai F, Nwankwo O, et al. A phase 1 study of everolimus plus docetaxel plus cisplatin as induction chemotherapy for patients with locally and/or regionally advanced head and neck cancer. Cancer. 2013;119(10):1823–31.

119. Saba NF, Hurwitz SJ, Magliocca K, Kim S, Owonikoko TK, Harvey D, et al. Phase 1 and pharmacokinetic study of everolimus in combination with cetuximab and carboplatin for recurrent/metastatic squamous cell carcinoma of the head and neck. Cancer. 2014;120(24):3940–51.

120. Geiger JL, Bauman JE, Gibson MK, Gooding WE, Varadarajan P, Kotsakis A, et al. Phase II trial of everolimus in patients with previously treated recurrent or metastatic head and neck squamous cell carcinoma. Head Neck. 2016; 38(12):1759–64.

121. Massarelli E, Lin H, Ginsberg LE, Tran HT, Lee JJ, Canales JR, et al. Phase II trial of everolimus and erlotinib in patients with platinum-resistant recurrent and/or metastatic head and neck squamous cell carcinoma. Ann Oncol. 2015;26(7):1476–80.

122. Cleary JM, Shapiro GI. Development of phosphoinositide-3 kinase pathway inhibitors for advanced cancer. Curr Oncol Rep. 2010;12(2):87–94.

123. Mahadevan D, Chiorean EG, Harris WB, Von Hoff DD, Stejskal-Barnett A, Qi W, et al. Phase I pharmacokinetic and pharmacodynamic study of the pan-PI3K/mTORC vascular targeted pro-drug SF1126 in patients with advanced solid tumours and B-cell malignancies. Eur J Cancer. 2012;48(18):3319–27.

124. Mallon R, Feldberg LR, Lucas J, Chaudhary I, Dehnhardt C, Santos ED, et al. Antitumor efficacy of PKI-587, a highly potent dual PI3K/mTOR kinase inhibitor. Clin Cancer Res. 2011;17(10):3193–203.

125. Venkatesan AM, Dehnhardt CM, Delos Santos E, Chen Z, Dos Santos O, Ayral-Kaloustian S, et al. Bis(morpholino-1,3,5-triazine) derivatives: potent adenosine 5′-triphosphate competitive phosphatidylinositol-3-kinase/mammalian target of rapamycin inhibitors: discovery of compound 26 (PKI-587), a highly efficacious dual inhibitor. J Med Chem. 2010;53(6):2636–45.

126. Liu T, Sun Q, Li Q, Yang H, Zhang Y, Wang R, et al. Dual PI3K/mTOR inhibitors, GSK2126458 and PKI-587, suppress tumor progression and increase radiosensitivity in nasopharyngeal carcinoma. Mol Cancer Ther. 2015;14(2):429–39.

127. Shapiro GI, Bell-McGuinn KM, Molina JR, Bendell J, Spicer J, Kwak EL, et al. First-in-human study of PF-05212384 (PKI-587), a small-molecule, intravenous, dual inhibitor of PI3K and mTOR in patients with advanced Cancer. Clin Cancer Res. 2015;21(8):1888–95.

128. Wainberg ZA, Alsina M, Soares HP, Brana I, Britten CD, Del Conte G, et al. A multi-arm phase I study of the PI3K/mTOR inhibitors PF-04691502 and Gedatolisib (PF-05212384) plus irinotecan or the MEK inhibitor PD-0325901 in advanced Cancer. Target Oncol. 2017;12(6):775–85.

129. Liu TJ, Koul D, LaFortune T, Tiao N, Shen RJ, Maira SM, et al. NVP-BEZ235, a novel dual phosphatidylinositol 3-kinase/mammalian target of rapamycin inhibitor, elicits multifaceted antitumor activities in human gliomas. Mol Cancer Ther. 2009;8(8):2204–10.

130. Massard C, Chi KN, Castellano D, de Bono J, Gravis G, Dirix L, et al. Phase Ib dose-finding study of abiraterone acetate plus buparlisib (BKM120) or dactolisib (BEZ235) in patients with castration-resistant prostate cancer. Eur J Cancer. 2017;76:36–44.

131. Fazio N, Buzzoni R, Baudin E, Antonuzzo L, Hubner RA, Lahner H, et al. A phase II study of BEZ235 in patients with Everolimus-resistant, advanced pancreatic neuroendocrine Tumours. Anticancer Res. 2016;36(2):713–9.

132. Wise-Draper TM, Moorthy G, Salkeni MA, Karim NA, Thomas HE, Mercer CA, et al. A phase Ib study of the dual PI3K/mTOR inhibitor Dactolisib (BEZ235) combined with Everolimus in patients with advanced solid malignancies. Target Oncol 2017.

133. Qian C, Lai CJ, Bao R, Wang DG, Wang J, Xu GX, et al. Cancer network disruption by a single molecule inhibitor targeting both histone deacetylase activity and phosphatidylinositol 3-kinase signaling. Clin Cancer Res. 2012; 18(15):4104–13.

134. Mondello P, Derenzini E, Asgari Z, Philip J, Brea EJ, Seshan V, et al. Dual inhibition of histone deacetylases and phosphoinositide 3-kinase enhances therapeutic activity against B cell lymphoma. Oncotarget. 2017;8(8):14017–28.

135. Sun K, Atoyan R, Borek MA, Dellarocca S, Samson ME, Ma AW, et al. Dual HDAC and PI3K inhibitor CUDC-907 downregulates MYC and suppresses growth of MYC-dependent cancers. Mol Cancer Ther. 2017;16(2):285–99.

136. Gupta M, Ansell SM, Novak AJ, Kumar S, Kaufmann SH, Witzig TE. Inhibition of histone deacetylase overcomes rapamycin-mediated resistance in diffuse large B-cell lymphoma by inhibiting Akt signaling through mTORC2. Blood. 2009;114(14):2926–35.

137. To KKW, Fu LW. CUDC-907, a dual HDAC and PI3K inhibitor, reverses platinum drug resistance. Investig New Drugs 2017.

138. Younes A, Berdeja JG, Patel MR, Flinn I, Gerecitano JF, Neelapu SS, et al. Safety, tolerability, and preliminary activity of CUDC-907, a first-in-class, oral, dual inhibitor of HDAC and PI3K, in patients with relapsed or refractory lymphoma or multiple myeloma: an open-label, dose-escalation, phase 1 trial. Lancet Oncol. 2016;17(5):622–31.

139. Okkenhaug K. Signaling by the phosphoinositide 3-kinase family in immune cells. Annu Rev Immunol. 2013;31:675–704.

140. Schmid MC, Avraamides CJ, Dippold HC, Franco I, Foubert P, Ellies LG, et al. Receptor tyrosine kinases and TLR/IL1Rs unexpectedly activate myeloid cell PI3kgamma, a single convergent point promoting tumor inflammation and progression. Cancer Cell. 2011;19(6):715–27.

141. Kaneda MM, Messer KS, Ralainirina N, Li H, Leem CJ, Gorjestani S, et al. PI3Kgamma is a molecular switch that controls immune suppression. Nature. 2016;539(7629):437–42.

142. Ali K, Soond DR, Pineiro R, Hagemann T, Pearce W, Lim EL, et al. Inactivation of PI(3)K p110delta breaks regulatory T-cell-mediated immune tolerance to cancer. Nature. 2014;510(7505):407–11.

143. Lucas CL, Chandra A, Nejentsev S, Condliffe AM, Okkenhaug K. PI3Kdelta and primary immunodeficiencies. Nat Rev Immunol. 2016;16(11):702–14.

144. Ferris RL, Blumenschein G, Jr., Fayette J, Guigay J, Colevas AD, Licitra L, et al. Nivolumab for recurrent squamous-cell carcinoma of the head and neck. N Engl J Med 2016;375(19):1856–1867.

145. Bauml J, Seiwert TY, Pfister DG, Worden F, Liu SV, Gilbert J, et al. Pembrolizumab for platinum- and Cetuximab-refractory head and neck Cancer: results from a single-arm, phase II study. J Clin Oncol. 2017;35(14):1542–9.

146. Lastwika KJ, Wilson W, 3rd, Li QK, Norris J, Xu H, Ghazarian SR, et al. Control of PD-L1 expression by oncogenic activation of the AKT-mTOR pathway in non-small cell lung Cancer. Cancer Res 2016;76(2):227–238.

147. Shayan G, Srivastava R, Li J, Schmitt N, Kane LP, Ferris RL. Adaptive resistance to anti-PD1 therapy by Tim-3 upregulation is mediated by the PI3K-Akt pathway in head and neck cancer. Oncoimmunology. 2017;6(1):e1261779.

148. Chamberlain MD, Chan T, Oberg JC, Hawrysh AD, James KM, Saxena A, et al. Disrupted RabGAP function of the p85 subunit of phosphatidylinositol 3-kinase results in cell transformation. J Biol Chem. 2008;283(23):15861–8.

149. Vanhaesebroeck B, Guillermet-Guibert J, Graupera M, Bilanges B. The emerging mechanisms of isoform-specific PI3K signalling. Nat Rev Mol Cell Biol. 2010;11(5):329–41.

150. Kapeller R, Prasad KV, Janssen O, Hou W, Schaffhausen BS, Rudd CE, et al. Identification of two SH3-binding motifs in the regulatory subunit of phosphatidylinositol 3-kinase. J Biol Chem. 1994;269(3):1927–33.

151. Jimenez C, Hernandez C, Pimentel B, Carrera AC. The p85 regulatory subunit controls sequential activation of phosphoinositide 3-kinase by Tyr kinases and Ras. J Biol Chem. 2002;277(44):41556–62.

18

HPV-driven oropharyngeal cancer: current knowledge of molecular biology and mechanisms of carcinogenesis

Cassie Pan[1], Natalia Issaeva[2] and Wendell G. Yarbrough[2]* (iD)

Abstract

Understanding of oropharyngeal squamous cell carcinoma has significantly progressed over the last decades, and the concept that this disease can be subdivided into two distinct entities based on human papilloma virus (HPV) status has gained acceptance. To combat the constantly growing epidemic of HPV+ oropharyngeal cancer, further investigation and characterization the unique features of the disease, along with the development and implementation of new, targeted therapies, is crucial. In this review, we summarize the etiology, pathogenesis, diagnosis, treatment, and molecular characteristics of HPV-associated oropharyngeal squamous cell carcinoma.

Keywords: Oropharyngeal cancer, HPV, Etiology, Treatment

Background

Head and neck squamous cell carcinomas comprise a diverse group of tumors, which are classified into anatomical subsites including oral cavity, oropharynx, hypopharynx, larynx, and nasopharynx. Cancers of different subsites are known to have unique epidemiology, anatomy, clinical behavior, and association with human papilloma virus (HPV) infection [1, 2]. In this review, we will focus on HPV-driven oropharyngeal squamous cell carcinoma (OPSCC), which has become a matter of growing clinical urgency as its incidence has dramatically increased in recent years. Unique epidemiological, molecular, biological and clinical differences have led to the increasing recognition of HPV-positive OPSCCs as distinct from HPV-negative OPSCCs. This review article will summarize clinical and molecular characteristics of HPV-driven OPSCCs, focusing on factors that distinguish HPV-positive and HPV-negative OPSCCs and examining differences between OPSCC and uterine cervical cancer with attention to an alternative mechanism of HPV carcinogenesis.

Epidemiology

In the late 20th and early twenty-first century, the campaign to reduce smoking decreased rates of tobacco-related cancers, including oral cavity and laryngeal cancers. During this same period, rates of oropharyngeal cancers increased [3–6]. With the growing number of OPSCCs, the etiologic role of HPV infection also burgeoned, and the percentage of OPSCCs associated with HPV increased from 20% in the 1980s to over 70% by 2005 [7–9]. CDC statistics from 2012 revealed that the incidence of HPV-associated OPSCCs exceeded that of HPV-associated uterine cervical cancers, making OPSCC the most frequently diagnosed cancer caused by HPV [10]. As opposed to HPV-negative cancers of the head and neck, HPV(+) OPSCCs occur in younger patients with minimal or no tobacco exposure [11–16]. HPV(+) OPSCC has a male predominance with men suffering a three to five times higher incidence than women worldwide [16, 17].

Over 90% of HPV(+) OPSCC is caused by the high-risk HPV genotype 16, with almost all oral HPV infections thought to be sexually acquired [14, 18, 19]. The prevalence of oral HPV16 infection in ages 14–69 in the US is ~ 1% (7% for all genotypes), with higher rates in men than in women [19]. The risk for oral HPV infection increases with the number of oral sexual partners, with the higher rates in men being possibly due to men performing oral sex on women and female genitalia

---

* Correspondence: dell@med.unc.edu; natalia.isaeva@med.uc.edu
[2]Department of Otolaryngology/Head and Neck Surgery; Lineberger Cancer Center, University of North Carolina at Chapel Hill, 170 Manning Drive, Campus Box 7070, Chapel Hill, NC 27599, USA
Full list of author information is available at the end of the article

carrying a higher HPV burden than male genitalia [17, 20]. Alternatively, since women have a higher seroconversion rate after genital HPV exposure, they may be relatively protected from oral infection [21].

Intense interest regarding the benefits of primary prevention of HPV infection has followed the introduction of HPV vaccines. The Gardasil four-valent vaccine covers HPV types 6, 11, 16, and 18 and received FDA approval for use in females in 2006 and in males in 2011. Since January 2017, the nine-valent Gardasil vaccine with expanded coverage, adding HPV types 31, 33, 45, 52, and 58, has been the only HPV vaccine available in the US. The CDC currently recommends routine vaccination for both girls and boys at age 11–12, with vaccination recommended for females through age 26 and for males through age 21 [22].

A US-based study that examined the effects of HPV vaccination on the burden of oral HPV16 infections found that between 2011 and 2014, vaccination potentially prevented almost one hundred thousand infections [23]. However, due to low vaccine uptake in males, less than half of this effect was seen in men, representing a gap in targeting the most at-risk population [23]. Due to the tepid HPV vaccine uptake and the long latency of developing OPSCC following exposure, it is estimated that the epidemic of HPV(+) OPSCC will continue until 2060 [17].

Diagnosis

The 2018 version of The National Comprehensive Cancer Network Clinical Practice Guidelines in Oncology (USA) directs that OPSCCs be tested for HPV by p16 immunohistochemistry (IHC) [24]. p16 (p16^{INK4a}) IHC has been widely adopted because it is cost effective, reliable, examines paraffin-embedded tissue, and has high sensitivity (94%) [25, 26]. IHC for p16 is particularly good for comparison of HPV(+) and HPV(–) HNSCC, because the protein is overexpressed in HPV(+) HNSCC and frequently lost in HNSCC not associated with HPV [27]. However, in various studies authors have reported that 8–33% of p16-positive OPSCCs lack HPV DNA, likely reflecting a combination of insensitive HPV detection techniques and that p16 overexpression occurs independently of HPV gene expression [28]. To more definitively identify HPV-associated OPSCC, multimodality HPV testing is increasing, with p16 IHC followed by HPV DNA PCR or in-situ hybridization (ISH) being the most common approaches [29]. In the UK, the National Institute for Health and Care Excellence (NICE) recommends reflexing to high-risk HPV DNA or RNA ISH in all p16-positive OPSCCs [30]. Because the specificity of HPV DNA PCR (87%) and ISH (88%) exceed that of p16, the use of these tests in tandem results in increased sensitivity and specificity for HPV detection as opposed to single-modality testing [26]. In addition,

HPV DNA testing is being used to diagnose cancer from fine needle aspirates from cervical lymph nodes and to help identify primary tumors [31]. However, the technical challenges and costs of HPV DNA PCR or ISH have limited their use for initial screening.

Next-generation sequencing (NGS) has emerged as an exciting new technology with the potential to identify HPV(+) tumors and provide rich mechanistic and prognostic information distinguishing subsets even within the HPV(+) group. A 2014 study using NGS found that HPV(+) tumors could be further categorized by presence of integrated versus nonintegrated HPV genes and that integration status corresponded with different patterns of DNA methylation and human and viral gene expression profiles in genes with known roles in carcinogenesis [32]. While implications of these findings are unknown, NGS will likely prove clinically useful in the future.

Prognosis

HPV-positive OPSCC carries a favorable prognosis compared to HPV-negative tumors. Five-year survival rates for patients with advanced stage HPV(+) OPSCC are 75–80%, versus survival rates of less than 50% among patients with similarly staged HPV(–) tumors [33]. The improved survival of patients with HPV(+) tumors can in part be attributed to their remarkable treatment sensitivity, as HPV(+) tumors have been shown to respond better to chemotherapy and radiation than HPV(–) tumors [16, 34]. The better prognosis conferred by HPV positivity is reflected in the updated AJCC 8th edition staging system, which for the first time separates staging for HPV(+) and HPV(–) OPSCCs and in general downgrades HPV(+) OPSCC staging [24, 35]. For example, HPV(+) OPSCC T3 N2, which was classified as Stage IVA in AJCC 7th edition, is newly classified as clinical Stage II in AJCC 8th edition.

Interest in identifying prognostic biomarkers in HPV-associated OPSCC has stemmed from the desire to decrease treatment morbidity while maintaining high cure rates. While a positive p16 by IHC predicts a favorable prognosis regardless of HPV status, recent data has shown that when used together with HPV status, further prognostic stratification is achieved [36]. A 2017 meta-analysis of both OPSCC and HNSCC patients found that the 5-year overall survival was best for patients with HPV(+)/p16(+) tumors, intermediate for HPV(–)/p16(+) tumors, and worst for HPV(+)/p16(–) and HPV(–)/p16(–) tumors [37].

Recent analysis of an HNSCC cohort in The Cancer Genome Atlas (TCGA) identified potential molecular biomarkers that can be used for prognostication [38, 39]. Deletion or mutation of two proteins that inhibit NF-kB and activate interferon, TNF receptor-associated factor 3 (TRAF3) and cylindromatosis (CYLD), were found in

28% of HPV(+) OPSCC [38]. Remarkably, survival for patients with HPV(+) tumors was better for those whose tumors carried defects in either TRAF3 or CYLD, while survival of HPV(+) patients without these mutations was similar to that of HPV(–) negative patients [38].

Treatment

Despite the prognostic significance of HPV in HNSCC, HPV status has not altered treatment guidelines. For the first time in 2018, The National Comprehensive Cancer Network Clinical Practice Guidelines in Oncology (NCCN, USA), separated treatment pathways for p16(+) and p16(–) OPSCCs [24]; however, recommendations for p16(+) and p16(–) OPSCCs are almost identical, with the only notable difference as follows: as an alternative to definitive radiation therapy (RT) alone or surgery alone, treatment with RT plus systemic therapy is a recommendation (category 2B) for T1 N1 p16-negative tumors, but is not recommended for p16-positive tumors until tumor size reaches T2 (with single node ≤3 cm). In general, regardless of p16 status, RT or surgery remain recommended treatment modalities for early-stage tumors, and combined therapy is recommended for advanced stages. The benefits of induction chemotherapy before concurrent chemoradiation are still being studied, with a recent meta-analysis demonstrating no survival advantage with induction chemotherapy [40].

Standard therapy for advanced OPSCC regardless of HPV status as either definitive or post-operative therapy includes chemotherapy and radiation, which is associated with dose-related adverse side effects, from acute toxicities like mucositis and loss of taste to long-term problems including dysphagia, renal dysfunction, hearing loss, xerostomia, osteoradionecrosis, accelerated arteriosclerosis, neck muscle fibrosis, and trismus. These side effects can lead to a cascade of events, including infections, difficulty eating, and increased hospitalizations, that can markedly erode quality of life. Based on analysis of long-term survivors from the RTOG 91–11 clinical trial, there is also the possibility that treatment-associated morbidity may impact 10-year or longer survival [41]. Given these concerns, minimizing side effects is especially important in advancing therapy for HPV(+) patients, who present at a younger age and have improved survival compared to patients with HPV(–) disease [11–13, 16].

The distinct tumor biology, higher treatment sensitivity, and better prognosis of HPV(+) OPSCCs has piqued interest in therapies that can minimize side effects, including new treatment approaches and de-escalation of current therapies. A single-arm phase II clinical trial, ECOG 1308, examined if response to induction chemotherapy could select stage III-IV (AJCC 7th edition) HPV(+) OPSCC patients for reduced-dose radiation

[42]. This trial found that patients with complete response to induction therapy maintained expected tumor control with reduced radiation doses of 54 Gy (compared to 69.3 Gy) but had fewer swallowing problems and nutritional deficiencies. A similar single institution trial also used induction chemotherapy, but stratified HPV(+) OPSCC patients to lower dose radiation (54 Gy) with similar survival and side effect findings [43]. The limited size of both studies as well as the recent changes to the AJCC staging criteria suggest the need for additional larger trials as are currently being considered through the National Clinical Trials Network (NCTN).

Several clinical trials (see Table 1 for currently active or recently completed clinical trials in HPV-associated OPSCC) are examining de-escalated treatments for HPV(+) OPSCCs, include reduced-dose radiation and/or chemotherapy (NCT03215719, NCT03323463, NCT01706939, NCT01898494, NCT02281955, NCT02048020, NCT02215265, NCT02048020), stratifying by responsiveness to induction chemotherapy to select subsequent loco-regional therapy (NCT02281955, NCT03107182), efficacy of chemotherapy or radiation as alternatives to surgery (NCT03210103, NCT03342911), minimally-invasive transoral robotic surgery using pathology to stratify patients for de-escalation (NCT02225496), treatment with surgery alone (NCT02072148), and using targeted therapies (NCT03 260023, NCT01855451, NCT02002182, NCT03410615, NCT02540928, NCT03342911).

In addition to de-escalation of standard therapy, new treatment modalities for HPV+ HNSCC are being developed with the hope of decreasing morbidity of current therapies. Early promising results from an ongoing clinical trial published in 2017 from the Yale Cancer Center examined molecular effects of DNA-demethylation using 5-azacytidine (5-azaC) for treatment of HPV(+) HNSCC patients [44], Table 1. Preclinical data revealed that 5-azaC inhibits growth and increases cell death of HPV(+) cancer cells associated with reduced expression of HPV genes, stabilization of p53, and activation of p53-dependent apoptosis. Evaluation of HPV(+) OPSCC tumor specimens from trial patients treated with 5-azaC (75 mg/m^2 for 5–7 days) reinforced the pre-clinical data, showing increased p53 expression, increased apoptosis and decreased expression of HPV genes. In a mouse xenograft model, 5-aza was also found to reduce the metastatic potential of HPV(+) tumors. A larger clinical trial is needed to fully characterize the therapeutic potential and safety of this promising therapy in HPV(+) HNSCC.

One mechanism of immune escape in HNSCCs is mediated by the receptor programmed death – 1 (PD-1) interacting with its ligand, PD-L1, which is expressed in 50–60% of HNSCC and 70% of HPV(+) HNSCCs [45]. PD-L1, found to be selectively expressed in tonsillar

Table 1 displays currently active or recently completed clinical trials in HPV-associated OPSCC (adapted from https://clinicaltrials.gov)

	NCT Number	Title	Interventions
1	NCT03656133	Use of a Proliferation Saturation Index to Determine Personalized Radiotherapy for HPV + Oropharyngeal Cancers	• Radiotherapy fractionation
2	NCT03618134	Stereotactic Body Radiation Therapy and Durvalumab With or Without Tremelimumab Before Surgery in Treating Participants With Human Papillomavirus Positive Oropharyngeal Squamous Cell Caner	• Durvalumab • Modified Radical Neck Dissection • Transoral Robotic Surgery • Tremelimumab
3	NCT03580070	Changes in the Microenvironment of HPV-induced Head and Neck Cancers in West Indies and Metropolitan Population	• Immunotherapy
4	NCT03578406	HPV-E6-Specific TCR-T Cells in the Treatment of HPV-Positive NHSCC or Cervical Cancer	• HPV E6-specific TCR-T cells
5	NCT03418480	HPV Anti-CD40 RNA Vaccine	• HPV vaccine
6	NCT03396718	De-escalation of Adjuvant Radio (Chemo) Therapy for HPV-positive Head-neck Squamous Cell Carcinomas	• De-escalation radio(chemo)therapy - Levels 1 and 2
7	NCT03342911	Nivolumab, Carboplatin, and Paclitaxel in Treating Patients With Stage III-IV Head and Neck Squamous Cell Carcinoma That Can Be Removed by Surgery	• Paclitaxel, Carboplatin, Nivolumab
8	NCT03260023	Phase Ib/II of TG4001 and Avelumab in HPV16 Positive R/M Cancers and Expansion Cohort to Oropharyngeal SCCHN	• TG4001, Avelumab
9	NCT03224000	Trial of Magnetic Resonance Imaging Guided Radiotherapy Dose Adaptation in Human Papilloma Virus Positive Oropharyngeal Cancer	• Modified Barium Swallow, MRI Guided Intensity Modulated Radiotherapy
10	NCT03162224	Safety and Efficacy of MEDI0457 and Durvalumab in Patients With HPV Associated Recurrent/Metastatic Head and Neck Cancer	• MEDI0457, CELLECTRA®5P device, Durvalumab
11	NCT03107182	Chemotherapy and Locoregional Therapy Trial (Surgery or Radiation) for Patients With Head and Neck Cancer	•Carboplatin, Nivolumab, Cisplatin, Hydroxyurea, 5-FU, Dexamethasone, Famotidine, Diphenhydramine, Paclitaxel
12	NCT03077243	P53 Mutational Status and cf HPV DNA for the Management of HPV-associated OPSCC	• Intensity Modulated Radiotherapy, Cisplatin (or alternative)
13	NCT02945631	Quarterback 2 - Sequential Therapy With Reduced Dose Chemoradiotherapy for HPV Oropharynx Cancer	• Radiation: PTV56
14	NCT02865135	Trial To Test Safety And Efficacy Of Vaccination For Incurable HPV 16-Related Oropharyngeal, Cervical And Anal Cancer	• DPX-E7 vaccine
15	NCT02827838	Durvalumab Before Surgery in Treating Patients With Oral Cavity or Oropharynx Cancer	• Durvalumab
16	NCT02784288	Phase II Treatment Stratification Trial Using Neck Dissection-Driven Selection to Improve Quality of Life for Low Risk Patients With HPV + Oropharyngeal Squamous Cell Cancer	•Radiation, Carboplatin, Paclitaxel
17	NCT02706691	BGJ398 in Treating Patients With FGFR Positive Recurrent Head and Neck Cancer	•BGJ398
18	NCT02686008	Pharmacodynamic Study to Assess the Anti-proliferative Activity of the PARP Inhibitor Olaparib in Patients With HPV Positive and HPV Negative HNSCC	• Olaparib
19	NCT02643550	Study of Monalizumab and Cetuximab in Patients With Recurrent or Metastatic Squamous Cell Carcinoma of the Head and Neck	• Monalizumab, Cetuximab
20	NCT02281955	De-intensification of Radiation and Chemotherapy for Low-Risk HPV-related Oropharyngeal SCC: Follow-up Study	• Radiation, cisplatin
21	NCT02215265	Post-operative Adjuvant Treatment for HPV-positive Tumours (PATHOS)	• Cisplatin, Postoperative radiotherapy
22	NCT02178072	Window Trial 5-aza in HNSCC, T-tare	• 5-Azacitadine
23	NCT02113878	Phase Ib Study of BKM120 With Cisplatin and XRT in High Risk Locally Advanced Squamous Cell Cancer of Head and Neck	• BKM120, Cisplatin, Intensity-modulated radiotherapy
24	NCT02002182	ADXS 11-001 Vaccination Prior to Robotic Surgery, HPV-Positive Oropharyngeal Cancer	• ADXS11-001 (ADXS-HPV)
25	NCT01716195	Induction Chemotherapy Followed by Chemoradiotherapy for Head and Neck Cancer	• Radiotherapy

Table 1 displays currently active or recently completed clinical trials in HPV-associated OPSCC (adapted from https://clinicaltrials.gov) (Continued)

	NCT Number	Title	Interventions
26	NCT01706939	The Quarterback Trial: Reduced Dose Radiotherapy for HPV+ Oropharynx Cancer	• Reduced Dose Radiation, Carboplatin
27	NCT01530997	De-intensification of Radiation & Chemotherapy in Low-Risk Human Papillomavirus-related Oropharyngeal Squamous Cell Ca	• Intensity Modulated Radiotherapy, Cisplatin
28	NCT01302834	Radiation Therapy With Cisplatin or Cetuximab in Treating Patients With Oropharyngeal Cancer	• cetuximab, cisplatin

crypts, may facilitate HPV infection at these sites, reflecting the potential for targeted therapy with PD-1 inhibitors in HPV(+) cancers [46]. Two PD-1 inhibitors, pembrolizumab (KEYTRUDA, Merck Sharp & Dohme) and nivolumab (OPDIVO, Bristol-Myers Squibb), were approved by the FDA for the treatment of recurrent or metastatic HNSCC that failed a platinum-based therapy [47, 48]. Studies examining the efficacy of these drugs in patients with recurrent or metastatic HNSCC revealed a relatively low overall response rate of 13–18% with no difference in response between HPV(+) and HPV(−) cancers [45]. Many clinical trials examining combinations of immune checkpoint inhibitors with other immune modulators, radiation, cytotoxic chemotherapy or epigenetic therapies are underway [49].

Molecular characteristics

In addition to the epidemiological, pathological, and clinical characteristics distinguishing HPV(+) and HPV(−) OPSCCs, TCGA and other efforts have elucidated molecular and epigenetic differences [50–52]. Here, we will explore heterogeneity between HPV(+) and HPV(−) HNSCC, as well as distinctions within OPSCC driven by HPV with particular attention on defects that correlate with tumor response and patient survival.

Altered DNA-repair pathways, differences in mitogenic signaling pathways, dysregulation of cell cycle control, and changes in the tumor micro-environment of HPV(+) tumors have all been proposed as possible explanations of their enhanced sensitivity to radiation [53]. SMG-1 (suppressor with morphogenetic effect on genitalia) is a member of the phosphoinositide 3-kinase-related kinases (PIKK) family and plays an important role in the DNA-damage response [54–56]. In OPSCCs, expression of SMG-1 was found to be decreased in HPV(+) tumors due to hypermethylation of its promotor [57]. This decreased expression of SMG-1 appears to be an important contributor to the radiosensitivity of HPV(+) cells, as depletion of SMG-1 in HPV(−) cells was shown to cause increased radiosensitivity while overexpression in HPV(+) protected cells from radiation [57]. Further evidence of the altered mechanisms in DNA repair in HPV(+) tumors was seen through reverse-phase protein array (RPPA) profiling of OPSCCs, which found that all eleven DNA repair proteins screened,

including BRCA2, MSH2, PARP-1, and ATM, were significantly upregulated in HPV(+) samples compared to HPV(−) samples [58]. This is particularly interesting, since HPV(+) oropharyngeal cancer cells have shown a partial deficiency in DNA double strand breaks repair mostly in the homologous recombination repair pathway [59, 60] that may also contribute to increased sensitivity to radiation or DNA damaging agents.

Differences in cell cycle regulation may also play a role in the remarkable treatment sensitivity of HPV(+) tumors. Amplification and overexpression of cyclin D1, inactivation of the cyclin-dependent kinase inhibitor p16, and mutations of the tumor suppressor p53 are common defects found in HPV(−) HNSCC, but are lacking in HPV(+) tumors [50, 61]. On the other hand, amplification and overexpression of E2F1, which is a driver of G1-to-S transition, is common in HPV(+) but not HPV(−) HNSCC [50, 61]. Given these differences in cell cycle regulation, it is not surprising that differences to treatment with cyclin-dependent kinase (CDK) inhibitors are observed. HPV-positivity has been shown to correlate with hypersensitivity of tumor cells to roscovitine, a cyclin-dependent kinase (CDK) inhibitor that inhibits CDK-1, 3, 5, 7, and 9 [62]. Treatment of HPV(+) OPSCC cells with roscovitine resulted in DNA-damage and induced a p53-dependent cell death [62]. Additionally, low-doses of roscovitine that did not cause weight loss in mice significantly inhibited growth of HPV(+) xenografted tumors.

In addition to differences distinguishing HPV(+) and HPV(−) head and neck tumors, significant molecular heterogeneity exists within HPV(+) tumors themselves. Gene expression profiling has classified HPV(+) tumors into two subgroups with one (HPV-KRT) having elevated expression of genes involved in keratinization, viral integrations, spliced E6, chr3q amplifications, and PIK3CA mutations, and the other subgroup (HPV-IMU) having more mesenchymal differentiation, full-length E6 activity, chr16q deletions, and a stronger immune response [63]. Although TCGA survival analysis showed a trend toward better survival in the HPV-IMU subgroup, the survival difference was not significant, warranting further investigation into the clinical implications of this HPV(+) stratification model [63].

Further proving the heterogeneity of HPV(+) HNSCCs, a 2014 study of HNSCCs from TCGA found that of the 35

HPV(+) tumors, 25 had integration of the viral genome while 10 tumors lacked integration [32]. The canonical paradigm of HPV carcinogenesis, which was developed through studies of uterine cervical cancer, highlights the importance of HPV genome integration as premalignant lesions transition to become malignant [64]. Discovering that nearly 30% of HPV(+) OPSCC contained only episomal HPV challenged this canonical theory of HPV carcinogenesis and presented an opportunity for understanding alternative mechanisms of HPV-driven tumorigenic conversion.

OPSCC with integrated versus nonintegrated HPV have differences in somatic gene methylation, gene expression patterns, mRNA processing, and inter- and intrachromosomal rearrangements [32]. For tumors with HPV integration, integration was not random, with many integration sites occurring within cancer-associated genes suggesting that even within tumors with integrated HPV, different molecular events may be involved in carcinogenesis [32, 65]. Given the molecular differences that are based on HPV integration status, it is not surprising that clinical parameters also differ. In support of this, absence of integration correlated with improved survival and with indications of increased immune infiltration [65]. Recently, defects in TRAF3 and CYLD were found as novel alterations in HNSCC that identified a subset of HPV(+) HNSCC with improved survival [38, 50]. TRAF3 and CYLD gene deletions or disruptive mutations were identified in 28% of HPV(+) specimens in the initial TCGA HNSCC cohort and correlated with the absence of HPV gene integration [38]. Consistent with known functions of TRAF3 and CYLD, tumors with altered TRAF3 or CYLD had activation of NF-kB and inactivation of innate immune signaling [38, 39]. These gene defects were nearly significant in correlating with decreased tobacco exposure in this cohort, raising the possibility that DNA damage, reactive oxygen species or other factors associated with tobacco smoke may increase the probability of HPV integration. In light of finding that TRAF3 or CYLD mutation or deletion identified a unique subset of HPV(+) patients, additional analysis of genes regulating the NF-kB pathway were examined in an independent Yale cohort (unpublished data). This analysis confirmed the existence of TRAF3 and CYLD mutations, but also found defects in additional NF-kB regulators (MAP3K14, BIRC3, TRAF2, and MYD88). This cohort is being followed, but time from treatment for this cohort is currently too short to draw survival conclusions. Identification of additional mutations in regulators of NF-kB suggest that NF-kB pathway defects in addition to TRAF3 and CYLD may be important for separating subtypes of HPV(+) OPSCC tumors.

Etiology

The mechanisms of HPV-driven OPSCC have not been intensely studied, as many have assumed that HPV carcinogenesis in OPSCC is identical to the accepted mechanism of HPV carcinogenesis in the uterine cervix; however, there are many differences between HPV(+) OPSCC and uterine cervical cancer. HPV(+) OPSCC and cervical cancer diverge in epidemiologic factors, molecular patterns, HPV type, mutational profile, cell-of-origin, treatment response, and clinical behavior (Table 2), suggesting that uterine cervical cancer and OPSCC are distinct [66]. While more than 85% of cervical cancer cases worldwide are from developing nations, the developing world has relatively fewer OPSCCs than higher-income countries [66]. Furthermore, over 90% of HPV(+) OPSCCs are caused by HPV16, whereas in cervical cancer, only 50% is attributable to HPV16 and up to 20% is caused by HPV18, which is rarely identified in OPSCC [14, 67]. HPV(+) OPSCC and uterine cervical cancer mutational landscapes also differ; for example, in an analysis of an expanded TCGA cohort, almost 30% of HPV(+) oropharyngeal tumors had TRAF3 or CYLD mutations or deletions, while these mutations were extremely rare in cervical cancer [38]. From a clinical standpoint, HPV(+) OPSCCs respond better to treatment than HPV(+) cervical cancer, possibly due to differences in the unique properties of their respective epithelial sites of infection, clinical presenting signs and symptoms, patterns of metastasis, and target populations, but also possibly due to molecular differences [66]. Clinical and molecular differences between OPSCC and uterine cervical cancer should caution against equating any aspect of these HPV-associated diseases including carcinogenesis, treatment response or outcome.

The productive HPV life cycle has been studied and is outlined here [68]. In the uterine cervix, HPV gains access through microabrasions to infect basal epithelial cells, and after infection, the HPV genome replicates to a low copy number to be maintained as nuclear episomes. HPV early genes are expressed at low levels, and after the initial low-level amplification, HPV episomes are maintained through replication in sync with cell division. These characteristics are thought to assist with immune evasion by minimizing activation of pattern recognition receptors, NF-kB, and downstream type I interferon signaling. Emphasizing the importance of immune system evasion in HPV life cycle, proteins encoded by HPV inhibit NF-kB and type I interferon signaling [69]. Cellular differentiation is critical for the final productive amplification stage of the HPV life cycle. As cells migrate toward the surface of the epithelium, differentiation triggers increased expression of E6 and E7 oncoproteins that in turn enables an expansion of DNA replication-competent cells and a several log amplification of HPV episomes, ultimately concluding with expression of late viral capsid genes, encapsidation of HPV genomes, and shedding of new viral particles from the epithelial surface [70, 71]. Most mucosal infections are cleared within two years through activation of innate and

Table 2 Major differences between cervical cancer and HPV-associated OPSCC

	OPSCC	Cervical Cancer
Incidence	Incidence increasing	Incidence decreasing
Prevalence	Increased in higher-income countries	Increased in lower-income countries
Sex	> 70% male	100% female
Etiology	Tobacco and alcohol remain important causes, along with HPV	Virtually all are caused by HPV
HPV genotype	> 95% HPV16 HPV18 rare	50% HPV16 20% HPV18
Premalignant lesions	Unknown	CIN1–3
Screening tests available	No	Yes
5-year survival rate	> 75%	< 70%
TRAF3/CYLD mutations	Approximately 30%	Rare
Treatment sensitivity to chemotherapy and radiation	High	Moderate

acquired immune mechanisms [72, 73]. The importance of acquired immunity in HPV clearance is supported by identification of HLA variants associated with decreased risk of both HPV(+) OPSCC and uterine cervical cancer [74]. On the other hand, persistent infection predisposes to malignant transformation that requires additional mutations and/or immune deficiency. The delay between HPV infection and detection of malignancy can be several decades [17, 70].

Studies of the transformation process initiated by HPV infection have relied heavily on the study of pre-malignant uterine cervical cells and have led to a canonical model of HPV carcinogenesis. In this model, initial infection, establishment and maintenance are thought to parallel the normal HPV life cycle; however, with persistent infection of basal or stem cells carcinogenesis can be initiated. The model details that as cells progress from early dysplasia (CIN1) to pre-malignant lesions (CIN3), the HPV genome integrates and disrupts the HPV E2 gene, which relieves negative feedback and increases expression of HPV oncoproteins, E6 and E7 [72, 75–77]. As opposed to the natural life cycle where E6 and E7 expression increases in the superficial layers of the epithelia, the carcinogenesis model establishes cells with high E6 and E7 expression at the basal layer of the epithelium where in the absence of immune clearance, these pre-malignant cells persist. Increased expression of HPV oncoproteins inactivates the major human tumor suppressor genes, p53 and RB leading to genomic instability, resistance to apoptosis, and dysregulated cell cycle control. One caveat of integration studies that contributed to the model is that methods for identification of integrated HPV frequently relied on loss of E2, and by design, these techniques exclude integrated forms that maintain E2 [77]. While integration of the HPV genome is part of the canonical HPV carcinogenesis model, it excludes a percentage of HPV

type 16-positive cervical cancers that lack detected HPV integration [77]. It is unclear if this model applies to a portion of OPSCC with integration, but it is evident that it does not describe carcinogenesis for HPV(+) OPSCC that lack integration of the HPV genome.

TCGA analysis of HPV-associated OPSCC provides some characterization of the role of HPV integration in tumors [32]. Genomic profiling revealed that HPV-driven carcinogenesis is more complex and heterogeneous than previously thought. In OPSCC, HPV integration was associated with breakpoints throughout the viral genome, with only breakpoints in E1 occurring more frequently than expected by chance. This finding contrasts with the canonical HPV carcinogenesis model, in which disruption of E2 through integration leads to enhanced expression of E6 and E7 [72]. Further complicating the picture, whole genome sequencing data identified a category of tumors containing both partially deleted HPV genomes and full-length genomes [78]. The status of HPV in these "mixed" tumors remains controversial, with some authors describing these tumors as containing both integrated and nonintegrated HPV, while others argue that these tumors represent viral-human hybrid episomes [79].

Direct analysis of the HPV carcinogenesis process in the tonsil is not possible due to the absence of a defined pre-malignant lesion. The area infected by HPV and prone to transformation within the tonsil – the tonsillar crypt – lacks tight epithelial junctions and is characterized by incomplete basement membranes making pathological distinction between invasive cancer and intra-epithelial neoplasia impossible [80, 81]. In fact, the College of American Pathologists 2017 Guidelines state that in-situ disease in HPV(+) oropharyngeal cancer is "non-existent" [82]. In addition, murine modeling of OPSCC may not re-create the human situation because mice do not have tonsils and therefore lack the tonsillar crypt cells that are the target of carcinogenic HPV infection.

Given the difficulties of studying progression of HPV pre-malignancies in the oropharynx, comparison of molecular characteristics of OPSCC and uterine cervical cancer may shed light on mechanisms of carcinogenesis in these distinct cancers. APOBEC (apolipoprotein B mRNA editing enzyme, catalytic polypeptide-like) is a cytidine deaminase whose mutations have been implicated in carcinogenesis. Both OPSCC and uterine cervical cancers have enrichment for APOBEC mutational signatures [50, 83, 84]. Consistent with finding APOBEC mutational signatures in each, both tumor types have a significant burden of APOBEC-driven PIK3CA mutations, and activating mutations of PI3KCA occur more frequently in HPV(+) than HPV(−) OPSCCs [50, 58, 84]. Enhanced PI3K signaling has been implicated in HNSCC tumorigenesis; however, the role of PI3K pathway activation by PIK3CA mutations in HPV(+) OPSCC needs to be further explored since AKT was not activated by mutant PIK3CA in the presence of HPV oncoproteins [58, 85, 86]. Cervical cancers and OPSCCs also share an absence of mutations in genes or pathways regulated by HPV oncoproteins such as p53 and p16^INK4a, confirming the importance of HPV oncogenes in tumorigenesis [50, 84]. Interestingly, EGFR (17%) and ERB2 (17%) amplifications were found in uterine cervical cancer, but not in HPV(+) OPSCC, while FGFR3 amplifications were found in 11% of HPV(+) OPSCC, but not in uterine cervical cancer, suggesting that these tumors rely differently on receptor tyrosine kinase signaling [50, 84].

For tumors caused by HPV type 16, integration of the HPV genome occurs at similar rates in OPSCC (72%) and cervical cancer (76%) [32, 84]. Despite the similar proportion of tumors lacking integration, the strong correlation of TRAF3 and CYLD defects with the absence of integration in OPSCC compared to the lack of these defects in uterine cervical cancer suggest that HPV carcinogenesis in tumors lacking integration may differ [38, 50, 84]. Although the reason for this difference is unknown, the function of TRAF3 and CYLD as inhibitors of NF-kB and activators of type I interferon signaling suggest that disruption of these genes may be critical for survival of infected cells and maintenance of unintegrated HPV DNA in oropharyngeal cells. A recent study confirmed that attenuated TRAF3 activated NF-kB and inhibited interferon in HPV(+) HNSCC cells [87]. The reason that TRAF3 or CYLD mutations are not required in uterine cervical cells is unknown but could relate to the differences in the infected cell. Unlike uterine cervical cells at the squamocolumnar junction, tonsillar crypt cells are closely associated with non-epithelial and lymphatic cells [88]. The lymphoepithelium of the tonsil is critical for initiation of immune responses with one role of the specialized crypt epithelial cells being endocytosis to deliver antigens to adjacent immune cells that initiate immune responses

through antigen processing and release of cytokines [88]. Several pathogens take advantage of the discontinuous epithelium and immune milieu to invade, including the Epstein-Barr Virus (EBV), which infects the lymphoepithelium of the nasopharynx and can result in nasopharyngeal cancer [88]. Like HPV, EBV infects many years before cancers develops and must be maintained for carcinogenic conversion. Unlike HPV, EBV is a herpesvirus, which does not integrate and therefore must be maintained in an episomal form [89]. Interestingly, EBV-associated nasopharyngeal cancer is one of the few solid tumor types other than HPV(+) OPSCC that has TRAF3 mutations [38, 90]. Inhibition of NF-kB signaling in EBV-associated nasopharyngeal cancer cells has been shown to inhibit their growth, suggesting that the cells are reliant on continuous NF-kB activity [90].

Together these data raise the intriguing possibility of an alternative mechanism of HPV carcinogenesis uncovered through the study of HPV(+) OPSCC. Instead of HPV integration as a driver for increased oncoprotein expression, a subset of OPSCC may rely on maintenance of unintegrated HPV that in turn requires molecular defects in TRAF3, CYLD or other genes to activate NF-kB and inhibit innate immune responses.

Conclusions

Recent studies of OPSCC are increasing our understanding of HPV-associated carcinogenesis, including the possibility of an alternative mechanism reliant on activation of NF-kB, inhibition of interferon and maintenance of non-integrated HPV. In addition, markers to identify HPV(+) OPSCC patients with improved prognosis are emerging. These insights are critical to improving our management of this rising disease and exploring effective new treatments and identification of patients for de-escalated therapy.

Abbreviations

5-azaC: 5-azacytidine; APOBEC: Apolipoprotein B mRNA editing enzyme, catalytic polypeptide-like; CDK: Cyclin-dependent kinase; CYLD: Cylindromatosis; EBV: Epstein-Barr Virus; HNSCC: Head and neck squamous cell carcinoma; HPV: Human papillomavirus; ISH: In-situ hybridization; NICE: National Institute for Health and Care Excellence; OPSCC: Oropharyngeal squamous cell carcinoma; PD-1: Programmed death − 1; PIKK: Phosphoinositide 3-kinase-related kinases; RPPA: Reverse-phase protein array; RT: Radiation therapy; SMG-1: Suppressor with morphogenetic effect on genitalia; TRAF3: TNF receptor-associated factor 3

Acknowledgements

The authors thank the Yale Department of Surgery, Otolaryngology Division; the Lineberger Cancer Center, and the UNC Department of Otolaryngology/ Head and Neck Surgery for support.

Funding

There was no funding for this review article; the financial support was provided by the Yale Department of Surgery Otolaryngology Division, the Lineberger Cancer Center, and the Deaprtment of Otolaryngology/Head and Neck Surgery at the University of North Carolina.

Authors' contributions

CP searched literature. CP, NI, and WGY wrote the manuscript. All authors read and approved the final manuscript.

Competing interests

The authors declare that they have no competing interest.

Author details

[1]Department of Surgery, Division of Otolaryngology, Yale University, New Haven, CT, USA. [2]Department of Otolaryngology/Head and Neck Surgery; Lineberger Cancer Center, University of North Carolina at Chapel Hill, 170 Manning Drive, Campus Box 7070, Chapel Hill, NC 27599, USA.

References

1. Dalla Torre D, Burtscher D, Soelder E, Offermanns V, Rasse M, Puelacher W. Human papillomavirus prevalence in a mid-European oral squamous cell cancer population: a cohort study. Oral Dis. 2018;24:948–56.
2. Götz C, Drecoll E, Straub M, Bissinger O, Wolff K-D, Kolk A. Impact of HPV infection on oral squamous cell carcinoma. Oncotarget. 2016;7:76704–12. https://doi.org/10.18632/oncotarget.12501.
3. Shiboski CH, Schmidt BL, Jordan RCK. Tongue and tonsil carcinoma: increasing trends in the U.S. population ages 20-44 years. Cancer. 2005;103:1843–9.
4. Frisch M, Hjalgrim H, Jaeger AB, Biggar RJ. Changing patterns of tonsillar squamous cell carcinoma in the United States. Cancer Causes Control CCC. 2000;11:489–95.
5. Mehta V, Yu G-P, Schantz SP. Population-based analysis of oral and oropharyngeal carcinoma: changing trends of histopathologic differentiation, survival and patient demographics. Laryngoscope. 2010;120: 2203–12. https://doi.org/10.1002/lary.21129.
6. Sturgis EM, Cinciripini PM. Trends in head and neck cancer incidence in relation to smoking prevalence. Cancer. 2007;110:1429–35. https://doi.org/10.1002/cncr.22963.
7. Chaturvedi AK, Engels EA, Pfeiffer RM, Hernandez BY, Xiao W, Kim E, et al. Human papillomavirus and rising oropharyngeal Cancer incidence in the United States. J Clin Oncol. 2011;29:4294–301. https://doi.org/10.1200/JCO.2011.36.4596.
8. Steinau M, Saraiya M, Goodman MT, Peters ES, Watson M, Cleveland JL, et al. Human papillomavirus prevalence in oropharyngeal cancer before vaccine introduction, United States. Emerg Infect Dis. 2014;20:822–8.
9. Singhi AD, Westra WH. Comparison of human papillomavirus in situ hybridization and p16 immunohistochemistry in the detection of human papillomavirus-associated head and neck cancer based on a prospective clinical experience. Cancer. 2010;116:2166–73.
10. CDC - How Many Cancers Are Linked with HPV Each Year? https://www.cdc.gov/cancer/hpv/statistics/cases.htm. Accessed 15 Mar 2018.
11. Pytynia KB, Dahlstrom KR, Sturgis EM. Epidemiology of HPV-associated oropharyngeal cancer. Oral Oncol. 2014;50:380–6. https://doi.org/10.1016/j.oraloncology.2013.12.019.
12. Gillison ML. Current topics in the epidemiology of oral cavity and oropharyngeal cancers. Head Neck. 2007;29:779–92.
13. Goon PKC, Stanley MA, Ebmeyer J, Steinsträsser L, Upile T, Jerjes W, et al. HPV & head and neck cancer: a descriptive update. Head Neck Oncol. 2009;1:36.
14. Gillison ML, Koch WM, Capone RB, Spafford M, Westra WH, Wu L, et al. Evidence for a causal association between human papillomavirus and a subset of head and neck cancers. J Natl Cancer Inst. 2000;92:709–20.
15. Dahlstrom KR, Calzada G, Hanby JD, Garden AS, Glisson BS, Li G, et al. an evolution in demographics, treatment, and outcomes of oropharyngeal cancer at a major cancer center. Cancer. 2013;119:81–9. https://doi.org/10.1002/cncr.27727.
16. Chaturvedi AK, Engels EA, Anderson WF, Gillison ML. Incidence trends for human papillomavirus-related and -unrelated oral squamous cell carcinomas in the United States. J Clin Oncol Off J Am Soc Clin Oncol. 2008;26:612–9.
17. Gillison ML, Chaturvedi AK, Anderson WF, Fakhry C. Epidemiology of human papillomavirus–positive head and neck squamous cell carcinoma. J Clin Oncol. 2015;33:3235–42. https://doi.org/10.1200/JCO.2015.61.6995.
18. Gillison ML, Alemany L, Snijders PJF, Chaturvedi A, Steinberg BM, Schwartz S, et al. Human papillomavirus and diseases of the upper airway: head and neck cancer and respiratory papillomatosis. Vaccine. 2012;30(Suppl 5):F34–54.
19. Gillison ML, Broutian T, Pickard RKL, Tong Z, Xiao W, Kahle L, et al. Prevalence of oral HPV infection in the United States, 2009-2010. JAMA. 2012;307:693–703.
20. D'Souza G, Agrawal Y, Halpern J, Bodison S, Gillison ML. Oral sexual behaviors associated with prevalent Oral human papillomavirus infection. J Infect Dis. 2009;199:1263–9. https://doi.org/10.1086/597755.
21. Kjaer SK, Chackerian B, van den Brule AJ, Svare EI, Paull G, Walbomers JM, et al. High-risk human papillomavirus is sexually transmitted: evidence from a follow-up study of virgins starting sexual activity (intercourse). Cancer Epidemiol biomark Prev Publ am Assoc Cancer res cosponsored am Soc Prev. Oncologia. 2001;10:101–6.
22. Clinician FAQs: CDC Recommendations for HPV Vaccine 2-Dose Schedule | Human Papillomavirus (HPV) | CDC. 2017. https://www.cdc.gov/hpv/hcp/2-dose/clinician-faq.html. Accessed 24 Feb 2018.
23. Chaturvedi AK, Graubard BI, Broutian T, Pickard RKL, Tong Z-Y, Xiao W, et al. Effect of Prophylactic Human Papillomavirus (HPV) Vaccination on Oral HPV Infections Among Young Adults in the United States. J Clin Oncol. 2017;36: 262–7. https://doi.org/10.1200/JCO.2017.75.0141.
24. DG Pfister, S Spencer. NCCN clinical practice guidelines in oncology: head and neck cancers (version 1. 2018). https://www.nccn.org/professionals/physician_gls/f_guidelines.asp. Accessed 11 Feb 2018.
25. Thavaraj S, Stokes A, Guerra E, Bible J, Halligan E, Long A, et al. Evaluation of human papillomavirus testing for squamous cell carcinoma of the tonsil in clinical practice. J Clin Pathol. 2011;64:308–12. https://doi.org/10.1136/jcp.2010.088450.
26. Schache AG, Liloglou T, Risk JM, Filia A, Jones TM, Sheard J, et al. Evaluation of human papilloma virus diagnostic testing in oropharyngeal squamous cell carcinoma: sensitivity, specificity, and prognostic discrimination. Clin Cancer Res. 2011;17:6262–71. https://doi.org/10.1158/1078-0432.CCR-11-0388.
27. Reed AL, Califano J, Cairns P, Westra WH, Jones RM, Koch W, et al. High frequency of p16 (CDKN2/MTS-1/INK4A) inactivation in head and neck squamous cell carcinoma. Cancer Res. 1996;56:3630–3.
28. Wasylyk B, Abecassis J, Jung AC. Identification of clinically relevant HPV-related HNSCC: in p16 should we trust? Oral Oncol. 2013;49:e33–7. https://doi.org/10.1016/j.oraloncology.2013.07.014.
29. Bishop JA, Lewis JS, Rocco JW, Faquin WC. HPV-related squamous cell carcinoma of the head and neck: an update on testing in routine pathology practice. Semin Diagn Pathol. 2015;32:344–51. https://doi.org/10.1053/j.semdp.2015.02.013.
30. Cancer of the upper aerodigestive tract: assessment and management in people aged 16 and over | Guidance and guidelines | NICE. https://www.nice.org.uk/guidance/NG36/chapter/Recommendations#hpvrelated-disease. Accessed 11 Feb 2018.
31. Baldassarri R, Aronberg R, Levi AW, Yarbrough WG, Kowalski D, Chhieng D. Detection and genotype of high-Risk human papillomavirus in fine-needle aspirates of patients with metastatic squamous cell carcinoma is helpful in determining tumor origin. Am J Clin Pathol. 2015;143:694–700. https://doi.org/10.1309/AJCPCZA4PSZCFHQ4.
32. Parfenov M, Pedamallu CS, Gehlenborg N, Freeman SS, Danilova L, Bristow CA, et al. Characterization of HPV and host genome interactions in primary head and neck cancers. Proc Natl Acad Sci. 2014;111:15544–9. https://doi.org/10.1073/pnas.1416074111.
33. Ang KK, Harris J, Wheeler R, Weber R, Rosenthal DI, Nguyen-Tân PF, et al. Human papillomavirus and survival of patients with oropharyngeal Cancer. N Engl J Med. 2010;363:24–35. https://doi.org/10.1056/NEJMoa0912217.
34. Fakhry C, Westra WH, Li S, Cmelak A, Ridge JA, Pinto H, et al. Improved survival of patients with human papillomavirus-positive head and neck squamous cell carcinoma in a prospective clinical trial. J Natl Cancer Inst. 2008;100:261–9.

35. Amin MB, Edge S, Greene F, Byrd DR, Brookland RK, Washington MK, et al. In: AJCC, editor. Cancer Staging Manual. 8th ed: Springer International Publishing; 2017. www.springer.com/us/book/9783319406176. Accessed 27 Feb 2018.

36. Lewis JS, Thorstad WL, Chernock RD, Haughey BH, Yip JH, Zhang Q, et al. p16 positive oropharyngeal squamous cell carcinoma: an entity with a favorable prognosis regardless of tumor HPV status. Am J Surg Pathol. 2010; 34:1088–96. https://doi.org/10.1097/PAS.0b013e3181e84652.

37. Albers AE, Qian X, Kaufmann AM, Coordes A. Meta analysis: HPV and p16 pattern determines survival in patients with HNSCC and identifies potential new biologic subtype. Sci Rep. 2017;7:16715.

38. Hajek M, Sewell A, Kaech S, Burtness B, Yarbrough WG, Issaeva N. TRAF3/ CYLD mutations identify a distinct subset of human papillomavirus-associated head and neck squamous cell carcinoma. Cancer. 2017;123:1778–90. https://doi.org/10.1002/cncr.30570.

39. Pan C, Yarbrough WG, Issaeva N. Advances in biomarkers and treatment strategies for HPV-associated head and neck cancer. Oncoscience. 2018;5:140–1.

40. Budach W, Bölke E, Kammers K, Gerber PA, Orth K, Gripp S, et al. Induction chemotherapy followed by concurrent radio-chemotherapy versus concurrent radio-chemotherapy alone as treatment of locally advanced squamous cell carcinoma of the head and neck (HNSCC): a meta-analysis of randomized trials. Radiother Oncol J Eur Soc Ther Radiol Oncol. 2016;118:238–43.

41. Forastiere AA, Zhang Q, Weber RS, Maor MH, Goepfert H, Pajak TF, et al. Long-term results of RTOG 91-11: a comparison of three nonsurgical treatment strategies to preserve the larynx in patients with locally advanced larynx cancer. J Clin Oncol Off J Am Soc Clin Oncol. 2013;31:845–52.

42. Marur S, Li S, Cmelak AJ, Gillison ML, Zhao WJ, Ferris RL, et al. E1308: phase II trial of induction chemotherapy followed by reduced-dose radiation and weekly Cetuximab in patients with HPV-associated Resectable squamous cell carcinoma of the oropharynx– ECOG-ACRIN Cancer research group. J Clin Oncol Off J Am Soc Clin Oncol. 2017;35:490–7.

43. Chen AM, Felix C, Wang P-C, Hsu S, Basehart V, Garst J, et al. Reduced-dose radiotherapy for human papillomavirus-associated squamous-cell carcinoma of the oropharynx: a single-arm, phase 2 study. Lancet Oncol. 2017;18:803–11. https://doi.org/10.1016/S1470-2045(17)30246-2.

44. Biktasova A, Hajek M, Sewell A, Gary C, Bellinger G, Deshpande HA, et al. Demethylation therapy as a targeted treatment for human papillomavirus-associated head and neck Cancer. Clin Cancer Res. 2017;23:7276–87. https://doi.org/10.1158/1078-0432.CCR-17-1438.

45. Saleh K, Eid R, Haddad FG, Khalife-Saleh N, Kourie HR. New developments in the management of head and neck cancer - impact of pembrolizumab. Ther Clin Risk Manag. 2018;14:295–303.

46. Lyford-Pike S, Peng S, Young GD, Taube JM, Westra WH, Akpeng B, et al. Evidence for a role of the PD-1:PD-L1 pathway in immune resistance of HPV-associated head and neck squamous cell carcinoma. Cancer Res. 2013; 73:1733–41. https://doi.org/10.1158/0008-5472.CAN-12-2384.

47. Pembrolizumab (KEYTRUDA). https://www.fda.gov/drugs/informationondrugs/approveddrugs/ucm515627.htm. Accessed 21 Mar 2018.

48. Nivolumab for SCCHN. https://www.fda.gov/drugs/informationondrugs/approveddrugs/ucm528920.htm. Accessed 21 Mar 2018.

49. ClinicalTrials.gov. https://www.clinicaltrials.gov/. Accessed 21 Mar 2018.

50. Cancer Genome Atlas Network. Comprehensive genomic characterization of head and neck squamous cell carcinomas. Nature. 2015;517:576–82.

51. Stransky N, Egloff AM, Tward AD, Kostic AD, Cibulskis K, Sivachenko A, et al. The mutational landscape of head and neck squamous cell carcinoma. Science. 2011;333:1157–60.

52. Agrawal N, Frederick MJ, Pickering CR, Bettegowda C, Chang K, Li RJ, et al. Exome sequencing of head and neck squamous cell carcinoma reveals inactivating mutations in NOTCH1. Science. 2011;333:1154–7. https://doi.org/10.1126/science.1206923.

53. Mirghani H, Amen F, Tao Y, Deutsch E, Levy A. Increased radiosensitivity of HPV-positive head and neck cancers: molecular basis and therapeutic perspectives. Cancer Treat Rev. 2015;41:844–52. https://doi.org/10.1016/j.ctrv.2015.10.001.

54. Brumbaugh KM, Otterness DM, Geisen C, Oliveira V, Brognard J, Li X, et al. The mRNA surveillance protein hSMG-1 functions in genotoxic stress response pathways in mammalian cells. Mol Cell. 2004;14:585–98. https://doi.org/10.1016/j.molcel.2004.05.005.

55. Gewandter JS, Bambara RA, O'Reilly MA. The RNA surveillance protein SMG1 activates p53 in response to DNA double-strand breaks but not exogenously oxidized mRNA. Cell Cycle. 2011;10:2561–7. https://doi.org/10.4161/cc.10.15.16347.

56. Shiloh Y. ATM and related protein kinases: safeguarding genome integrity. Nat Rev Cancer. 2003;3:155–68.

57. Gubanova E, Brown B, Ivanov SV, Helleday T, Mills GB, Yarbrough WG, et al. Downregulation of SMG-1 in HPV-positive head and neck squamous cell carcinoma due to promoter hypermethylation correlates with improved survival. Clin Cancer res off J am Assoc Cancer Res. 2012;18:1257–67.

58. Sewell A, Brown B, Biktasova A, Mills GB, Lu Y, Tyson DR, et al. Reverse-phase protein array profiling of oropharyngeal cancer and significance of PIK3CA mutations in HPV-associated head and neck cancer. Clin Cancer Res Off J Am Assoc Cancer Res. 2014;20:2300–11.

59. Dok R, Kalev P, Van Limbergen EJ, Asbagh LA, Vázquez I, Hauben E, et al. p16INK4a impairs homologous recombination-mediated DNA repair in human papillomavirus-positive head and neck tumors. Cancer Res. 2014;74:1739–51.

60. Weaver AN, Cooper TS, Rodriguez M, Trummell HQ, Bonner JA, Rosenthal EL, et al. DNA double strand break repair defect and sensitivity to poly ADP-ribose polymerase (PARP) inhibition in human papillomavirus 16-positive head and neck squamous cell carcinoma. Oncotarget. 2015;6:26995–7007.

61. Slebos RJC, Jehmlich N, Brown B, Yin Z, Chung CH, Yarbrough WG, et al. Proteomic analysis of oropharyngeal carcinomas reveals novel HPV-associated biological pathways. Int J Cancer J Int Cancer. 2013;132:568–79. https://doi.org/10.1002/ijc.27699.

62. Gary C, Hajek M, Biktasova A, Bellinger G, Yarbrough WG, Issaeva N. Selective antitumor activity of roscovitine in head and neck cancer. Oncotarget. 2016;7:38598–611.

63. Zhang Y, Koneva LA, Virani S, Arthur AE, Virani A, Hall PB, et al. Subtypes of HPV-positive head and neck cancers are associated with HPV characteristics, copy number alterations, PIK3CA mutation, and pathway signatures. Clin Cancer Res Off J Am Assoc Cancer Res. 2016;22:4735–45.

64. Muñoz N, Castellsagué X, de González AB, Gissmann L. Chapter 1: HPV in the etiology of human cancer. Vaccine. 2006;24:S1–10. https://doi.org/10.1016/j.vaccine.2006.05.115.

65. Koneva LA, Zhang Y, Virani S, Hall PB, McHugh JB, Chepeha DB, et al. HPV integration in HNSCC correlates with survival outcomes, immune response signatures, and candidate drivers. Mol Cancer Res MCR. 2018;16:90–102.

66. Berman Tara A, Schiller John T. Human papillomavirus in cervical cancer and oropharyngeal cancer: one cause. two diseases Cancer. 2017;123:2219–29. https://doi.org/10.1002/cncr.30588.

67. Stanley M. Pathology and epidemiology of HPV infection in females. Gynecol Oncol. 2010;117(2 Suppl):S5–10.

68. Nakahara T, Kiyono T. Interplay between NF-κB/interferon signaling and the genome replication of HPV. Future Virol. 2016;11:141–55. https://doi.org/10.2217/fvl.16.2.

69. Hong S, Laimins LA. Manipulation of the innate immune response by human papillomaviruses., manipulation of the innate immune response by human papillomaviruses. Virus res Virus Res 2017;231, 231:34, 34–240. doi: https://doi.org/10.1016/j.virusres.2016.11.004, https://doi.org/10.1016/j.virusres.2016.11.004.

70. Thomas M, Narayan N, Pim D, Tomaić V, Massimi P, Nagasaka K, et al. Human papillomaviruses, cervical cancer and cell polarity. Oncogene. 2008;27:7018–30.

71. Maglennon GA, McIntosh P, Doorbar J. Persistence of viral DNA in the epithelial basal layer suggests a model for papillomavirus latency following immune regression. Virology. 2011;414:153–63.

72. Stanley MA, Pett MR, Coleman N. HPV: from infection to cancer. Biochem Soc Trans. 2007;35:1456–60. https://doi.org/10.1042/BST0351456.

73. Moscicki A-B, Schiffman M, Kjaer S, Villa LL. Chapter 5: updating the natural history of HPV and anogenital cancer. Vaccine. 2006;24(Suppl 3):S3/42–51.

74. Lesseur C, Diergaarde B, Olshan AF, Wünsch-Filho V, Ness AR, Liu G, et al. Genome-wide association analyses identify new susceptibility loci for oral cavity and pharyngeal cancer. Nat Genet. 2016;48:1544–50.

75. Cullen AP, Reid R, Campion M, Lörincz AT. Analysis of the physical state of different human papillomavirus DNAs in intraepithelial and invasive cervical neoplasm. J Virol. 1991;65:606–12.

76. Hudelist G, Manavi M, Pischinger KID, Watkins-Riedel T, Singer CF, Kubista E, et al. Physical state and expression of HPV DNA in benign and dysplastic cervical tissue: different levels of viral integration are correlated with lesion grade. Gynecol Oncol. 2004;92:873–80.

77. Woodman CBJ, Collins SI, Young LS. The natural history of cervical HPV infection: unresolved issues. Nat Rev Cancer. 2007;7:11–22.

78. Nulton TJ, Olex AL, Dozmorov M, Morgan IM, Windle B, Nulton TJ, et al. Analysis of the Cancer genome atlas sequencing data reveals novel properties of the human papillomavirus 16 genome in head and neck

squamous cell carcinoma. Oncotarget. 2017;8:17684–99. https://doi.org/10.18632/oncotarget.15179.

79. Morgan IM, DiNardo LJ, Windle B. Integration of human papillomavirus genomes in head and neck Cancer: is it time to consider a paradigm shift? Viruses. 2017;9:208. https://doi.org/10.3390/v9080208.

80. Gelwan E, Malm I-J, Khararjian A, Fakhry C, Bishop JA, Westra WH. Nonuniform distribution of high-risk human papillomavirus in squamous cell carcinomas of the oropharynx: rethinking the anatomic boundaries of Oral and oropharyngeal carcinoma from an oncologic HPV perspective. Am J Surg Pathol. 2017;41:1722–8.

81. Perry ME. The specialised structure of crypt epithelium in the human palatine tonsil and its functional significance. J Anat. 1994;185(Pt 1):111–27.

82. Marur S, D'Souza G, Westra WH, Forastiere AA. HPV-associated head and neck Cancer: a virus-related Cancer epidemic – A Review of Epidemiology, Biology, Virus Detection and Issues in Management. Lancet Oncol. 2010;11:781–9. https://doi.org/10.1016/S1470-2045(10)70017-6.

83. Henderson S, Chakravarthy A, Su X, Boshoff C, Fenton TR. APOBEC-mediated cytosine deamination links PIK3CA helical domain mutations to human papillomavirus-driven tumor development. Cell Rep. 2014;7:1833–41.

84. The Cancer Genome Atlas Research Network. Integrated genomic and molecular characterization of cervical cancer. Nature. 2017;543:378–84. https://doi.org/10.1038/nature21386.

85. Bancroft CC, Chen Z, Yeh J, Sunwoo JB, Yeh NT, Jackson S, et al. Effects of pharmacologic antagonists of epidermal growth factor receptor, PI3K and MEK signal kinases on NF-κB and AP-1 activation and IL-8 and VEGF expression in human head and neck squamous cell carcinoma lines. Int J Cancer. 2002;99:538–48. https://doi.org/10.1002/ijc.10398.

86. Lui VWY, Hedberg ML, Li H, Vangara BS, Pendleton K, Zeng Y, et al. Frequent mutation of the PI3K pathway in head and neck cancer defines predictive biomarkers. Cancer Discov. 2013;3:761–9.

87. Zhang J, Chen T, Yang X, Cheng H, Späth SS, Clavijo PE, et al. Attenuated TRAF3 fosters alternative activation of NF-κB and reduced expression of anti-viral interferon, TP53, and RB to promote HPV-positive head and neck cancers. Cancer Res. 2018;78(16):4613–4626. https://doi.org/10.1158/0008-5472.CAN-17-0642.

88. Nave H, Gebert A, Pabst R. Morphology and immunology of the human palatine tonsil. Anat Embryol (Berl). 2001;204:367–73.

89. Young LS, Dawson CW. Epstein-Barr virus and nasopharyngeal carcinoma. Chin J Cancer. 2014;33:581–90. https://doi.org/10.5732/cjc.014.10197.

90. Chung GT-Y, Lou WP-K, Chow C, To K-F, Choy K-W, Leung AW-C, et al. Constitutive activation of distinct NF-κB signals in EBV-associated nasopharyngeal carcinoma. J Pathol. 2013;231:311–22.

19

Sex differences in patients with high risk HPV-associated and HPV negative oropharyngeal and oral cavity squamous cell carcinomas

Hong Li[1], Henry S. Park[1,2,4], Heather A. Osborn[1,3,4] and Benjamin L. Judson[1,3,4*]

Abstract

Background: Human papilloma virus (HPV)-associated head and neck cancer is now recognized as a distinct clinical entity from HPV-negative tumors, which are primarily associated with tobacco and alcohol exposure.Little is known, however, about the behavior of HPV-associated oropharynx (OP) and oral cavity (OC) SCCs as two distinct cancers and how sex affects the overall survival (OS) in these two cancers. The objective of our study is to determine if sex is associated with overall survival (OS) in patients with high-risk human papillomavirus (HPV)-positive and HPV-negative squamous cell carcinomas (SCC) in the oropharynx and oral cavity sites.

Methods: This is a retrospective cohort study using a national database. Data were extracted from the National Cancer Database (NCDB) of patients diagnosed with OP or OC SCC from 2010 to 2014. Univariate and multivariate survival analyses were conducted with chi-square tests, Kaplan-Meier estimates, log-rank tests, and Cox proportional hazards multivariable modeling.

Results: A total of 30,707 patients (13,694 OP HPV-associated, 7933 OP HPV-, 1220 OC HPV-associated, 7860 OC HPV-) were identified. In all four groups, women tended to be older and have lower T and N clinical classification than men. Though there were no significant differences in OS between the sexes in OP HPV-associated cancers, female sex was associated with worse OS in OP HPV- cancers (HR: 1.15; 95% CI 1.04–1.28, $p = 0.004$), whereas it was associated with improved OS in OC HPV-associated and HPV- cancers (HPV-associated: HR: 0.71; 95% CI 0.50–0.99, $p = 0.048$; HPV-: HR: 0.87; 95% CI 0.78–0.95, $p = 0.004$).

Conclusion: The effect of sex on OS in OC and OP SCC appears to vary based on tumor location and HPV status. While the source of this difference in prognostic association is unclear, it may be related to an emerging difference in the biology of HPV carcinogenesis in these locations.

Keywords: Human papilloma virus, Sex difference, Head and neck cancer, Oropharyngeal cancer, Oral cavity cancer

Background

In the last 15 years, evidence has amassed on the human papilloma virus (HPV) as an important cause of head and neck squamous cell carcinomas (HNSCC). HPV-associated HNSCC is now recognized as a distinct clinical entity from HPV-negative HNSCC tumors [1], which are primarily associated with tobacco and alcohol exposure [2].

Given this recent discovery, many questions still remain regarding the epidemiology and management of patients with HPV-associated HNSCC. A subset of HNSCCs occurs in the oropharynx (OP). Chaturvedi and colleagues found that the incidence of OP cancers have been rising ~1–2% every year from 1973 to 2004 [3]. Despite HPV infection being common in both men and women, the incidence of HPV-associated OPSCCs is more than two-fold higher among men than women [4]. This sex-specific finding raises questions regarding possible differences in the biological presentation of the cancer between men and women.

* Correspondence: benjamin.judson@yale.edu
[1]Yale School of Medicine, New Haven, CT, USA
[3]Department of Surgery (Section of Otolaryngology), Yale New Haven Hospital, New Haven, CT, USA
Full list of author information is available at the end of the article

OPSCCs are now hypothesized to behave distinctly compared to HNSCCs at other sites. HPV DNA has been discovered in tumors from other head and neck sites such as cancers of the oral cavity (OC) [5–7]. A recent study found that HPV-associated non-OPSCCs display a distinct immune microenvironment and clinical behavior compared to HPV-associated OPSCCs [8].

To date, few studies have alluded to the sex-related differences in the prognosis for OPSCCs and other HNSCCs. One retrospective, multi-institutional study [9] found sex to be a significant prognostic factor for overall survival (OS) in OPSCCs even after accounting for HPV status. Interestingly, the same study found that in non-OPSCCs, sex did not have any prognostic significance for OS.

Many studies in HPV-associated HNSCCs have examined all HNSCCs as a whole entity [10, 11]. Little is known, however, about the behavior of HPV associated OP and OC SCCs as two distinct cancers and how sex affects the OS in these two cancers. Therefore, this study aims to classify patient characteristics and investigate survival differences by sex in patients with HPV-associated and HPV- OPSCCs and OCSCCs.

Methods
Data
Data were extracted from the National Cancer Database (NCDB) from 2010 to 2014. The NCDB is a joint project of the Commission on Cancer and the American Cancer Society [12]. Cases are recorded from over 1500 accredited hospitals in the United States and Puerto Rico. The database represents over 70% of incident cases of cancer in the United States. Each hospital that participates in the registry is responsible for submitting and tracking patient and tumor level data on patients with malignant neoplastic diseases.

Patient population
Our study population includes patients whose primary malignancy was diagnosed as squamous cell carcinoma of the oropharynx or oral cavity. The following *Internal Classification of Disease for Oncology, Third Edition* (ICD-O-3) histology codes were used for squamous cell carcinoma M8070–8073 and the following topography codes were used for oropharynx (OP): C09.0–09.1, C09.8–09.9 (tonsil) C10.0, C10.2–10.4 (other oropharynx) and C-01.9 (base of tongue), for oral cavity (OC) cancer C00.0–00.9 (lip), C02.0–02.4, C02.8–02.9 (other/unspecified parts of the tongue), C03.0–03.1, C03.9 (gum), C04.0–04.1, C04.8–04.9 (floor of mouth), C05.0–05.1, C05.8–05.9 (palate), C06.0–06.2, C06.8–06.9 (other/unspecified parts of the mouth).

HPV status was available for cases diagnosed 2010–2014 and was categorized as negative, positive for low-risk HPV types, positive for high-risk HPV types (HPV 16 and/or 18) and HPV status unknown. For our study, patients were classified as 'HPV-positive' if they tested positive for high-risk HPV types, and 'HPV-negative' if they received a negative HPV test. Patients with low-risk HPV types or unknown HPV status were excluded.

We examined patient demographic and tumor data (age at diagnosis, race, Charlson/Deyo score, primary tumor site, American Joint Commission on Cancer T and N classification, lymph node metastasis, primary treatment type, insurance status, median income quartiles, treatment facility type and location, and rural/urban classification of

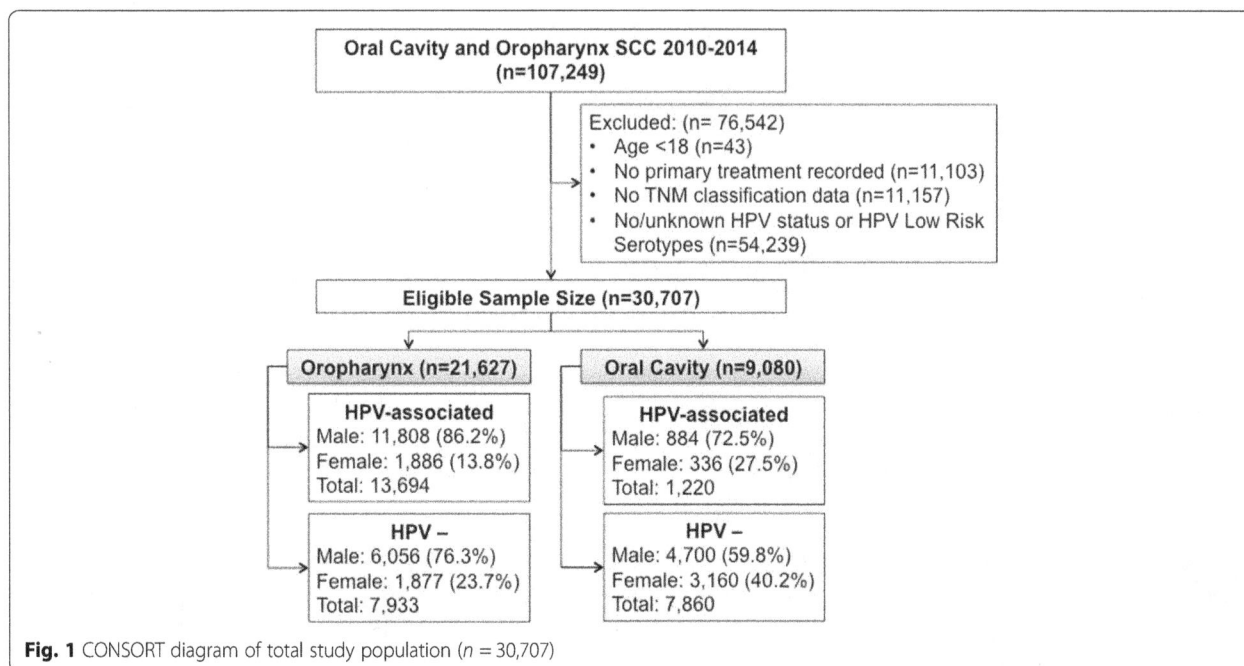

Fig. 1 CONSORT diagram of total study population (*n* = 30,707)

Table 1 Patient characteristics among those with oropharyngeal squamous cell carcinoma based on sex and HPV status

	Oropharynx HPV-associated					Oropharynx HPV -				
	Male		Female			Male		Female		
	Count	%	Count	%	p-value	Count	%	Count	%	p-value
Mean age (years)	58,69		59,65		< 0.001	60,74		61,66		< 0.001
Ethnicity					0.006					0.32
White	10,997	94.0%	1717	91.9%		5167	86.0%	1566	84.2%	
Black	538	4.6%	107	5.7%		709	11.8%	243	13.1%	
American Indian/Eskimo	22	0.2%	5	0.3%		13	0.2%	7	0.4%	
Asian/Pacific Islander	103	0.9%	28	1.5%		87	1.4%	32	1.7%	
Other	45	0.4%	12	0.6%		32	0.5%	11	0.6%	
Charlson/Deyo Score					< 0.001					0.72
0	9957	84.3%	1530	81.1%		4817	79.5%	1477	78.7%	
1	1486	12.6%	272	14.4%		942	15.6%	304	16.2%	
2	365	3.1%	84	4.5%		297	4.9%	96	5.1%	
AJCC Clinical Staging										
T Staging					< 0.001					0.002
T0	85	0.7%	13	0.7%		16	0.3%	6	0.3%	
T1	3225	27.4%	582	31.1%		1221	20.3%	428	23.0%	
T2	4834	41.1%	770	41.2%		2097	34.9%	671	36.0%	
T3	1925	16.4%	254	13.6%		1319	22.0%	339	18.2%	
T4	1354	11.5%	190	10.2%		1180	19.7%	380	20.4%	
TX	326	2.8%	61	3.3%		170	2.8%	38	2.0%	
N Staging					< 0.001					< 0.001
N0	1336	11.3%	318	16.9%		1410	23.4%	594	31.7%	
N1	1874	15.9%	424	22.5%		997	16.5%	344	18.3%	
N2	8023	68.1%	1088	57.8%		3298	54.6%	877	46.8%	
N3	522	4.4%	49	2.6%		293	4.9%	50	2.7%	
NX	33	0.3%	3	0.2%		37	0.6%	10	0.5%	
M Staging					0.812					0.013
M0	11,042	97.7%	1763	98.0%		5435	95.4%	1718	96.7%	
M1	265	2.3%	36	2.0%		264	4.6%	58	3.3%	
Primary Site					< 0.001					0.005
Base of Tongue	4845	41.0%	611	32.4%		2543	42.0%	745	39.7%	
Tonsil	6258	53.0%	1150	61.0%		2615	43.2%	796	42.4%	
Other OP	705	6.0%	125	6.6%		898	14.8%	336	17.9%	
Insurance Status					< 0.001					< 0.001
Not Insured	437	3.7%	71	3.8%		383	6.4%	111	6.0%	
Private Insurance/Managed Care	7264	62.2%	989	52.9%		2601	43.8%	732	39.5%	
Medicaid	753	6.4%	162	8.7%		703	11.8%	240	13.0%	
Medicare	2940	25.2%	634	33.9%		2121	35.7%	750	40.5%	
Other Government	290	2.5%	12	0.6%		132	2.2%	18	1.0%	
Median Income Quartiles 2008–2012					0.002					0.043
< $38,000	1472	12.5%	274	14.6%		1184	19.7%	389	20.9%	
$38,000–$47,999	2443	20.8%	435	23.1%		1335	22.2%	451	24.2%	

Table 1 Patient characteristics among those with oropharyngeal squamous cell carcinoma based on sex and HPV status *(Continued)*

| | Oropharynx HPV-associated | | | | | Oropharynx HPV - | | | | |
| | Male | | Female | | | Male | | Female | | |
	Count	%	Count	%	p-value	Count	%	Count	%	p-value
$48,000–$62,999	3265	27.7%	488	25.9%		1606	26.7%	491	26.4%	
$63,000 +	4588	39.0%	685	36.4%		1900	31.5%	530	28.5%	
Urban/Rural 2013					0.190					0.27
Metro	9826	85.3%	1573	84.8%		5053	85.5%	1539	84.0%	
Urban	1488	12.9%	259	14.0%		775	13.1%	265	14.5%	
Rural	200	1.7%	24	1.3%		80	1.4%	28	1.5%	
Facility Type					0.214					0.346
Community Cancer Program	743	6.4%	128	7.0%		531	8.9%	159	8.6%	
Comprehensive Community Cancer Program	3719	31.8%	596	32.7%		2153	36.0%	632	34.3%	
Academic/Research Program	5810	49.7%	907	49.8%		2618	43.8%	851	46.2%	
Integrated Network Cancer Program	1407	12.0%	192	10.5%		671	11.2%	199	10.8%	
Other specified types of cancer programs	0	0.0%	0	0.0%		0	0.0%	0	0.0%	
Facility Location					0.110					0.130
East	2440	20.9%	419	23.0%		1223	20.5%	398	21.6%	
South	3915	33.5%	610	33.5%		2454	41.1%	704	38.2%	
Midwest	3196	27.4%	493	27.0%		1408	23.6%	467	25.4%	
West	2128	18.2%	301	16.5%		888	14.9%	272	14.8%	
Treatment Group					< 0.001					< 0.001
No treatment	210	1.8%	31	1.6%		286	4.7%	90	4.8%	
Radiation only	868	7.4%	158	8.4%		508	8.4%	186	9.9%	
Radiation and Chemo	7185	60.8%	1011	53.6%		3571	59.0%	1004	53.5%	
Surgery and Radiation	726	6.1%	155	8.2%		240	4.0%	94	5.0%	
Surgery, Chemotherapy and Radiation	2027	17.2%	341	18.1%		725	12.0%	210	11.2%	
Surgery only	572	4.8%	155	8.2%		464	7.7%	218	11.6%	
Chemotherapy Only	220	1.9%	35	1.9%		262	4.3%	75	4.0%	

patient's primary country of residence). Patients were excluded if they were younger than 18 years old, if TNM classification or primary treatment type was unknown. Primary treatment type was classified into the following groups: no treatment, radiation only, chemoradiation therapy, surgery and radiation, surgery and chemoradiation, surgery only and chemotherapy only.

Statistical analysis

Data analyses were performed using SPSS 19.0 (IBM Corp., Armonk, NY). The comparison of mean age at diagnosis was analyzed using the Student's t-test. Proportional distribution of race, Charleson/Deyo score, primary tumor site, T and N classification, lymph node metastasis, primary treatment type, insurance status, median income quartiles, treatment facility type and location, and rural/urban classification of patient's primary country of residence were compared using chi-squared tests. Survival analysis was performed using Kaplan-Meier

analysis. The comparison of survival rates among the groups was performed using the two-tailed log-rank test. The average follow up time for survival analysis in the dataset was 31.7 months. Cox proportional hazards regression model was used for multivariable survival analysis. Age, sex, race, Charleson/Deyo score (for OPSCCs only), T and N classification, site of primary tumor (for OPSCCs only), primary treatment type, insurance status and median income were entered a priori into the model. A two-sided p-value < 0.05 was considered statistically significant.

Our study is exempt from review by the Yale Human Research Protection Program because it uses a pre-existing, de-identified public database.

Results

Our study population (n = 30,707) included 13,694 OP HPV-associated; 7933 OP HPV- cancers; 1220 OC HPV-associated and 7860 OC HPV- cancers (Fig. 1).

Table 2 Patient characteristics among those with oral cavity squamous cell carcinoma based on sex and HPV status

| | Oral Cavity HPV-associated | | | | | Oral Cavity HPV - | | | | |
| | Male | | Female | | | Male | | Female | | |
	Count	%	Count	%	p-value	Count	%	Count	%	p-value
Mean age (years)	58,85		59,72		< 0.001	61,35		63,95		< 0.001
Ethnicity					0.502					0.512
White	804	91.6%	296	88.9%		4093	87.7%	2777	88.7%	
Black	44	5.0%	25	7.5%		371	7.9%	218	7.0%	
American Indian/Eskimo	2	0.2%	1	0.3%		15	0.3%	7	0.2%	
Asian/Pacific Islander	20	2.3%	9	2.7%		151	3.2%	103	3.3%	
Other	8	0.9%	2	0.6%		39	0.8%	26	0.8%	
Charlson/Deyo Score					0.11					0.92
0	689	77.9%	259	77.1%		3607	76.7%	2434	77.0%	
1	165	18.7%	57	17.0%		837	17.8%	552	17.5%	
2	30	3.4%	20	6.0%		256	5.4%	174	5.5%	
AJCC Clinical Staging										
T Staging					0.005					< 0.001
T0	4	0.5%	0	0.0%		8	0.2%	5	0.2%	
T1	251	29.3%	129	40.1%		1579	34.6%	1292	42.3%	
T2	277	32.4%	101	31.4%		1409	30.8%	914	29.9%	
T3	96	11.2%	32	9.9%		506	11.1%	271	8.9%	
T4	216	25.2%	56	17.4%		1039	22.7%	551	18.1%	
TX	12	1.4%	4	1.2%		29	0.6%	19	0.6%	
N Staging					0.003					< 0.001
N0	420	47.5%	198	59.5%		3001	64.0%	2226	70.7%	
N1	130	14.7%	46	13.8%		552	11.8%	332	10.5%	
N2	313	35.4%	86	25.8%		1038	22.2%	551	17.5%	
N3	15	1.7%	2	0.6%		57	1.2%	14	0.4%	
NX	6	0.7%	1	0.3%		38	0.8%	27	0.9%	
M Staging					0.939					0.004
M0	833	97.9%	313	97.8%		4339	97.7%	2959	98.6%	
M1	18	2.1%	7	2.2%		102	2.3%	41	1.4%	
Insurance Status					0.09					< 0.001
Not Insured	51	5.8%	23	6.9%		236	5.1%	132	4.2%	
Private Insurance/Managed Care	420	48.1%	145	43.5%		1935	41.9%	1197	38.5%	
Medicaid	90	10.3%	30	9.0%		515	11.1%	260	8.4%	
Medicare	286	32.8%	131	39.3%		1850	40.0%	1480	47.6%	
Other Government	26	3.0%	4	1.2%		85	1.8%	38	1.2%	
Median Income Quartiles 2008–2012					0.22					0.010
< $38,000	137	15.6%	47	14.0%		843	18.0%	512	16.3%	
$38,000–$47,999	206	23.4%	93	27.8%		1171	25.0%	725	23.0%	
$48,000–$62,999	264	30.0%	85	25.4%		1250	26.7%	863	27.4%	
$63,000 +	272	30.9%	110	32.8%		1426	30.4%	1046	33.2%	
Urban/Rural 2013					0.510					0.072
Metro	741	85.2%	287	87.8%		3799	82.8%	2579	83.9%	

Table 2 Patient characteristics among those with oral cavity squamous cell carcinoma based on sex and HPV status *(Continued)*

| | Oral Cavity HPV-associated | | | | | Oral Cavity HPV - | | | | |
| | Male | | Female | | | Male | | Female | | |
	Count	%	Count	%	*p*-value	Count	%	Count	%	*p*-value
Urban	114	13.1%	35	10.7%		708	15.4%	461	15.0%	
Rural	15	1.7%	5	1.5%		81	1.8%	35	1.1%	
Facility Type					0.507					0.967
Community Cancer Program	64	7.6%	20	6.6%		274	6.1%	188	6.3%	
Comprehensive Community Cancer Program	239	28.3%	75	24.8%		1226	27.3%	823	27.6%	
Academic/Research Program	466	55.2%	176	58.1%		2487	55.3%	1643	55.0%	
Integrated Network Cancer Program	75	8.9%	32	10.6%		507	11.3%	331	11.1%	
Other specified types of cancer programs	0	0.0%	0	0.0%		0	0.0%	0	0.0%	
Facility Location					0.990					0.026
East	178	21.1%	64	21.1%		995	22.1%	662	22.2%	
South	278	32.9%	98	32.3%		1660	36.9%	1014	34.0%	
Midwest	240	28.4%	87	28.7%		1149	25.6%	793	26.6%	
West	148	17.5%	54	17.8%		690	15.4%	516	17.3%	
Treatment Group					< 0.001					< 0.001
No treatment	29	3.3%	11	3.3%		163	3.5%	120	3.8%	
Radiation only	56	6.3%	26	7.7%		282	6.0%	217	6.9%	
Radiation and Chemo	269	30.4%	62	18.5%		717	15.3%	356	11.3%	
Surgery and Radiation	100	11.3%	37	11.0%		573	12.2%	396	12.5%	
Surgery, Chemotherapy and Radiation	146	16.5%	55	16.4%		806	17.1%	408	12.9%	
Surgery only	264	29.9%	139	41.4%		2072	44.1%	1620	51.3%	
Chemotherapy Only	20	2.3%	6	1.8%		87	1.9%	43	1.4%	

The presence of HPV was correlated with higher proportion of disease burden among men. Among the OP HPV-associated and HPV- cohorts, 86.2 and 76.3% of patients were men respectively. Among the OC HPV-associated and HPV- cohorts, 76.3 and 59.8% were men respectively. Each group was further analyzed for baseline characteristic differences by sex (Tables 1 and 2).

Baseline characteristic differences
Within all four groups, women were on average older at age of diagnosis ($p < 0.001$ for each group). Women were generally diagnosed with cancers in earlier T and N clinical classification than men. In OP, this difference was most pronounced in N classification; in OP HPV-associated cancers, 39.4% women vs. 27.2% men had N0–1 cancers ($p < 0.001$), in OP HPV- cancers, 50.0% women vs. 39.9% men had N0–1 cancers ($p < 0.001$). In OC HPV-associated cancers, 40.1% women had T0–1 cancers vs. 29.8% men and in OC HPV- cancers ($p = 0.005$), 42.3% vs. 34.8% in women and men respectively ($p < 0.001$). Women in all four groups were more likely to be treated with a modality including surgery (surgery only, surgery and radiation, or surgery and chemo-radiation; p < 0.001 in each group). For

insurance coverage, more women were covered by Medicare than men across all four study populations.

Factors associated with survival in OPSCCs
Kaplan-Meier survival analysis showed no difference in OS between the two sexes in OP HPV-associated cancers ($p = 0.64$; Figs. 2a). On multivariate analysis, after accounting for age at diagnosis, ethnicity, clinical T and N classification, primary disease site, primary treatment, insurance status and median income, female sex (HR: 0.93; 95% CI 0.79–1.009, $p = 0.412$) did not prove to be an independent prognostic factor for OS.

In OP HPV- cancers, men had a statistically significant better OS than women on Kaplan Meier survival analysis ($p = 0.035$, Fig. 2b). In multivariate analysis, female sex (HR: 1.15; 95% CI 1.04–1.28, $p = 0.004$) continued to be an independent prognostic factor for worse OS in OP HPV- cancers even after controlling for other variables (as described previously, Table 3).

The hazard of death was notably higher for both OP HPV-associated and HPV- cohorts with increasing age, higher T and N classification, cancers at sites other than base of tongue or tonsils and patients with no primary treatment (Table 3).

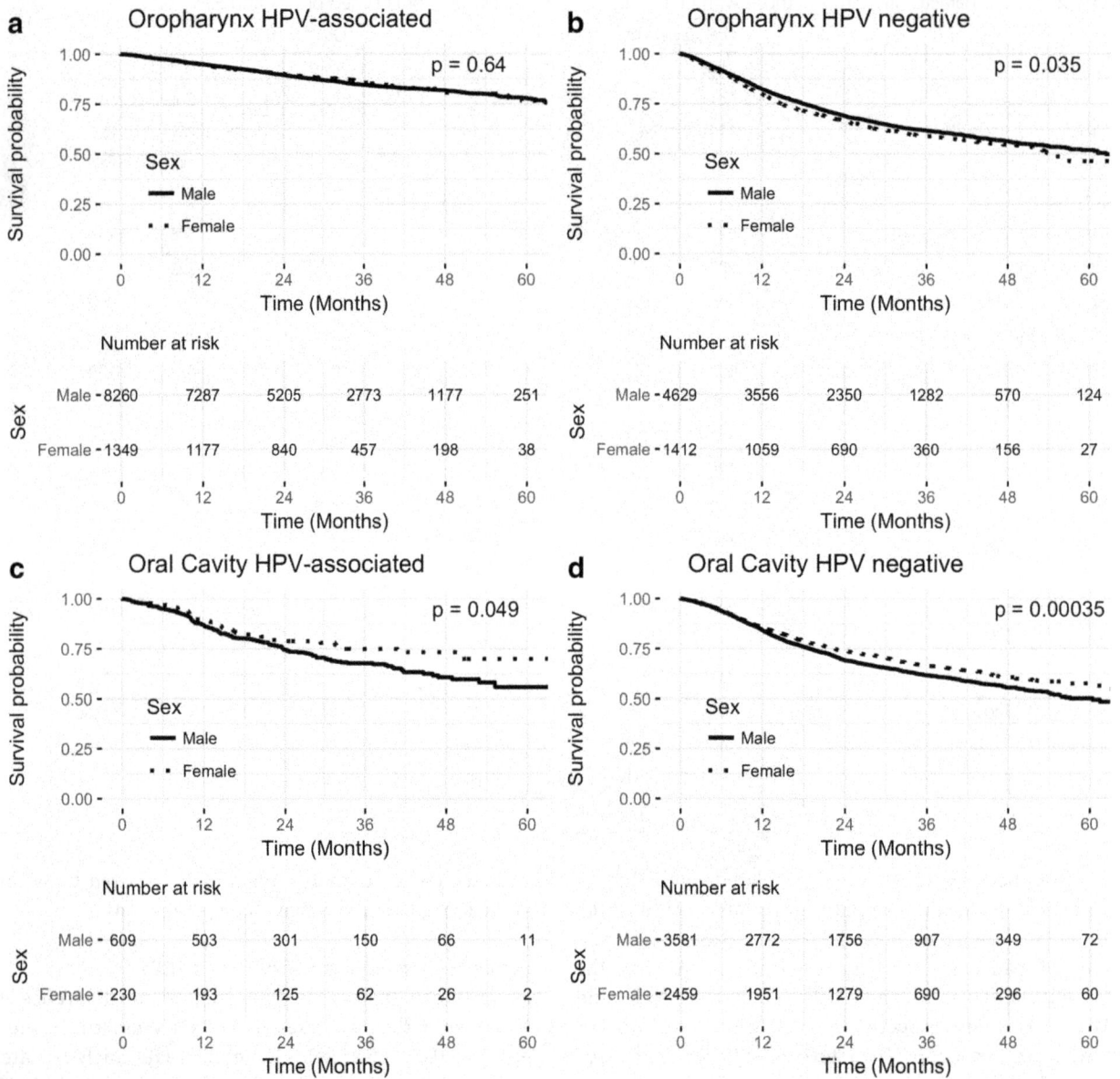

Fig. 2 Kaplan-Meier survival and number at risk **a** OP HPV-associated: $p = 0.638$, **b** OP HPV negative: $p = 0.035$, **c** OC HPV-associated: $p = 0.049$, **d** OC HPV negative: $p < 0.001$

Factors associated with survival in OCSCCs

Kaplan-Meier survival analysis showed that among OC cancers, women had better OS than men in both HPV-associated and HPV- cancers ($p = 0.049$, $p < 0.001$ respectively, Fig. 2c, d).

In contrast to the varying prognostic roles of female sex in OPSCCs, in OCSCCs, female sex remained a strong prognostic factor for better OS in both HPV-associated and HPV- cancers (HPV-associated: HR: 0.71; 95% CI 0.0.50–0.99, $p = 0.048$; HPV-: HR: 0.87; 95% CI 0.78–0.95, $p = 0.004$; Table 4) after controlling for over variables. In OC HPV-associated cancers, age (HR: 1.02; 95% CI 1.00–1.04, $p = 0.01$) and black race (HR: 1.88; 95% CI 1.14–3.11,

$p = 0.013$) were significant predictors of OS in patients. In OC HPV- cancers, age (HR: 1.02; 95% CI 1.02–1.02, $p < 0.001$), N classification ($p < 0.001$) and having higher median income \$63,000+ ((HR: 0.77; 95% CI 0.67–0.88, $p < 0.001$), and having treatment (over no treatment; $p < 0.001$ for all except chemotherapy only group $p = 0.31$) were all significant predictors of OS.

Discussion

HPV status and its importance as a prognostic marker in oropharyngeal SCCs has been well established [13, 14]. The prognostic associations of HPV status with other clinical factors such as sex and primary tumor

Table 3 Cox proportional hazards regression analysis for patients with oropharyngeal squamous cell carcinoma

	Oropharynx HPV-associated		Oropharynx HPV -	
	HR (95% CI)	P	HR (95% CI)	P
Mean age	1.02 (1.01–1.03)	< 0.001	1.01 (1.00–1.02)	< 0.001
Ethnicity				
White	1.00		1.00	
Black	0.86 (0.67–1.10)	0.25	1.14 (1.01–1.30)	0.03
American Indian/Eskimo	0.61 (0.15–2.47)	0.49	0.22 (0.03–1.58)	0.13
Asian/Pacific Islander	0.52 (0.24–1.10)	0.09	0.75 (0.50–1.14)	0.19
Other	0.63 (0.15–2.52)	0.51	1.29 (0.67–2.49)	0.44
Sex				
Men	**1.00**		**1.00**	
Women	**0.93 (0.79–1.09)**	**0.412**	**1.15 (1.04–1.28)**	**0.004**
Charlson/Deyo Score				
0	1.0		1.0	
1	1.42 (1.23–1.65)	< 0.001	1.31 (1.17–1.46)	< 0.001
2	1.97 (1.56–2.48)	< 0.001	1.49 (1.25–1.77)	< 0.001
AJCC Clinical Staging				
T Staging				
T0	1.00		1.00	
T1	2.61 (0.64–10.5)	0.18	1.31 (0.32–5.30)	0.70
T2	4.24 (1.05–17.0)	0.04	1.93 (0.48–7.79)	0.35
T3	6.47 (1.60–26.1)	0.01	3.26 (0.81–13.1)	0.10
T4	9.92 (2.45–40.0)	0.00	4.35 (1.08–17.5)	0.04
TX	3.93 (0.93–16.4)	0.06	2.65 (0.64–10.9)	0.18
N Staging				
N0	1.00		1.00	
N1	0.81 (0.64–1.01)	0.07	0.95 (0.82–1.10)	0.53
N2	1.14 (0.95–1.37)	0.14	1.10 (0.98–1.24)	0.09
N3	2.06 (1.58–2.67)	< 0.001	1.76 (1.45–2.15)	< 0.001
NX	0.73 (0.29–1.83)	0.51	1.47 (0.91–2.36)	0.11
Primary Site				
Base of Tongue	1.00		1.00	
Tonsil	1.03 (0.91–1.16)	0.63	0.87 (0.79–0.96)	0.01
Other OP	1.48 (1.21–1.81)	< 0.001	1.15 (1.02–1.30)	0.02
Insurance Status				
Not Insured	1.00		1.00	
Private Insurance/Managed Care	0.53 (0.41–0.68)	< 0.001	0.61 (0.51–0.72)	< 0.001
Medicaid	1.04 (0.78–1.38)	0.77	1.11 (0.93–1.34)	0.23
Medicare	0.99 (0.76–1.30)	0.98	0.94 (0.78–1.13)	0.55
Other Government	0.96 (0.63–1.46)	0.85	0.96 (0.67–1.36)	0.83
Median Income Quartiles 2008–2012				
< $38,000	1.00		1.00	
$38,000–$47,999	0.89 (0.75–1.06)	0.21	0.9 (0.79–1.02)	0.11
$48,000–$62,999	0.78 (0.65–0.93)	0.01	0.83 (0.73–0.94)	0.01
$63,000 +	0.65 (0.54–0.77)	< 0.001	0.73 (0.64–0.83)	< 0.001

Table 3 Cox proportional hazards regression analysis for patients with oropharyngeal squamous cell carcinoma *(Continued)*

	Oropharynx HPV-associated		Oropharynx HPV -	
	HR (95% CI)	P	HR (95% CI)	P
Treatment Group				
No treatment	1.00		1.00	
Radiation only	0.34 (0.24–0.48)	< 0.001	0.44 (0.35–0.54)	< 0.001
Radiation and Chemo	0.22 (0.16–0.29)	< 0.001	0.27 (0.23–0.33)	< 0.001
Surgery and Radiation	0.16 (0.10–0.24)	< 0.001	0.20 (0.14–0.28)	< 0.001
Surgery, Chemotherapy and Radiation	0.21 (0.15–0.29)	< 0.001	0.29 (0.23–0.35)	< 0.001
Surgery only	0.21 (0.14–0.32)	< 0.001	0.37 (0.29–0.47)	< 0.001
Chemotherapy Only	1.08 (0.76–1.54)	0.64	0.94 (0.76–1.18)	0.64

location have not been well investigated. Given that HNSCCs affect the two sexes disproportionately (80% men), we hypothesized that sex will be a prognostic factor for survival in HNSCCs. Our study found that sex does appear to play a distinct role in predicting OS and that the prognostic value of sex is dependent on HPV status and location of primary tumor. This finding is consistent with the idea that HPV-driven cancers in non-OP locations exhibit distinct clinical behavior and possess unique risk factors than HPV-driven cancers in OP [8, 9].

Molecular underpinnings of the HPV infection between the two sexes also vary. One Finnish study examining the clearance of HPV DNA using oral rinses between spouses found earlier virus clearance in men than in women as well as significantly different cumulative clearance rates (5% vs. 0% clearance in men and women respectively over 24 months) [15]. In a long-term prospective 6 year study of asymptomatic HPV infections, Syrjänen and colleagues found a 5.5 fold number of viral HPV copies in women than in men who were able to clear the infection [16]. Although similar copy numbers were found between sexes for those with persistent infections, 71% of the HPV DNA was integrated or mixed in women vs. 57% in men. Full integration of the HPV episome into human chromosomes has been shown to be an early event in cervical carcinogenesis [17, 18], though its role in oral mucosal carcinogenesis is still debated. Nonetheless, these studies reflect a distinction in HPV's molecular behavior between sexes that needs to be further categorized.

Prior studies have been inconclusive on the significance of sex as a prognostic marker for overall survival. A recent two-institution retrospective study found sex to be prognostic in OPSCCs even after accounting for HPV-status [9]. The authors examined 860 patients with OPSCCs (including HPV-associated and HPV- patients) and performed a multivariate regression model. Our study utilizes more targeted patient subgroups that specifically examines the role of sex among HPV-associated or HPV- patients. To our knowledge, our study is the

largest study with patients and their HPV status spanning across the entire U.S. As a result, our sample provides the power for the subgroup analyses for the detection of differences in sex. However, due to the nature of the national cancer registry, there is inherent uncertainty to the nature of our data as the quality of the data relies on the accuracy of data entry, diagnosis and treatment at over 1500 hospitals. In comparison, Fakhry et al.'s two-institution study limits their data inaccuracies due to a smaller sample size.

Existing research has shown that women have a significant survival benefit in many cancers outside of the head and neck region [19]. However, for HPV-OPSCCs, we found the opposite where men have better survival than women. This similar trend also exists in patients with bladder cancer [20, 21]. The reason for this observed survival advantage is unknown. Preclinical studies support a role for sex hormones as cofactors for HPV-related malignancies [22, 23] though other unidentified factors may also be responsible for this unique sex-specific finding. One study found the progesterone antagonists and nuclease-resistant oligomers containing HPV-16 response element are able to abrogate cell growth and E6/E7 gene transcription [22]. Another study examining HPV-induced laryngeal tumors found estradiol stimulated proliferation while 2-hydroxyestrone was anti-proliferative [23]. Both preclinical studies found hormonal interactions using HPV-associated tumor models, thus this does not fully explain our findings in the HPV- OPSCC cohort. Perhaps there exists an interaction between HPV and sex hormones in the OP sub-site, which improves the survival of women thus equalizing overall survival between the two sexes. Nonetheless, we acknowledge the proximity of the Kaplan-Meier survival curve between the two sexes in the HPV- OPSCC cohort. Given the absence of tobacco and alcohol data, it is possible that the two sexes may have no survival difference in HPV- OPSCCs.

Table 4 Cox proportional hazards regression analysis for patients with oral cavity squamous cell carcinoma

	Oral Cavity HPV-associated		Oral Cavity HPV -	
	HR (95% CI)	P	HR (95% CI)	P
Mean age	1.02 (1.00–1.04)	0.010	1.02 (1.02–1.02)	< 0.001
Ethnicity				
White	1.00		1.00	
Black	1.88 (1.14–3.11)	0.013	0.93 (0.79–1.09)	0.41
American Indian/Eskimo	a		1.18 (0.52–2.64)	0.68
Asian/Pacific Islander	1.60 (0.64–4.00)	0.312	0.93 (0.71–1.22)	0.63
Other	0.65 (0.09–4.78)	0.678	0.54 (0.30–0.99)	0.05
Sex				
Men	**1.00**		**1.00**	
Women	**0.71 (0.50–0.99)**	**0.048**	**0.87 (0.78–0.95)**	**0.004**
AJCC Clinical Staging				
T Staging				
T0	1.00		1.00	
T1	0.36 (0.07–1.65)	0.189	0.45 (0.14–1.43)	0.18
T2	0.61 (0.13–2.80)	0.529	0.79 (0.25–2.49)	0.70
T3	0.90 (0.19–4.21)	0.903	1.07 (0.34–3.38)	0.90
T4	1.33 (0.29–5.98)	0.707	1.19 (0.37–3.73)	0.76
TX	0.67 (0.11–4.00)	0.666	1.36 (0.39–4.70)	0.63
N Staging				
N0	1.00		1.00	
N1	1.07 (0.70–1.63)	0.743	1.54 (1.34–1.77)	< 0.001
N2	1.08 (0.75–1.55)	0.651	1.72 (1.52–1.94)	< 0.001
N3	0.88 (0.26–2.93)	0.836	2.12 (1.49–3.03)	< 0.001
NX	1.30 (0.17–9.88)	0.795	1.19 (0.75–1.89)	0.45
Insurance Status				
Not Insured	1.00		1.00	
Private Insurance/Managed Care	0.74 (0.42–1.32)	0.319	0.81 (0.65–1.00)	0.06
Medicaid	1.82 (0.96–3.43)	0.064	1.27 (1.00–1.60)	0.043
Medicare	1.32 (0.72–2.41)	0.355	1.04 (0.83–1.30)	0.72
Other Government	0.83 (0.31–2.19)	0.713	1.17 (0.78–1.76)	0.44
Median Income Quartiles 2008–2012				
< $38,000	1.00		1.00	
$38,000–$47,999	1.38 (0.88–2.17)	0.160	0.84 (0.73–0.96)	0.02
$48,000–$62,999	1.49 (0.96–2.33)	0.075	0.90 (0.79–1.03)	0.14
$63,000 +	1.37 (0.87–2.16)	0.169	0.77 (0.67–0.88)	< 0.001
Treatment Group				
No treatment	1.00		1.00	
Radiation only	0.56 (0.25–1.23)	0.151	0.49 (0.37–0.63)	< 0.001
Radiation and Chemo	0.42 (0.22–0.82)	0.011	0.44 (0.35–0.55)	< 0.001
Surgery and Radiation	0.23 (0.10–0.50)	< 0.001	0.33 (0.26–0.43)	< 0.001
Surgery, Chemotherapy and Radiation	0.59 (0.30–1.15)	0.127	0.42 (0.33–0.53)	< 0.001
Surgery only	0.48 (0.24–0.94)	0.033	0.37 (0.29–0.45)	< 0.001
Chemotherapy Only	1.18 (0.49–2.82)	0.710	0.84 (0.61–1.16)	0.31

[a]Insufficient sample size

Interestingly, in our OCSCC study population, women were shown to have better survival than men in both the HPV-associated and HPV- group. This finding contrasts with the role that sex plays in OPSCCs and is consistent with the developing hypothesis that OP and non-OP SCCs are distinct cancers. Risk factors for OCSCC are well established: alcohol, tobacco and betel nut chewing [2, 24]. Current rates of tobacco usage in the US are lower in women than in men [25]. As a result, a lower overall lifetime exposure to tobacco may partly explain the survival advantage among women in OCSCC. There is a new growing body of research interested in characterizing HPV in non-OP sites. A molecular study of 520 HNSCCs profiling the gene-expression signature of HPV-associated OP and non-OP sites found there to be two distinct tumor immune microenvironments [8].

While our study did not directly test for the role of HPV within the OCSCC group, the similarity in risk factors between the HPV-associated and HPV- OCSCC groups infers that HPV may only play a minor prognostic role in OC cancers. A recent study by our group [26] found HPV to be associated with improved survival at the OCSCC subsite, though the survival advantage noted at the oral cavity subsite was not as great as that at the oropharynx subsite.

In our study, we found women were generally diagnosed with earlier T and N staged cancers than men. Earlier detection of cancers would lead to better prognosis [27]. From a health behavior perspective, this finding may be explained by the consistent underutilization of preventative healthcare by men leading to a delay in early diagnosis [28, 29]. It has been hypothesized that women have more frequent contact with healthcare professionals due to pregnancy, childcare and hormone replacement therapy as well as women having more interest in health [28, 30].

The NCDB database, as a source, has well-documented limitations [31]. We were unable to account for every variable that may influence survival (e.g. alcohol, tobacco use, and other comorbidities), as these data were not captured by NCDB. In addition, the database does not capture other causes of OC and OP cancers that may influence survival. Specifically, studies have shown that patients with cancer from previous leukoplakia [32] or oral mucositis [33] leading to earlier cancer detection is associated with improved survival, where as patients with cancer from immunosuppression [34] tend to have worse survival. The type of testing (PCR, ISH for HPV DNA vs. p16) for HPV status may vary depending on each institution and reporting agency. Furthermore, the source of the sample may not necessarily derive from the primary site. There are likely low rates of misclassification due to the nature of the registry of the data; however, any misclassification is likely to have been evenly distributed across our four subgroups. Our retrospective study focuses on OS, not cancer-specific survival. The absence of cause-specific

survival data in NCDB makes in plausible that other causes of death such as treatment derived toxicities, secondary primary cancer and comorbid cardiovascular, pulmonary and metabolic syndrome causes which are more prominent in men may contribute to the difference in mortality seen between the two sexes. In addition, other general cancer risk factors such as tobacco and alcohol as well as high-risk sex behavior associated with HPV+ transmission [35] may also influence the survival difference seen.

Conclusion

In summary, the effect of sex on outcomes of OP and OC SCCs appears to vary based on primary tumor location and HPV status. Notably, sex does not appear to affect the prognosis of HPV-associated OPSCCs after accounting for other risk factors. Men with HPV- OPSCCs appear to have a better prognosis for survival than women, though women appear to have a better prognosis in OCSCCs regardless of HPV-status. Given these results, we recommend further studies to investigate the clinical behavior and the sex-specific pathophysiological biology of HPV-associated HNSCCs and explore opportunities to further eliminate disparities in our patients.

Abbreviations

HNSCC: Head and neck squamous cell carcinomas; HPV: Human papilloma virus; NCDB: National Cancer Database; OC: Oral cavity; OP: Oropharynx; OS: Overall survival; SCC: Squamous cell carcinomas

Funding

William U. Gardner Memorial Student Research Fellowship at Yale University School of Medicine.

Authors' contributions

HL: Conceptualization, methodology, software, validation, formal analysis, investigation, resources, data curation, writing–original draft, and visualization. HSP: Writing–review and editing, visualization. HAO: Writing–review and editing. BLJ: Conceptualization, methodology, formal analysis, investigation, writing–review and editing, supervision, project administration, and funding acquisition. All authors read and approved the final manuscript.

Competing interests

The authors declare that they have no competing interests.

Author details

[1]Yale School of Medicine, New Haven, CT, USA. [2]Department of Therapeutic Radiology, Yale New Haven Hospital, New Haven, CT, USA. [3]Department of Surgery (Section of Otolaryngology), Yale New Haven Hospital, New Haven, CT, USA. [4]Yale Cancer Center, 330 Cedar Street, PO Box 208062, New Haven, CT 06520-8062, USA.

References

1. Gillison ML. Human papillomavirus-associated head and neck cancer is a distinct epidemiologic, clinical, and molecular entity. Semin Oncol. 2004;31: 744–54. https://doi.org/10.1053/j.seminoncol.2004.09.011.

2. Blot WJ, McLaughlin JK, Winn DM, Austin DF, Greenberg RS, Preston-Martin S, et al. Smoking and drinking in relation to oral and pharyngeal Cancer. Cancer Res. 1988;48:3282. http://cancerres.aacrjournals.org/content/48/11/3282.abstract

3. Chaturvedi AK, Engels EA, Anderson WF, Gillison ML. Incidence trends for human papillomavirus-related and -unrelated oral squamous cell carcinomas in the United States. J Clin Oncol Off J Am Soc Clin Oncol. 2008;26:612–9.

4. D'Souza G, Westra WH, Wang SJ, van Zante A, Wentz A, Kluz N, et al. Differences in the prevalence of human papillomavirus (HPV) in head and neck squamous cell cancers by sex, race, anatomic tumor site, and HPV detection method. JAMA Oncol. 2017;3:169. https://doi.org/10.1001/jamaoncol.2016.3067.

5. Chung CH, Zhang Q, Kong CS, Harris J, Fertig EJ, Harari PM, et al. p16 protein expression and human papillomavirus status as prognostic biomarkers of nonoropharyngeal head and neck squamous cell carcinoma. J Clin Oncol. 2014;32:3930–8. https://doi.org/10.1200/JCO.2013.54.5228.

6. Herrero R, Castellsagué X, Pawlita M, Lissowska J, Kee F, Balaram P, et al. Human papillomavirus and oral cancer: the International Agency for Research on Cancer multicenter study. J Natl Cancer Inst. 2003;95:1772–83.

7. Lassen P, Primdahl H, Johansen J, Kristensen CA, Andersen E, Andersen LJ, et al. Impact of HPV-associated p16-expression on radiotherapy outcome in advanced oropharynx and non-oropharynx cancer. Radiother Oncol J Eur Soc Ther Radiol Oncol. 2014;113:310–6.

8. Chakravarthy A, Henderson S, Thirdborough SM, Ottensmeier CH, Su X, Lechner M, et al. Human papillomavirus drives tumor development throughout the head and neck: improved prognosis is associated with an immune response largely restricted to the oropharynx. J Clin Oncol. 2016; 34:4132–41. https://doi.org/10.1200/JCO.2016.68.2955.

9. Fakhry C, Westra WH, Wang SJ, van Zante A, Zhang Y, Rettig E, et al. The prognostic role of sex, race, and human papillomavirus in oropharyngeal and nonoropharyngeal head and neck squamous cell cancer: role of sex, race, and HPV in HNSCC prognosis. Cancer. 2017;123:1566–75. https://doi.org/10.1002/cncr.30353.

10. Fakhry C, Westra WH, Li S, Cmelak A, Ridge JA, Pinto H, et al. Improved survival of patients with human papillomavirus-positive head and neck squamous cell carcinoma in a prospective clinical trial. J Natl Cancer Inst. 2008;100:261–9.

11. Gillison ML, Chaturvedi AK, Anderson WF, Fakhry C. Epidemiology of human papillomavirus-positive head and neck squamous cell carcinoma. J Clin Oncol Off J Am Soc Clin Oncol. 2015;33:3235–42.

12. About the National Cancer Database. American College of Surgeons. https://www.facs.org/quality-programs/cancer/ncdb/about. Accessed 20 Sep 2017.

13. Goon PKC, Stanley MA, Ebmeyer J, Steinsträsser L, Upile T, Jerjes W, et al. HPV & head and neck cancer: a descriptive update. Head Neck Oncol. 2009;1:36.

14. Ang KK, Harris J, Wheeler R, Weber R, Rosenthal DI, Nguyen-Tân PF, et al. Human papillomavirus and survival of patients with oropharyngeal cancer. N Engl J Med. 2010;363:24–35.

15. Rintala M, Grénman S, Puranen M, Syrjänen S. Natural history of oral papillomavirus infections in spouses: a prospective Finnish HPV family study. J Clin Virol Off Publ Pan Am Soc Clin Virol. 2006;35:89–94.

16. Lorenzi A, Rautava J, Kero K, Syrjänen K, Longatto-Filho A, Grenman S, et al. Physical state and copy numbers of HPV16 in oral asymptomatic infections that persisted or cleared during the 6-year follow-up. J Gen Virol. 2017;98: 681–9. https://doi.org/10.1099/jgv.0.000710.

17. Tsakogiannis D, Kyriakopoulou Z, Ruether IGA, Amoutzias GD, Dimitriou TG, Diamantidou V, et al. Determination of human papillomavirus 16 physical status through E1/E6 and E2/E6 ratio analysis. J Med Microbiol. 2014;63(Pt 12):1716–23.

18. Briolat J, Dalstein V, Saunier M, Joseph K, Caudroy S, Prétet J-L, et al. HPV prevalence, viral load and physical state of HPV-16 in cervical smears of patients with different grades of CIN. Int J Cancer. 2007;121:2198–204.

19. Cook MB, McGlynn KA, Devesa SS, Freedman ND, Anderson WF. Sex disparities in cancer mortality and survival. Cancer Epidemiol Biomark Prev Publ Am Assoc Cancer Res Cosponsored Am Soc Prev Oncol. 2011;20:1629–37.

20. Scosyrev E, Noyes K, Feng C, Messing E. Sex and racial differences in bladder cancer presentation and mortality in the US. Cancer. 2009;115:68–74.

21. Shariat SF, Sfakianos JP, Droller MJ, Karakiewicz PI, Meryn S, Bochner BH. The effect of age and gender on bladder cancer: a critical review of the literature. BJU Int. 2010;105:300–8.

22. Yuan F, Auborn K, James C. Altered growth and viral gene expression in human papillomavirus type 16-containing cancer cell lines treated with progesterone. Cancer Investig. 1999;17:19–29.

23. Newfield L, Goldsmith A, Bradlow HL, Auborn K. Estrogen metabolism and human papillomavirus-induced tumors of the larynx: chemo-prophylaxis with indole-3-carbinol. Anticancer Res. 1993;13:337–41.

24. Warnakulasuriya S, Trivedy C, Peters TJ. Areca nut use: an independent risk factor for oral cancer. BMJ. 2002;324:799–800. https://www.ncbi.nlm.nih.gov/pmc/articles/PMC1122751/. Accessed 18 Oct 2017

25. Health CO on S and. Smoking and Tobacco Use; Fact Sheet; Adult Cigarette Smoking in the United States; Smoking and Tobacco Use. http://www.cdc.gov/tobacco/data_statistics/fact_sheets/adult_data/cig_smoking/. Accessed 18 Oct 2017.

26. Li H, Torabi S, Yarbrough WG, Mehra S, Osborn HA, Judson BL. Association of Human Papillomavirus Status with Overall Survival at head and neck carcinoma subsites. JAMA Otolaryngol Neck Surg. 144:1–7.

27. Cancer Screening Overview. National Cancer Institute https://www.cancer.gov/about-cancer/screening/hp-screening-overview-pdq. Accessed 22 Apr 2018.

28. Green CA, Pope CR. Gender, psychosocial factors and the use of medical services: a longitudinal analysis. Soc Sci Med. 1999;48:1363–72.

29. Bertakis KD, Azari R, Helms LJ, Callahan EJ, Robbins JA. Gender differences in the utilization of health care services. J Fam Pract. 2000;49:147–52.

30. Evans R, Brotherstone H, Miles A, Wardle J. Gender differences in early detection of cancer. J Men's Health Gend. 2:209–17.

31. Boffa DJ, Rosen JE, Mallin K, Loomis A, Gay G, Palis B, et al. Using the National Cancer Database for outcomes research: a review. JAMA Oncol. 2017; https://doi.org/10.1001/jamaoncol.2016.6905.

32. Yanik EL, Katki HA, Silverberg MJ, Manos MM, Engels EA, Chaturvedi AK. Leukoplakia, oral cavity Cancer risk, and Cancer survival in the U.S. elderly. Cancer Prev Res Phila Pa. 2015;8:857–63.

33. Rastogi M, Dwivedi RC, Kazi R. Oral mucositis in head and neck cancer. Eur J Cancer Care (Engl). 2011;20:144.

34. Deeb R, Sharma S, Mahan M, Al-Khudari S, Hall F, Yoshida A, et al. Head and neck cancer in transplant recipients. Laryngoscope. 2012;122:1566–9.

35. Giuliano AR, Tortolero-Luna G, Ferrer E, Burchell AN, de Sanjose S, Kjaer SK, et al. Epidemiology of human papillomavirus infection in men, cancers other than cervical and benign conditions. Vaccine. 2008;26:K17–28. https://doi.org/10.1016/j.vaccine.2008.06.021.

20

Investigating adherence to Australian nutritional care guidelines in patients with head and neck cancer

Sophie Hofto[1]* (ID), Jessica Abbott[2], James E. Jackson[1,3] and Elisabeth Isenring[1]

Abstract

Background: Significant weight loss and malnutrition are common in patients with head and neck cancer, despite advances in treatment and development of evidenced-based guidelines. The aim of this study was to assess adherence to evidenced-based guidelines and investigate nutrition outcomes during and post radiation treatment in head and neck cancer patients.

Methods: This was a two-year retrospective cohort study of 209 head and neck cancer patients (85% male) treated with ≥20 fractions of radiation (mean dose = 64.8 Gy delivered over 31.9 fractions) at an Australian tertiary hospital.

Results: Regarding guideline adherences, 80% of patients were seen by a dietitian weekly during treatment and 62% of patients were seen bi-weekly for six-weeks post-treatment. Average weight loss was 6.7% during treatment and 10. 3% three-months post treatment. At the end of treatment, oropharyngeal and oral cavity patients had lost the most weight (8.8, 10.9%), with skin cancer and laryngeal patients losing the least weight (4.8, 2.9%). Gastrostomy patients (n = 60) had their tube in-situ for an average of 150 days and lost an average of 7.7 kg (9.4%) during treatment and 11. 5 kg (13.5%) from baseline to three-months post treatment. The number of malnourished patients increased from 15% at baseline to 56% at the end of treatment, decreasing to 30% three-months post treatment.

Conclusions: Despite high adherence to evidenced-based guidelines, large discrepancies in weight loss and nutritional status between tumor sites was seen. This highlights the opportunity for further investigation of the relationship between tumor site, nutritional status and nutrition interventions, which may then influence future evidenced-based guidelines.

Keywords: Head and neck cancer, Nutrition, Dietitian, Radiation therapy, Gastrostomy, PG-SGA

Background

As the global incidence of head and neck cancer (HNC) increases, there is a corresponding rise in clinician concern for maximising patient nutritional status [1]. The proximity of tumors to structures vital in mastication and deglutition often result in patients being unable to meet their nutrition and hydration requirements orally [2]. Complications of HNC can include dysphagia, odynophagia, impaired saliva production and changes in speech and breathing [3, 4]. Approximately 25–50% of HNC patients have a significant decrease in dietary intake prior to the commencement of anti-cancer therapy,

due to the cancer directly affecting function of the upper aero-digestive tract [5]. In addition, most patients lose in excess of 5% body weight prior to the commencement of treatment [6] and are likely to lose at least 10% of their body weight during treatment, contributing to high rates of protein-energy malnutrition (PEM) [5]. PEM is associated with decreased quality of life, decreased effectiveness of treatment (due to treatment disruptions), increased healthcare costs associated with unplanned hospital admissions, and may negatively impact survival in HNC [7, 8].

Dietetic interventions can help HNC patients meet their nutrition requirements while they are experiencing toxicities of radiotherapy or chemo-radiotherapy [9, 10]. Interventions may include high energy-high protein diets, oral nutrition supplementation and enteral tube feeding. There

* Correspondence: soph_hofto@live.com.au
[1]Faculty of Health Sciences and Medicine, Bond University, 2 Promethean Way, Robina, QLD 4226, Australia
Full list of author information is available at the end of the article

are two main strategies for enteral feeding in HNC patients, a nasogastric tube (NGT) and a gastrostomy tube, both of which have demonstrated effectiveness in achieving optimal nutritional intake in this population [11]. Proactive placement of a gastrostomy tube is seen as the optimal method to reduce unplanned hospital admissions and treatment interruptions [3], with early intervention associated with improved treatment tolerance, nutritional status, and fewer unplanned hospital admissions [2]. To assist clinicians in achieving the best possible outcomes for HNC patients, both the Clinical Oncology Society of Australia (COSA) and the Royal Brisbane Women's Hospital (RBWH) have developed evidenced-based guidelines [12, 13]. These guidelines include care pathways for HNC patients based on proposed treatments and severity of malnutrition and dysphagia at diagnosis, and provide recommendations for frequency of dietetic care, goals and nutrition interventions.

Despite the introduction of HNC nutritional management guidelines, there is still debate among clinicians as to what the best nutrition interventions for patients are, due to differences in professional judgement and difficulties adopting evidenced-based guidelines into practice [13, 14]. It is also unclear how well institutions are able to implement and follow evidence-based guidelines in clinical practice. The aims of this study were to determine local adherence to the RBWH 'Swallowing and Nutrition Management Guidelines for Patients with Head and Neck Cancer' [12] and the COSA 'Evidence-based practice guidelines for the nutritional management of adult patients with Head and Neck Cancer' [13], and to determine local nutrition outcomes pre-treatment, at the completion of treatment, one-month post and three-months post treatment.

Methods

Study design

Data were retrieved from electronic medical records of HNC patients treated at a single tertiary facility. Participants were eligible for inclusion if they were 18 years or older and received ≥20 fractions of definitive or high dose palliative intent radiation treatment to the head and neck area. Treatment was scheduled on 5 days per week, within a two-year period between the 1st April 2014 and the 31st of March 2016. Ethical clearance was received from the Gold Coast Hospital and Health Service Human Research Ethics and University Committees.

Standard care

The facility has a HNC multidisciplinary clinic that is attended by surgical specialists, medical and radiation oncologists, cancer care nurses, speech pathologists and dietitians. All patients attending the clinic underwent baseline swallow and communication screening by a speech pathologist, and baseline nutrition risk was assessed by a dietitian using a validated malnutrition risk screening tool. All patients recommended for radiotherapy +/- systemic therapy with any head and neck cancer diagnosis irrespective of subtype are referred to the hospital's joint radiation oncology speech pathologist and dietitian HNC clinic. Patients having 20 or more fractions of radiotherapy (i.e. 4 weeks or more) are invited to attend the allied health multidisciplinary pre-treatment education session, followed by weekly individual consultations in the joint speech pathologist and dietitian clinic during treatment. Patient's having shorter courses of radiation (i.e. < 20 fractions) are offered consultation in the clinic, however frequency of consultations is on an individual basis. In the post treatment setting, patients were scheduled for bi-weekly review appointments for the first 6 weeks and could remain in the service for up to 12 months post treatment.

Measures

Local clinical practice was assessed against four selected recommendations from the COSA guidelines. These were: 1) the use of a validated malnutrition screening tool (MST) [15, 16], 2) nutrition assessment using the Patient-Generated Subjective Global Assessment (PG-SGA), 3) weekly contact with a dietitian during treatment and 4) post treatment dietitian follow up bi-weekly for 6 weeks. Prophylactic gastrostomy placement was assessed against the risk classification of the RBWH guidelines.

Nutritional status was assessed by dietitians using the global rating of the PG-SGA [17], and weight was measured on calibrated digital scales. The PG-SGA is a nutrition assessment tool that was adapted from the Subjective Global Assessment (SGA), specifically for cancer patients. It is based on patients using a check box format to answer questions regarding recent food intake, nutrition impact symptoms, activities and function and short-term weight loss. A physical examination is then performed by a health professional to assess muscle wasting, loss of subcutaneous fat and oedema [18].

Measures were taken at baseline (initial contact with radiation dietitian and speech pathologist), end of treatment, 1 month post treatment (± 1 week) and 3 months post treatment (± 2 weeks). Gastrostomy dependence was defined as patients who relied on their gastrostomy for any nutrition or hydration intake at 6 and 12 months post completion of treatment. At each assessment, clinicians documented a Functional Oral Intake Scale (FOIS) score that was determined from patient reported typical intake prior to attending their appointment. This is a 7-point ordinal scale that quantifies restrictions on oral intake [19, 20].

Data analysis

All data were de-identified and stored in Microsoft Excel. Statistical analysis of the data was completed using SPSS (version 22.0, 2013, IBM Corp) and Microsoft Excel. Chi-square tests were used to compare categorical variables, and t tests were used for continuous variables. Significance was reported at the $P = < 0.05$ level.

Results

From the 273 patients referred to the joint dietitian and speech pathologist clinic over the two-year period, 231 were eligible for inclusion. A further 22 patients were excluded due to missing data, mainly from patients declining the speech and dietetics service ($n = 9$), failing to attend multiple appointments (resulting in discharge from service as per local guidelines) ($n = 8$) or not completing treatment ($n = 5$). The sample population ($N = 209$) was predominantly male (85%), over the age of 65 years (range 28–93 years). Common cancer primary sites included skin (32%), oropharynx (27%) and oral cavity (22%) (Table 1). The mean dose of radiation treatment received was 64.8 Gy delivered over 31.9 fractions with 92.3% of patients receiving a dose between 60 and 70 Gy. In the 6 months before treatment, a total of 77 (36.8%) patients reported prior weight loss, with 2.9% experiencing > 10% loss of body weight prior to treatment.

Regarding adherence to guideline recommendations, use of a validated malnutrition screening tool pre-treatment was met in 86% of cases and the use of a validated nutrition assessment tool during treatment (PG-SGA) was met for 100% of patients. Weekly review by a dietitian during treatment occurred 80% of the time and 62% of patients were reviewed bi-weekly for 6 weeks post treatment. In patients for whom nutrition screening was not completed, this was mainly due to patient non-attendance at the hospital's multidisciplinary HNC clinic where screening takes place. The main reason ($n = 37$, 90%) patients were not seen weekly during treatment was due to failure to attend scheduled appointments. In the post-treatment setting, the main reasons patients were not seen fortnightly included failure to attend appointments ($n = 42$, 70%) or clinicians deeming a review was not clinically indicated ($n = 8$, 13%). Of the patients who were not seen fortnightly post treatment, 53% had primary tumors of the larynx or skin, who together lost the least amount of weight in the cohort (Table 2).

Of the 72 patients who were identified as high risk as per the RBWH guidelines, 58 (81%) received a prophylactic gastrostomy. Fourteen patients did not receive a gastrostomy as they declined the procedure ($n = 5$) or the procedure was medically contraindicated and not offered to the patient ($n = 9$). Of these patients, 86% ($n = 12$) were malnourished at the end of treatment, 3 patients accepted reactive nasogastric feeding tubes, and 4 patients had nutrition-related hospital admissions. An additional 2 patients in the overall cohort ($N = 209$) received a reactive gastrostomy (1 oral cavity patient, 1 oropharynx patient) and 8 patients required reactive

Table 1 Baseline patient characteristics of head and neck cancer patients treated with radiation therapy at Gold Coast University Hospital between 1st April 2014 and the 31st of March 2016

Patient characteristics	No. of patients [N, (%)]
Gender	
Male	177 (85)
Female	32 (15)
Age (years)	
< 50	26 (12.5)
50–65	86 (41)
> 65	97 (46.5)
Prior weight loss	
0%	133 (64)
< 5%	51 (24)
5- < 10%	19 (9)
> 10%	6 (3)
Site	
Oral cavity	22 (10.5)
Oropharynx	56 (27)
Nasopharynx	8 (4)
Hypopharynx	7 (3)
Larynx	21 (10)
Salivary	19 (9)
Skin primary	67 (32)
Unknown primary	6 (3)
Other	3 (1.5)
T Stage	
T0	24 (11.5)
T1	35 (17)
T2	51 (24.5)
T3	37 (17.5)
T4	48 (23)
Tx	12 (5.5)
Other	2 (1)
N Stage	
0	54 (25.5)
1	35 (17)
2	112 (53.5)
3	5 (2.5)
Unknown	3 (1.5)
M Stage	
0	206 (97.5)
1	3 (1.5)
Treatment	
Radiation therapy	50 (24)
Radiation therapy + chemotherapy	96 (46)
Surgery + radiation therapy	54 (26)
Surgery + radiation therapy and chemotherapy	10 (4)

Table 2 Average weight loss and percentage weight loss by tumor subsite at the end of treatment and three-months post treatment

Cancer Site	End of treatment [kg, (SD), (%)]	3 months post treatment [kg, (SD), (%)]
Oral Cavity	7.9 (4.6) (10.1%)	11.7 (5.3) (14.0%)
Oropharynx	7.5 (4.5) (8.9%)	11.0 (5.9) (12.5%)
Hypopharynx	5.9 (5.0) (7.0%)	7.9 (1.7) (10.9%)
Salivary	4.3 (4.1) (5.7%)	7.1 (3.8) (11%)
Nasopharynx	3.6 (3.0) (4.8%)	3.5 (2.0) (4.8%)
Skin	4.1 (3.9) 5.6 (4.8%)	6.0 (6.1) (6.8%)
Larynx	2.6 (3.6) (2.9%)	4.5 (4.9) (4.7%)

nasogastric feeding tube placement (4 oropharynx patients, 2 salivary patients, 1 nasopharynx patient, 1 unknown primary).

The average weight loss from baseline at the end of treatment was 5.6 kg (SD 4.5) (6.7%) ($p = < 0.001$), 7.9 kg (SD 5.5) (8.6%) at one-month post treatment ($p = < 0.001$) and 8.9 kg (SD 6.4) (10.3%) 3 months post treatment ($p = < 0.001$) (Fig. 1). The average weight loss was greatest for patients with oral cavity and oropharynx cancers both at the end of treatment (10.9, 8.8%), and three-months post treatment (14.7, 12.5%) (Table 2). Weight loss was statistically significant between oropharyngeal and skin primary cancers at all time points ($p = < 0.001$). Additionally, at the end of treatment, malnutrition rates were statistically higher ($p = < 0.001$) in oropharynx patients ($n = 41$, 77%) in comparison to skin primary cancer patients ($n = 22$, 38%).

Weight loss was not significantly different between patients who received Cetuximab ($n = 32$) and patients who received Cisplatin ($n = 64$) both at the end of treatment ($p = 0.210$) and three-months post treatment ($p = 0.954$). The average weight loss for Cetuximab patients at the end of treatment was 7.3 kg (SD 5.0) (8.9%) and 9.7 kg (SD 6.0) (11.4%) three-months post treatment, compared to 7.4 kg (SD 5.1) (8.6%), and 10.7 kg (SD 6.1) (12.1%) three-months post treatment for Cisplatin patients. A total of 18 (28%) patients who received Cisplatin required a change to Cetuximab during treatment due to toxicity and 23 (36%) of Cisplatin patients planned for 3 high dose cycles either had their dose reduced or third cycle cancelled.

As seen in Table 3, malnutrition rates increased throughout treatment. There was a statistically significant difference in the number of patients malnourished at baseline and the number of patients malnourished at the end of treatment ($p = < 0.001$), the number of patients malnourished one-month post treatment ($p = < 0.001$) and the number of patients malnourished 3 months' post treatment ($p = 0.006$).

Changes in type of oral intake as reported by patients and classified by clinicians completing the FOIS were significant between baseline and end of treatment ($p = < 0.001$) and baseline to one-month post treatment ($p = < 0.001$). FOIS scores were not significantly different from baseline to three-months post treatment ($p = 0.538$). The average FOIS score at baseline was 7 (i.e. total oral intake with no restrictions), 4.6 at the end of treatment (i.e. heavily texture-modified diet), 5.6 (texture modified diet) at one–month post treatment and 6 (i.e. near normal diet with special preparation of some foods) three-months post treatment.

Gastrostomy patients ($n = 60$) had their tube in-situ for an average of 150 days (range 44–751 days), with 8 (13%) patients being dependent on their tubes at

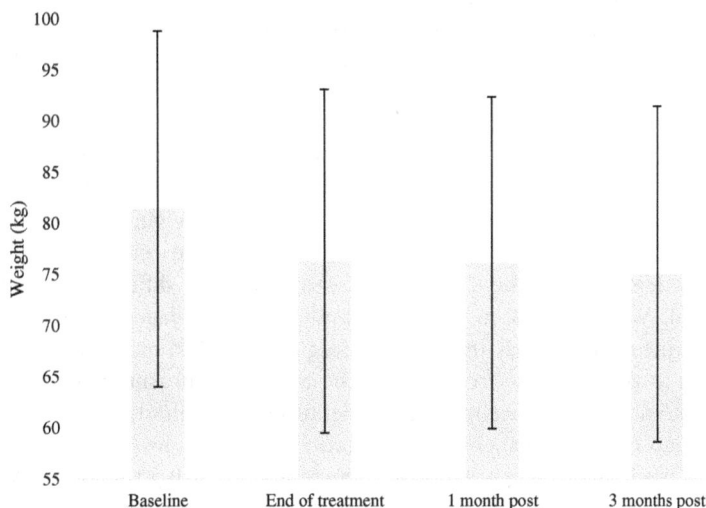

Fig. 1 Average weight change for HNC patients from baseline to three months post treatment. Relationship between time and weight loss over a period of three months in head and neck cancer patients over the duration of radiation treatment. Weight change was measure in kilos (kg), with large variations seen at each time point

Table 3 Patient Generated-Subjective Global Assessment (PG-SGA) global ratings of head and neck cancer patients from baseline to three-months post treatment

Time point	Well-nourished (PG-SGA A) [N, (%)]	Malnourished (PG-SGA B + C) [N, (%)]
Baseline (n = 209)	177 (85)	32 (15)
End of Treatment (n = 183)	80 (44)	103 (56)
One month post treatment (n = 144)	66 (46)	79 (54)
Three months post treatment (n = 124)	87 (70)	37 (30)

6 months post treatment and 2 patients (3%) dependent 12 months post treatment. Gastrostomy patients lost an average of 7.7 kg (9.4%) whilst on treatment and 11.5 kg (13.5%) from baseline to three-months post treatment.

A total of 55 (26%) patients in the cohort had an unplanned hospital admission during treatment, of which 14 (25%) were nutrition-related. The average length of stay was 4.6 days, with common admission reasons including decreased oral intake and anorexia. Of the 60 gastrostomy patients, 24 (40%) required unplanned admissions during treatment, of which 5 (21%) were nutrition-related.

Discussion

Significant weight loss and malnutrition still occur in HNC patients, despite the introduction of best-practice nutritional guidelines and treatment advances in radiation oncology. Little is known however, how well guidelines are able to be integrated into clinical practice. This study shows that despite good adherence to guidelines selected for comparison, clinically significant weight loss and malnutrition are still highly prevalent. This raises the question as to whether current recommendations for dietetic care both during and post-treatment should be reviewed, particularly for tumor sites which are known to put patients at higher risk for nutritional inadequacy, including those which originate in the oropharynx and oral cavity region.

This study reports an 81% adherence rate to the RBWH HNC risk category guidelines for prophylactic gastrostomy placement, interestingly higher than the 75% reported in 2008 by RBWH [5]. With regards to patient attendance, it was apparent in the current study the main reason patients were not seen as per guideline frequency was due to patient failure to attend. Compliance with appointments in this patient group has previously been reported to be poor [21], with some dietetic clinics stating a non-attendance rate as high as 27% [7]. Non-compliance is more common in patients with mental illnesses, substance abuse, and those who do not feel that dietetic care is a central component of treatment [21].

The average time gastrostomy patients had their feeding tube in-situ (5 months) was substantially shorter than that reported in other studies, with Crombie et al., [22] reporting the average length a patient had their tube in-situ was 7 months and Jack et al., [23] greater than 21 months. This may be due to some services having protocols that recommend gastrostomy tubes remain in for various amounts of time, depending on the treating institutions services and specialist support [13]. Gastrostomy tube dependence is also linked with swallowing outcomes, with literature demonstrating those who are tube-dependent long-term often having minimal swallow function [13]. Stimulation of musculature involved in swallowing has demonstrated to assist patients in returning to a full and non-texture modified diet more quickly post treatment [24]. Although patients in this study showed a decline in their reported ability to consume a full-textured diet during treatment, at three-months post treatment, patient reported dietary restrictions had almost returned to baseline levels in the majority of patients. Decline in the ability to consume a full-textured diet during intensive treatment may reflect a decline in swallow function. Diet restrictions returning to baseline may be in part attributable to the intensive support and prophylactic swallowing exercises patients received as part of the joint dietetic and speech pathologist service.

Weight loss prior to treatment is a prognostic factor for overall survival and is one of the biggest indicators of malnutrition [25]. Malnutrition is strongly related to decreased quality of life, increased unplanned hospital admissions and decreased effectiveness of treatment [7] [8]. The number of patients malnourished both at the end of treatment (56%) and three-months post treatment (30%) is comparable to that demonstrated in the literature. A study by Jager-Wittenaar et al., [26] on oral cavity and oropharyngeal cancer patients, reported that during treatment overall malnutrition rates were 16, and 25% 3 months post treatment [26]. This is similar to van de Berg et al., [27] who conducted a study with squamous cell carcinoma patients, demonstrating even with individual dietary care, 18% of patients were malnourished while receiving treatment and 10.5% were malnourished in the rehabilitation phase two-months post treatment. The differences seen between the current study and both Jager-Wittenaar et al., [26] and van de Berg et al. [27] in malnutrition rates may be due to both the timing of measured outcomes and the difference in definition of malnutrition, with both studies using percentage weight loss to define malnutrition and the current study using the PG-SGA tool.

Clinically significant weight loss (> 10%) prior to treatment was reported by 2.9% of the cohort, less than the 6.6% reported by Brown et al., [5] and the 5% reported by Languis et al., [25]. Weight loss during treatment (average 6.7%) was similar to a study by Langius et al., [25] where patients lost 6.1% body weight during treatment, although greater than that reported by Paccagnella et al., [28] where patients had lost 4.6% of body weight at the end of treatment. The current study also demonstrates that despite continued dietetic intervention, at 3 months post treatment, patients continued to lose weight. This highlights the potential need for increased length of intensive monitoring (bi-weekly) post treatment or additional community support. Weight loss between patients in the current study who received Cisplatin and Cetuximab was not statistically significant both during and post-treatment. It should however be noted, that a large proportion of patients who were planned to receive Cisplatin either did not complete their full course of chemotherapy or changed to Cetuximab to due treatment-related toxicities.

There are currently few studies that demonstrate the difference in weight loss between tumor sites in HNC, despite it being recognised that some tumor sites are at higher risk nutritionally [26]. Weight loss for skin primary HNC patients in particular, is underrepresented in the literature, with some studies not including these tumors in the classification of HNC or grouping these into the 'other' category [13, 22, 24, 25, 29]. Consistent with the RBWH guidelines, this demonstrates that those with HNC skin cancer tumors are generally not considered to be at high risk nutritionally. A study by Jager-Wittenaar et al., [29] demonstrated that critical weight loss (> 5% in 1 month or > 10% in 6 months) was seen in 8% of patients with skin, salivary and thyroid tumors, compared to 34% of patients with oropharynx/oral cavity tumors. These results are comparable to those presented in the current study with oropharynx patients losing on average 12.5%, oral cavity patients losing 14.7% and skin cancer patients losing 6.0% of body weight at three-months post treatment. Significant differences ($p = < 0.001$) in weight loss for oral cavity (10%) and oropharynx (11%) patients compared to weight loss in patients with laryngeal tumors (5%) has also been demonstrated in a study by Ehrsson et al., [30]. Likewise, in a study by Nourissat et al., [31] critical weight loss (> 5% during radiation therapy) was reported in 62.9% of oral cavity or oropharynx patients. These studies did not include skin cancer tumors in analysis. Tumor location can then be seen to have a significant impact on both weight loss and nutritional status. As nutritional status exerts its effects not only on the patient, but the healthcare system and dietetic services as well, the relationship between tumor location and weight loss warrants further investigation. Additionally, a review of current guidelines to include more intense nutritional care and updated care pathways for patients at higher risk of clinically significant weight loss (e.g. oropharyngeal and oral cavity tumors)

may be justified. Streaming care by tumor site may also reduce unneeded or unnecessary appointments and allow specialised clinicians more time with high risk patients.

The strengths of this study are that the primary researcher who reviewed the outcomes of patients treated at the hospital was not involved in any clinical care of patients, reducing potential researcher bias. The study also had a relatively large sample size and a representative sample of patients recruited. This study is inherently limited by its retrospective, single-institution design. Furthermore, we do not have data on all patients across all the time points, for reasons that include patients transferring back to a local service, thus making it difficult to draw stronger conclusions. A prospective study could overcome this by gathering data of enrolled patients ongoing from outside institutions, should enrolled patients choose to receive follow-up care closer to home. The study is also limited in that it does not address patient adherence to dietary optimization at home or quantify energy and protein intake in comparison to best practice guidelines. Non-adherence to dietetic recommendations may have resulted in higher rates of malnutrition and more significant weight loss. Data on energy and protein intake quantified against guideline recommendations would also demonstrate if patients were meeting their nutrition requirements and still experiencing significant weight loss or malnutrition.

Conclusion

The use of evidenced-based guidelines for HNC enables the early identification of patients at nutritional risk and provides care pathways for clinicians to follow. Our study supports the use of current Australian guidelines as a method of identifying patients who may need enteral feeding, however suggests that streaming care, in particular for dietetic monitoring by tumor site has the potential to further improve patient outcomes and could be a better use of finite healthcare resources. Continued weight loss in this population post treatment also suggests that perhaps bi-weekly follow up should continue to occur for greater than 6 weeks post treatment. Suggestions for future studies include the trial of care pathways by tumor site to explore weight loss and malnutrition in subgroups of the HNC population, and assessing patient adherence to nutrition recommendations (energy and protein intake) as directed by the dietitian.

Abbreviations
COSA: Clinical Oncology Society of Australia; FOIS: Functional Oral Intake Scale; HNC: Head and neck cancer; MST: Malnutrition Screening Tool; NGT: Nasogastric Tube; PEG: Percutaneous Gastrostomy Tube; PEM: Protein Energy Malnutrition; PG-SGA: Patient Generated Subjective Global Assessment; RBWH: Royal Brisbane Women's Hospital.

Acknowledgements

The authors thank the staff of the combined Head and Neck Clinic at the Gold Coast University Hospital for their support and the speech pathologist and nutrition and dietetic departments for data collection.

Authors' contributions

SH, JA and JJ gathered, interpreted and analysed all patient data. EI provided guidance for statistics and interpretation. All authors read and approved the final manuscript.

Competing interests

The authors declare that they have no competing interests. The authors acknowledge that we have full control of all primary data and agree to allow the journal to review the data upon request.

Author details

[1]Faculty of Health Sciences and Medicine, Bond University, 2 Promethean Way, Robina, QLD 4226, Australia. [2]Gold Coast University Hospital, Southport, QLD, Australia. [3]Radiation Oncology Centres, Gold Coast University Hospital, Southport, QLD, Australia.

References

1. Madhoun MF, et al. Prophylactic PEG placement in head and neck cancer: how many feeding tubes are unused (and unnecessary)? World J Gastroenterolo. 2011;17(8):1004–8.
2. Zhang Z, et al. Comparative effects of different enteral feeding methods in head and neck cancer patients receiving radiotherapy or chemoradiotherapy: a network meta-analysis. Onco Targets Ther. 2016;9: 2897–909.
3. Epstein JB, et al. Quality of life and oral function following radiotherapy for head and neck cancer. Head Neck. 1999;21(1):1–11.
4. Sroussi HY, et al. Common oral complications of head and neck cancer radiation therapy: mucositis, infections, saliva change, fibrosis, sensory dysfunctions, dental caries, periodontal disease, and osteoradionecrosis. Cancer Med. 2017;6(12):2918–31.
5. Brown TE, et al. Validated swallowing and nutrition guidelines for patients with head and neck cancer: identification of high-risk patients for proactive gastrostomy. Head Neck. 2013;35(10):1385–91.
6. Baxi SS, Schwitzer E, Jones LW. A review of weight loss and sarcopenia in patients with head and neck cancer treated with chemoradiation. Cancers Head Neck. 2016;1(1):9.
7. Kiss NK, et al. A dietitian-led clinic for patients receiving (chemo)radiotherapy for head and neck cancer. Support Care Cancer. 2012; 20(9):2111–20.
8. Brookes GB. Nutritional status--a prognostic indicator in head and neck cancer. Otolaryngol Head Neck Surg. 1985;93(1):69–74.
9. Isenring E, et al. Updated evidence-based practice guidelines for the nutritional management of patients receiving radiation therapy and/or chemotherapy. Nutr Diet. 2013;70(4):312–24.
10. Arends J, et al. ESPEN guidelines on nutrition in cancer patients. Clin Nutr. 2017;36(1):11–48.
11. Wang J, et al. Percutaneous endoscopic gastrostomy versus nasogastric tube feeding for patients with head and neck cancer: a systematic review. J Radiat Res. 2014;55(3):559–67.
12. Brown T, et al. Nutrition outcomes following implementation of validated swallowing and nutrition guidelines for patients with head and neck cancer. Support Care Cancer. 2014;22(9):2381–91.
13. Findlay, M., J. Bauer, and T. Brown, Evidenced-based guidelines for the nutritional management of adult patients with head and neck cancer head and neck guideline steering Comittee, editor. 2014.
14. Nugent B, Lewis S, O'Sullivan JM. Enteral feeding methods for nutritional management in patients with head and neck cancers being treated with radiotherapy and/or chemotherapy. Cochrane Database Syst Rev. 2013;1
15. Ferguson ML, et al. Validation of a malnutrition screening tool for patients receiving radiotherapy. Australas Radiol. 1999;43(3):325–7.
16. Shaw C, et al. Comparison of a novel, simple nutrition screening tool for adult oncology inpatients and the malnutrition screening tool (MST) against the patient-generated subjective global assessment (PG-SGA). Support Care Cancer. 2015;23(1):47–54.
17. Ottery FD. Definition of standardized nutritional assessment and interventional pathways in oncology. Nutrition. 1996;12(1 Suppl):S15–9.
18. Jager-Wittenaar H, Ottery FD. Assessing nutritional status in cancer: role of the patient-generated subjective global assessment. Curr Opin Clin Nutr Metab Care. 2017;20(5):322–9.
19. van der Molen L, et al. Pretreatment organ function in patients with advanced head and neck cancer: clinical outcome measures and patients' views. BMC Ear, Nose Throat Disord. 2009;9(1):1–9.
20. Crary MA, Mann GD, Groher ME. Initial psychometric assessment of a functional oral intake scale for dysphagia in stroke patients. Arch Phys Med Rehabil. 2005;86(8):1516–20.
21. Britton B, et al. Eating as treatment (EAT) study protocol: a stepped-wedge, randomised controlled trial of a health behaviour change intervention provided by dietitians to improve nutrition in patients with head and neck cancer undergoing radiotherapy. BMJ Open. 2015;5(7)
22. Crombie JM, et al. Swallowing outcomes and PEG dependence in head and neck cancer patients receiving definitive or adjuvant radiotherapy +/− chemotherapy with a proactive PEG: a prospective study with long term follow up. Oral Oncol. 2015;51(6):622–8.
23. Jack DR, et al. Guideline for prophylactic feeding tube insertion in patients undergoing resection of head and neck cancers. J Plast Reconstr Aesthet Surg. 2012;65(5):610–5.
24. Ames JA, et al. Outcomes after the use of gastrostomy tubes in patients whose head and neck cancer was managed with radiation therapy. Head Neck. 2011;33(5):638–44.
25. Langius JAE, et al. Critical weight loss is a major prognostic indicator for disease-specific survival in patients with head and neck cancer receiving radiotherapy. Br J Cancer. 2013;109(5):1093–9.
26. Jager-Wittenaar H, et al. Malnutrition in patients treated for oral or oropharyngeal cancer—prevalence and relationship with oral symptoms: an explorative study. Support Care Cancer. 2011;19(10):1675–83.
27. van den Berg MGA, et al. Comparison of the effect of individual dietary counselling and of standard nutritional care on weight loss in patients with head and neck cancer undergoing radiotherapy. Br J Nutr. 2010;104(6):872–7.
28. Paccagnella A, et al. Early nutritional intervention improves treatment tolerance and outcomes in head and neck cancer patients undergoing concurrent chemoradiotherapy. Support Care Cancer. 2010;18(7):837–45.
29. Jager-Wittenaar H, et al. Critical weight loss in head and neck cancer—prevalence and risk factors at diagnosis: an explorative study. Support Care Cancer. 2007;15(9):1045–50.
30. Ehrsson YT, Langius-Eklöf A, Laurell G. Nutritional surveillance and weight loss in head and neck cancer patients. Support Care Cancer. 2012;20(4):757–65.
31. Nourissat A, et al. Predictors of weight loss during radiotherapy in patients with stage I or II head and neck cancer. Cancer. 2010;116(9):2275–83.

Survival and associated factors among patients with oral squamous cell carcinoma (OSCC) in Mulago hospital

Juliet Asio[1*], Adriane Kamulegeya[2] and Cecily Banura[3]

Abstract

Background: Despite improvements in diagnosis and patient management, survival and prognostic factors of patients with oral squamous cell carcinoma (OSCC) remains largely unknown in most of Sub Saharan Africa.

Objective: To establish survival and associated factors among patients with oral squamous cell carcinoma treated at Mulago Hospital Complex, Kampala.

Methods: We conducted a retrospective cohort study among histologically confirmed oral squamous cell carcinoma (OSCC) patients seen at our centre from January 1st 2002 to December 31st 2011. Survival was analysed using Kaplan-Meier method and comparison between associated variables made using Log rank-test. Cox proportional hazards model was used to determine independent predictors of survival. P-values of less than 0.05 were considered statistically significant.

Results: A total of 384 patients (229 males and 155 females) were included in this analysis. The overall mean age was 55.2 (SD 4.1) years. The 384 patients studied contributed a total of 399.17 person-years of follow-up. 111 deaths were observed, giving an overall death rate of 27.81 per 100 person-years [95% CI; 22.97–32.65]. The two-year and five-year survival rates were 43.6% (135/384) and 20.7% (50/384), respectively. Tumours arising from the lip had the best five-year survival rate (100%), while tumours arising from the floor of the mouth, alveolus and the gingiva had the worst prognosis with five-year survival rates of 0%, 0% and 15.9%, respectively. Independent predictors of survival were clinical stage ($p = 0.001$), poorly differentiated histo-pathological grade ($p < 0.001$), male gender ($p = 0.001$), age > 55 years at time of diagnosis ($p = 0.02$) and moderately differentiated histo-pathological grade ($p = 0.027$). However, tobacco & alcohol consumption, tumour location and treatment group were not associated with survival ($p > 0.05$).

Conclusions: The five-year survival rate of OSCC was poor at 20.7%. Male gender, late clinical stage at presentation, poor histo-pathological types and advanced age were independent prognostic factors of survival. Early detection through screening and prompt treatment could improve survival.

Keywords: Oral squamous cell carcinoma, Uganda, Survival, Clinical-pathological presentation

* Correspondence: julietasio@yahoo.com
[1]HIV Reference Laboratory, Uganda Virus Research Institute, P. O. Box 49, Entebbe, Uganda
Full list of author information is available at the end of the article

Background

Oral squamous cell carcinoma (OSCC) is a potentially disfiguring and debilitating disease that affects the physical appearance of patients and devastates their self-esteem. Globally, over 175,000 cases are diagnosed annually [1]. The age-adjusted incidence and mortality rates of OSCC increases with age and are greater in males than females [2]. It is well established that tobacco use and alcohol consumption are significant risk factors [3]. Some studies suggest that among people living with HIV, the risk of oral cancer is elevated [4].

The risk factors for Human Papilloma Virus (HPV) positive OSCC are mainly related to sexual habits rather than to tobacco and alcohol use in HPV negative OSCC [5]. Furthermore, over the past decade, oncogenic HPV type 16 has been linked to the development of some oral pharyngeal cancers but the association with oral cancer proper was not evident [6]. The detection of HPV DNA in some oral pharyngeal cancers has been linked to a favourable prognosis particularly among males [7]. Sub Saharan Africa (SSA) having a high burden of infection related cancers may provide unique circumstances in oral cancers worth researching.

Despite improvements in diagnostic facilities and patient management, survival and prognostic factors of OSCC remain unknown in most of SSA. Data from the Kampala Cancer Registry showed that oral cancer (ICD-10 C00-C06) was a rare disease that contributed 1.1% cases in Uganda [8]. However, there is paucity of data on survival and prognostic factors of oral cancers in Uganda. Therefore, the purpose of this study was to establish survival rates and determine independent prognostic factors of survival among patients with OSCC.

Methods

Study design and setting

Records of patients with histologically confirmed OSCC seen at Mulago Hospital Complex from January 1st 2002 to December 31st 2011 were reviewed.

Mulago hospital is a national referral hospital, which has the only functional oral and maxillofacial surgery unit and the only radiotherapy unit serving the whole of Uganda and the neighbouring countries. Additionally, Mulago Hospital Complex shares location with the Uganda Cancer Institute (UCI) that provides chemotherapy treatment and care of cancer patients in Uganda and neighbouring countries. Records of patients with OSCC were retrieved from the Oral and Maxillofacial department and their socio-demographic, clinical and pathological data was abstracted. At both UCI and the Radiotherapy department, registers were used to identify patients with OSCC. Records of patients with OSCC were then retrieved and their details recorded.

Study population

The sample size was determined using the following assumptions: the log rank comparisons of the probability of experiencing death in 5 years between patients with early disease and those with advanced disease at 0.47, power of 80%, 5% significance level, an effect size of 1.595 and adjusting for loss to follow-up of 10%. The total number of (events) deaths that were required was 149 and at least 270 participants were required for this study.

Consecutive records of 384 index patients with a histological diagnosis of OSCC seen at Mulago Hospital Complex were retrieved for assessment. Records with missing important variables (e.g. date of diagnosis, site of lesion) or those with vague histological diagnosis (such as 'moderately-well' differentiated, 'poorly-well' differentiated), those of patients who presented with second primaries and patients who were referred to Hospice Uganda for terminal care, were excluded from the study. To eliminate duplicate recruits, patient demographic characteristics at different entry points of care were compared using hospital identification numbers and patient details. From each eligible record, demographic characteristics, pre-operative tumour characteristics, TNM stage, tobacco and alcohol usage, treatment instituted, length of follow-up and survival status were abstracted. To determine the nodal status in TNM staging, both clinical and radiological findings were assessed whenever available, while the evaluation of metastases was based on chest x-ray reports. In some cases, follow-up phone calls were made to patients or their next of kin with recorded telephone contacts in order to ascertain the status of the patient.

Statistics and analysis

Statistical analyses were performed using STATA Version 12. The length of follow-up was defined as the period in months between the date of histological diagnosis and time to death or censoring. Cases were classified as alive, dead (if date of death was recorded) or lost to follow-up (date of last visit as recorded in patient's file). Baseline characteristics for the patients were described using percentages for categorical variables and medians for continuous variables.

Survival was calculated using the Kaplan-Meier analysis and the significance of the difference between survival curves for each variable was determined using the Breslow-test. P-values less than 0.05 were considered statistically significant. The Cox proportional hazards model was used to obtain independent predictors of survival. Construction of the final model was done in stages. Initially, all variables with a p value < 0.25 at univariate analysis were included in the multivariable model. To test for goodness of fit of the multivariable model a plot of

Nelson–Aalen cumulative hazard estimate against Cox Snell residuals was plotted.

Results

Records of 512 patients were retrieved. One hundred twenty eight (25.0%) records were excluded due to missing data including: vague or no histological diagnosis, patients with second primaries, and patients referred to Hospice Uganda for terminal care. Therefore, 384 (75.0%) records were included in the analysis. In addition, 70 (13.7%) records with no data on clinical stage at presentation were excluded from survival analysis.

Socio-demographic characteristics, alcohol consumption and tobacco use

The mean age of the 384 patients included in this study was 55.2 years with a standard deviation of 4.1 years. There were 229 (59.6%) males and 155 (40.4%) females. Males had a mean age of 55.8 years (SD = 19.9 years), whereas females had a mean age of 55.6 years (SD = 15.9 years). Most patients were in their sixth decade 104 (27.1%). Most patients came from the western region of the country 130 (33.9%). Of the 214 patients with a history of education background, less than 40% had attained secondary level education (Table 1). Compared to females, more males reported use of tobacco and alcohol.

Sub-site tumour presentation, histopathological grading and clinical stage

The distribution of primary tumour sites, spread and clinical stage of OSCC is presented in Table 2. In descending order, the tongue (34.1%), palate (13.5%), buccal mucosa (13.3%) and floor of the mouth (12.2%) were the commonest primary sites.

Majority 51.6% ($n = 198$) of patients had well differentiated tumours, and about one-fifth (21.9%, $n = 84$) had poorly differentiated tumours. Majority (61%) of the identified OSCC were in TNM stage III and IV (Table 1).

Survival pattern of 384 patients with OSCC

The 384 patients studied contributed a total of 399.17 person–years of follow-up. One hundred eleven deaths were observed, giving an overall death rate of 27.81 per 100 person–years [95% CI; 22.97–32.65]. The overall average survival time for patients with OSCC was 375 days. The two-year and five-year survival rates were respectively 43.6% (135/384) and 20.7% (50/384), (Table 3).

The two-year and five-year survival rates were significant for age ($p = 0.001$), clinical stage ($p < 0.001$) and pathological stage ($p < 0.001$). There was no difference in gender, tumour localisation, treatment group and in

Table 1 Demographic, clinical and pathological characteristics of 384 OSCC patients

Characteristic	n(%)
Gender	
Male	229(59.6)
Female	155(40.4)
Age (years)	
Mean (SD)	55.2(4.1)
Tobacco use	
User	147(54.7)
Non-User	122(45.4)
Alcohol use	
User	140(52.6)
Non-User	126(47.4)
Geographical region	
Central	132(34.4)
Eastern	72(18.7)
Northern	41(10.7)
Western	109(28.4)
Non-Ugandan	30(7.8)
Education level	
Tertiary	27(12.6)
Secondary	44(20.6)
Primary	68(31.8)
None	75(35.0)
Histo-pathological grade	
Well differentiated	198(51.5)
Moderately differentiated	102(26.6)
Poorly differentiated	84(21.9)
Treatment modality	
Surgery	38(9.9)
Radiotherapy	224(58.3)
Chemotherapy	4(1.0)
Surgery + Radiotherapy	41(10.7)
Surgery + Chemotherapy	8(2.1)
Surgery + Radiotherapy +Chemotherapy	8(2.1)
Radiotherapy + Chemotherapy	3(0.8)
None	58(15.1)

patients with or without a history of either tobacco or alcohol consumption ($p > 0.05$), (Table 4). Kaplan–Meier analysis and log-rank test were used for bivariate analysis. Kaplan–Meier curves were constructed for all patients and for significant variables (Figs. 1, 2, 3, 4 and 5).

Predictors of survival among OSCC patients

Construction of the final model containing variables found to be independently associated with survival of

Table 2 Sub-site distribution, TNM classification and clinical stage at presentation of 384 patients with OSCC

Variable	Number	Percentage
Site		
Alveolus	18	4.7
Buccal Mucosa	51	13.3
Floor of mouth	47	12.2
Gingiva	43	11.2
Lip	16	4.2
Palate	52	13.5
Tongue	131	34.1
Other[a]	26	6.8
T (Tumour)		
1	41	10.7
2	142	37.0
3	91	23.7
4	62	16.1
X	48	12.5
N (Nodal involvement)		
0	151	39.3
1	63	16.5
2	106	27.6
3	22	5.7
X	42	10.9
M (Metastasis)		
0	228	59.4
1	86	22.4
X	70	18.2
Clinical Stage (Based on TNM staging system)		
I	23	6.0
II	57	14.8
III	148	38.5
IV	86	22.5
X	70	18.2

[a]Other includes Commissure, Buccal sulcus, Retromolar trigone, Sublingual salivary glands
X Missing data

oral cancer was made using Cox proportional hazards model. A model which included all variables that had a P–value of less than 0.25 at univariate analysis was formed (Table 5). These included clinical stage, pathological variant, treatment group, gender, age and tobacco use. The variable tumour site ($p = 0.26$) was included on the basis of previous studies.

The model was tested to verify whether the assumption of proportionality between early-stage and late stage disease patient categories. The proportionality of hazards assumption of the model was tested as a whole, and for each variable using the global test and the extended Cox model. The model was not significant based on the Schoenfeld's test ($p = 0.838$) and the extended Cox model indicating that the data did not violate the proportional hazards assumption. There model was tested for interaction and confounding, using clinical stage as the main predictor of survival. The final model was thus determined as:

$$h(t, x) = h_0 \ \exp \ (1.098 \text{clinical stage}(IIIIV) \\ + 0.027 \text{moderately differentiated tumour} \\ + 01.094 \text{poorly differentiated tumour} \\ + 0.023 \text{age} - 0.731 \text{female})$$

The model itself was significant ($p < 0.001$). It was also tested for goodness of fit using a plot of Nelson–Aalen cumulative hazard estimate against Cox Snell residuals which gave a good model.

Assessment of selection bias on participants lost to follow-up

A total of 141 (44.9%) participants were lost to follow-up during the study. This rate is higher than the acceptable 15%. The characteristics of these patients were assessed to determine the possibility of selection bias. The patients who were lost to follow-up had similar characteristics to those who remained in the study except with reference to treatment group, as shown in Table 6 below.

Table 3 Survival Pattern of 384 patients with OSCC

Time (years)	Total number	Deaths	Censored	Survival	95% Confidence Interval
0	384	50	199	0.824	0.775 0.864
1	135	40	45	0.531	0.450 0.606
2	50	8	11	0.436	0.347 0.521
3	31	10	6	0.280	0.189 0.378
4	15	0	2	0.280	0.189 0.378
5	13	3	3	0.207	0.117 0.314

Table 4 Univariate Analysis of 384 Patients with OSCC

Variable	Survival rate (%)		P value (log-rank)
	2-year	5-year	
Gender			
Male	43.3	22.9	0.053
Female	59.2	30.1	
Age (years)			
≤ 55	69.7	53.7	0.001
> 55	34.0	8.8	
Tobacco Use			
User	47.7	15.8	0.091
Non-User	49.6	29.8	
Alcohol Use			
User	46.6	26.3	0.460
Non-User	50.7	21.0	
Tumour Location			
Alveolus	59.3	0.0	0.255
Buccal mucosa	47.0	19.6	
Floor of mouth	34.5	0.0	
Gingiva	39.7	15.9	
Lip	100.0	100.0	
Palate	52.3	43.6	
Tongue	53.3	21.2	
Other	53.9	53.9	
Clinical Stage			
I	100.0	100.0	< 0.001
II	69.1	61.5	
III	41.7	14.5	
IV	35.4	0.0	
Histo-pathological grade			
Well differentiated	64.9	42.2	< 0.001
Moderately differentiated	50.1	21.7	
Poorly differentiated	26.4	0.0	
Treatment Group			
Surgery	73.8	61.5	0.103
Radiotherapy	47.5	27.6	
Chemotherapy	100.0	0.0	
At least 2	55.3	12.3	

Other – Commissure, Buccal sulcus, Retromolar trigone, Sublingual salivary glands
At least 2 – Surgery and Radiotherapy or Surgery and Chemotherapy
P value is for 5-year survival

Discussion

This study, to the best of our knowledge presents one of a few on survival of OSCC patients in Sub Saharan Africa. It showed poor survival of patients with OSCC (20.7%) after five years and almost half of them (43.6%) had died within 2 years of diagnosis. Our findings are similar to the low five-year survival rate observed in Egypt for intra oral cancers (20.8%) [9]. However, better survival especially for stages III and IV has been reported in resource rich countries like Taiwan 26.6% and 11.8% [10], Brazil 32.6% and 24.5% [11] and the USA [12]. This discrepancy may be a reflection of better screening programs for early detection of cases and better treatment modalities, which ultimately improves survival, in the better resourced countries. The case for standardised treatment and its effect on survival irrespective of the difference in ethnicity and economic status has already been made for all head and neck squamous cell carcinomas [13].

Gender had a significant effect on survival in our study with the risk of death two times greater in males compared to females (Table 5 and Fig. 2). The effect of gender on survival remains mixed and unclear. Whereas some studies suggest a greater survival for females [14, 15], Mehta et al. reported lesser improvement in survival for females with oral cavity and oral pharyngeal carcinomas [16]. Other studies have reported no significant difference in survival between males and females [10]. It is believed that more males than females are affected by OSCC and have worse survival because of their increased exposure to tobacco and alcohol [2]. Furthermore, the males have poor health seeking behaviours, which may translate into delayed diagnosis and treatment initiation [17].

Age was a significant prognostic factor for survival in this study (Table 5 and Fig. 3). Patients who presented with OSCC and were above 55 years had a significantly shorter survival time as compared to those who were younger ($p = 0.001$). Our findings are consistent with studies conducted in Brazil [11], USA [16], Taiwan [10] and Egypt [9]. There seems to be a general agreement that the lower survival among older patients may be related to the higher rates of co-morbidities associated with ageing. It is also possible that these co-morbidities preclude the older patients from long surgical interventions which disadvantages their survival yet radiotherapy alone has been reported to lead to worse prognosis [11, 18]. In addition, with the emerging role of HPV, in oral and oral pharyngeal cancers, it may be that the younger population has a different causative factor hence better outcomes. However, a study from Mbarara in western Uganda showed a low prevalence of HPV among the head and neck cancers [19].

Education level, alcohol consumption and tobacco smoking were not significant predictors of survival. However, determination of cigarette smoking and tobacco and alcohol use, post event, may not be accurate thus making determination of their influence on patient survival hard to establish [20]. Education level is a surrogate for socio-economic status which has been shown

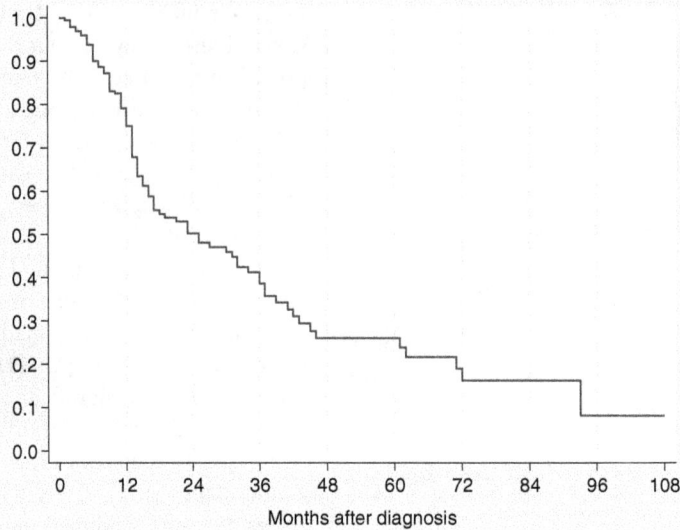

Fig. 1 Kaplan–Meier estimates for 384 patients with OSCC

to affect survival. Therefore, more research needs to be done to establish why it had no effect in our study.

Tumour site was not an independent predictor of survival. This was consistent with other studies [21] but different from others [9, 11, 14]. The possibility of misclassification of original OSCC site is high given the complex anatomy of the oral cavity coupled with delayed presentation seen among our patients [22]. In advanced stages, there could be an overlap of oral tumours that arise from adjacent structures leading to misclassification. In this study, about two-thirds of patients presented with late stage disease making misclassification of the original site of OSCC highly likely.

OSCC arising from the lip had the best five-year survival rate (100%) consistent with results from other studies [9, 14]. This may be because lip cancer is noticed earlier by patients and so they tend to seek care earlier. On the other hand, the floor of the mouth, alveolus and the gingiva had the worst five-year survival rates of 0%, 0% and 15.9%, respectively. Our results are different from those obtained from other studies which showed that the tongue had the lowest survival rate [11, 12]. The differences in survival by tumour site could arise from the ease of early diagnosis, accessibility for excision of the tumour with sufficient surgical margin and the different lymph node involvement that

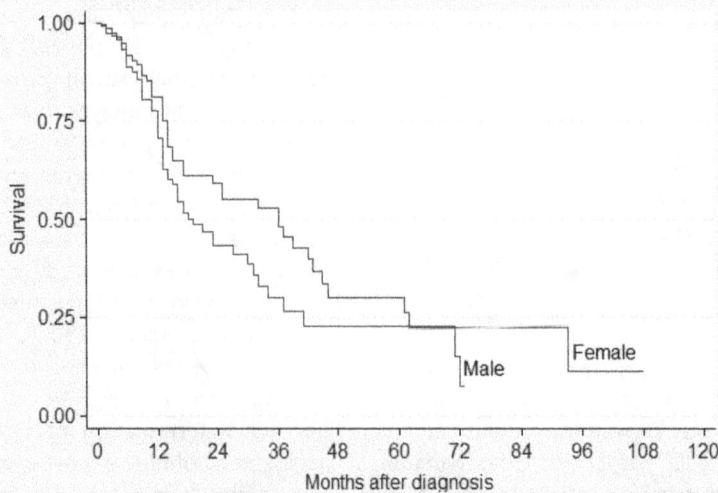

Fig. 2 Kaplan–Meier estimates by Gender for patients with OSCC

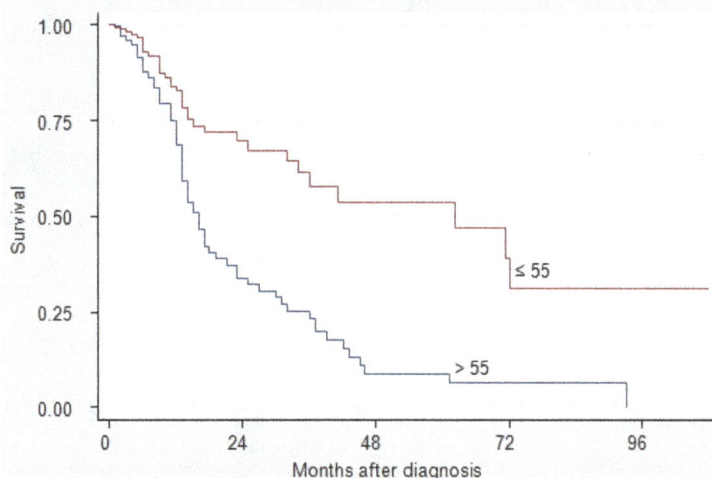

Fig. 3 Kaplan–Meier survival estimates by Age for patients with OSCC

each site presents. However, given the previously reported late presentation among our patients [22], tongue carcinomas may progress into the floor of the mouth making it hard to know the original site. In addition, some anatomic sites manifest greater metastatic capacity due to high lymphatic drainage [17].

We found an inverse relationship between tumour stage and survival ($p <$ 0.001), which was consistent with other studies [9, 11, 18, 21, 23]. The five-year survival rates were 100%, 61.5%, 14.5% and 0% for patients with stages I, II, III and IV, respectively. A study conducted in Egypt found similar survival rates of 100%, 65.5%, 42.2% and 0% for stages I, II, III and IV disease, respectively [9]. However, the rates in our study are much lower than those reported by two studies that investigated the outcomes of OSCC after surgical and/or radiation therapy in America [24] and

Taiwan [21]. The much lower survival rates reported in this study could be a reflection of the study population that comprised more of patients in clinical stages III and IV than those in stages I and II at presentation, which was much higher than those reported by other studies.

Histo-pathological grading was a significant predictor of survival in this study. It is widely reported that prognosis is better with early stage well differentiated disease than other histo-pathological types [21]. In fact, the risk of death increased with less well differentiated tumours in this study. Patients with poorly and moderately differentiated tumours had three fold and almost two fold risk of death, respectively, compared to those who had well differentiated tumours. However, it is worth noting that some reports have not shown tumour grade to have an effect on survival [11, 23].

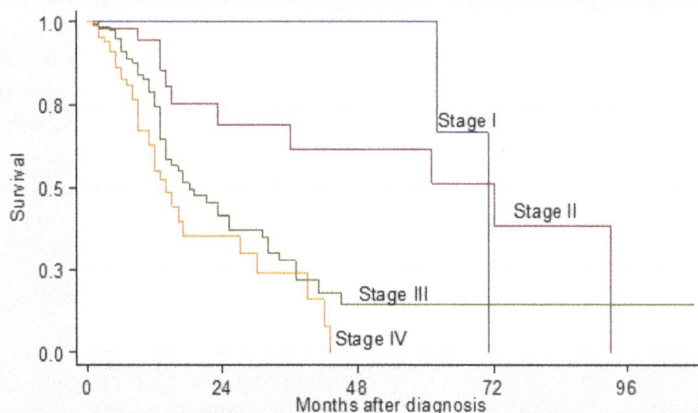

Fig. 4 Kaplan–Meier survival estimates by Clinical Stage for patients with OSCC

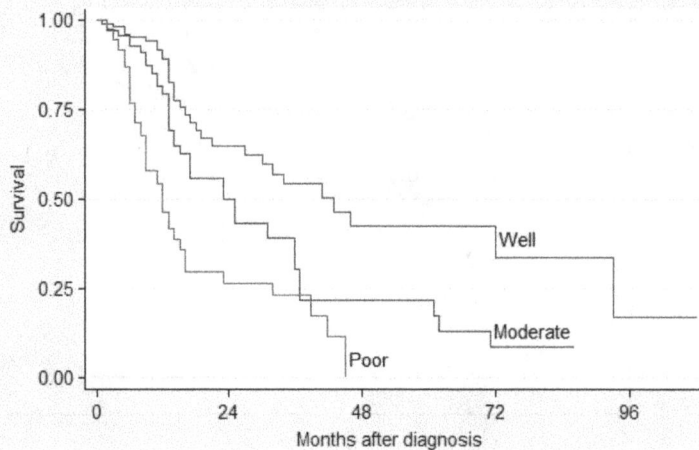

Fig. 5 Kaplan–Meier survival estimates by Histo-pathological Grade for patients with OSCC

The type of treatment received by the patient was not a predictor of survival in this study. Of the 384 patients, about two-thirds (67.3%) received at least one form of treatment (Table 3). Radiotherapy, either alone or in combination with surgery was the most common treatment modality. Patients treated with surgery showed the highest two-year and five-year survival rates followed by surgery and radiotherapy. However, most untreated patients died within 5 years and so did many of the patients treated with radiotherapy alone or chemotherapy alone. However, several studies where surgery was the primary mode of treatment found treatment modality as a significant predictor of survival [10–12, 21]. The treatment modality is dependent on stage of disease and other parameters such as anatomical site, tumour size, distant metastasis, histological type and lymph node involvement [12]. While surgery alone may be recommended for patients with early stage disease, adjuvant radiotherapy or chemotherapy is indicated for patients with advanced stages [12].

The large number of patients lost to follow up could also explain why treatment modality was not a significant predictor of survival since patients who were lost to follow-up had a borderline difference ($p = 0.057$) from those who were not, with respect to treatment group. Patients who were lost to follow-up were most likely those who were assigned to treatment modalities that required repeated visits such as chemotherapy and radiotherapy for advanced stage disease. It is also possible that many of the patients lost to follow-up were travelling long distances to access these treatment modalities, which would make re-visits expensive. Furthermore, patients were classified solely on their treatment status without taking into consideration the dosage, duration and compliance with treatment received. In our setting sometimes surgery is not an option due limited surgical space. Sometimes this may lead to significant delays in accessing the service thus disease progression and change in stage [25]. This does have a significant effect on outcomes. It is not any different when it comes to radiotherapy were machine breakdowns and patient load likewise lead to delayed treatment compromising outcomes [26].

Table 5 Model showing the combined effect of significant variables

Variables	Hazard Ratio	95% Confidence Interval		P value
Clinical stage				
I & II	1			
III & IV	2.998	1.584	5.674	0.001
Histo-pathological grade				
Well differentiated	1			
Moderately differentiated	1.756	1.065	2.897	0.027
Poorly differentiated	2.985	1.798	4.957	< 0.001
Age				
≤ 55	1			
> 55	1.022	1.008	1.036	0.002
Gender				
Male	1			
Female	0.482	0.310	0.749	0.001

Limitations

Our study was a hospital and not population-based study. It may therefore not be a representative sample of all the OSCC in Uganda. Data on HIV status of the patients and detection of HPV DNA in the tumours was not available.

Table 6 Comparison of characteristics of patients enrolled and those lost to follow-up

Variable	Alive/Dead		Lost to follow-up		P value
	Total (n = 173)	%	Total (n = 141)	%	
Gender					
Male	105	60.7	81	57.4	0.560
Female	68	39.3	60	42.6	
Age (years)					
Median (IQR)	56	(44.5–66)	60	(47.5–66)	0.284
Tobacco use					
User	79	51.6	68	58.6	0.254
Non-user	74	48.4	48	41.4	
Alcohol use					
User	85	55.9	55	48.2	0.215
Non-user	67	44.1	59	51.8	
Tumour location					
Alveolus	6	3.6	10	7.1	0.764
Buccal mucosa	17	9.8	18	12.8	
Floor of mouth	22	12.7	13	9.2	
Gingiva	23	13.3	15	10.6	
Lip	7	4.0	9	6.4	
Palate	24	13.9	21	14.9	
Tongue	62	35.8	47	33.3	
Other	12	6.9	8	5.7	
Clinical stage					
I	16	9.2	7	5.0	0.410
II	31	17.9	26	18.4	
III	79	45.7	69	48.9	
IV	47	27.2	39	27.7	
Histo-pathological grade					
Well differentiated	80	45.8	89	63.1	9.351
Moderately differentiated	46	26.8	32	22.7	
Poorly differentiated	47	27.4	20	14.2	
Treatment group					
Surgery	18	11.8	17	15.0	0.057
Radiotherapy	110	71.9	72	63.7	
Chemotherapy	2	1.3	1	0.9	
At least 2	23	15	23	20.4	

Seventy (13.7%) records with no data on clinical stage at presentation were excluded from survival analysis. However, this did not affect the power of the study given that we sampled 384 records, compared to 270 required for this study.

Conclusion

Poor survival rates of oral cancer were recorded in this study, with two-year and five-year survival rates at 43.6% and 20.7% respectively. Male gender, late clinical stage at presentation due to delay in seeking medical care, poor histo-pathological types and advanced age were independent predictors of survival. Early detection through screening and prompt treatment could improve survival.

Abbreviations
CI: Confidence Interval; CMV: Cytomegalovirus; EBV: Epstein barr virus; HIV: Human immunodeficiency virus; HPV: Human Papilloma Virus; HR: Hazard Ratio; HSSP: Health sector strategic plan; IQR: Inter-quartile range; LTC: Lymphoma treatment centre; MoH: Ministry of Health; NCD: Non-communicable disease; OSCC: Oral Squamous Cell Carcinoma; SD: Standard deviation; SSA: Sub-Saharan Africa; STC: Solid tumour treatment centre;

TNM: Tumour node metastasis; UCI: Uganda Cancer Institute; WHO: World Health Organisation

Acknowledgements

The authors are very grateful to Professor Charles Karamagi (PhD) and Ass Prof Joan Kalyango (PhD) of the Clinical Epidemiology Unit, College of Health Sciences, Makerere University Kampala Uganda, for mentoring JA and for their invaluable input during the study.

Funding

This study was personally funded.

Authors' contributions

JA contributed to the conception and design of the study, collected data, analysed and interpreted the data, drafted and revised the manuscript. CB participated in the design of the study, interpreted the data, and revised the manuscript. AK interpreted the data, and revised the manuscript. All authors have given their final approval of the version to be published.

Competing interests

The authors declare that they have no competing interests.

Author details

[1]HIV Reference Laboratory, Uganda Virus Research Institute, P. O. Box 49, Entebbe, Uganda. [2]Department of Dentistry, College of Health Sciences, Makerere University, P. O. Box 6717, Kampala, Uganda. [3]Child Health and Development Centre, College of Health Sciences, Makerere University, P. O. Box 6717, Kampala, Uganda.

References

1. Parkin DM, Bray F, Ferlay J, Pisani P. Global Cancer statistics, 2002. CA Cancer J Clin. 2005;55:74–108.
2. Lambert R, Sauvaget C, de Camargo Cancela M, Sankaranarayanan R. Epidemiology of cancer from the oral cavity and oropharynx. Eur J Gastroenterol Hepatol. 2011 Aug;23:633–41.
3. Johnson N. Tobacco use and Oral Cancer: a global perspective. J Dent Educ. 1991;65:328–39.
4. Shiels MS, Pfeiffer RM, Gail MH, Hall HI, Li J, Chaturvedi AK, et al. Cancer burden in the HIV-infected population in the United States. J Natl Cancer Inst. 2011;103:753–62.
5. Termine N, Panzarella V, Falaschini S, Russo A, Matranga D, Muzio LL, et al. HPV in oral squamous cell carcinoma vs head and neck squamous cell carcinoma biopsies : a meta-analysis. Ann Oncol. 2008;19:1681–90.
6. Schwartz SR, Yueh B, Mcdougall JK, Daling JR, Schwartz SM. Human papillomavirus infection and survival in oral squamous cell cancer:a population based study. Otolarygol Head Neck Surg. 2001;125:1–9.
7. Fakhry C, Westra WH, Li S, Cmelak A, Ridge JA, Pinto H, et al. Improved survival of patients with human papillomavirus – positive head and neck squamous cell carcinoma in a prospective clinical trial. J Natl Cancer Inst. 2008;100:261–9.
8. Wabinga HR, Nambooze S, Amulen PM, Okello C, Mbus L, Parkin DM. Trends in the incidence of cancer in Kampala Uganda 1991-2010. Int J Cancer. 2014;135:432–9.
9. Ibrahim NK, Al Ashakar MS, Gad ZM, Warda MH, Ghanem H. An epidemiological study on survival of oropharyngeal cancer cases in Alexandria, Egypt. East Mediterr Heal J. 2009;15:369–77.
10. Chen YK, Huang HC, Lin LM, Lin CC. Primary oral squamous cell carcinoma: an analysis of 703 cases in southern Taiwan. Oral Oncol. 1999;35:173–9.
11. Leite ICG, Koifman S. Survival analysis in a sample of oral cancer patients at a reference hospital in Rio de Janeiro, Brazil. Oral Oncol. 1998;34:347–52.
12. Hoffman HT, Karnell LH, Funk GF, Robinson RA, Menck HR. The National Cancer Data Base report on cancer of the head and neck. Arch Otolaryngol Head Neck Surg. 1998 Sep;124:951–62.
13. Chen LM, Li G, Reitzel LR, Pytynia KB, Zafereo ME, Wei Q, et al. Matched-pair analysis of race or ethnicity in outcomes of head and neck Cancer patients receiving similar multidisciplinary care. [Phila Pa]. Cancer Prev Res (Phila). 2009;2:782–91.
14. Boing AF, Peres MA, Antunes JLF. Mortality from oral and pharyngeal cancer in Brazil : trends and regional patterns , 1979 – 2002. Rev Panam Salud Publica. 2006;20:1–8.
15. Cook MB, Mcglynn KA, Devesa SS, Freedman ND, Anderson WF. Sex disparities in Cancer mortality and survival. Canncer Epidemiol Biomarkers Prev. 2009;20:1–9.
16. Mehta V, Yu G, Schantz SP. Population-based analysis of Oral and oropharyngeal carcinoma: changing trends of histopathologic differentiation , survival and patient demographics. Laryngoscope. 2010;120:2203–12.
17. Massano J, Regateiro SF, Januario G, Ferreira A. Oral squamous cell carcinoma : review of prognostic and predictive factors. Oral Surg Oral Med Oral Pathol Oral Radiol Endod. 2006;102:67–76.
18. Morris LGT, Ganly I. Outcomes of oral cavity squamous cell carcinoma in pediatric patients. Oral Oncol. 2011;46:292–6.
19. Nabukenya J, Hadlock TA, Arubaku W. Head and neck squamous cell carcinoma in Western Uganda: disease of uncertainty and poor prognosis. Oto Open. 2018;1:7.
20. Christensen AJ, Moran PJ, Ehlers SL, Raichle K, Karnell L, Funk G. Smoking and drinking behavior in patients with head and neck Cancer: effects of behavioral self-blame and perceived control. J Behav Med. 1999;22:407–8.
21. Lo W, Kao S, Chi L, Wong Y, Chang CR. Outcomes of Oral squamous cell carcinoma in Taiwan after surgical therapy: factors affecting survival. J Oral Maxillofac Surg. 2003;61:751–8.
22. Kakande E, Byaruhaga R, Kamulegeya A. Head and neck squamous cell carcinoma in a Ugandan population: a descriptive epidemiological study. J Afr Cancer. 2010;2:219–25.
23. Kantola S, Parikka M, Jokinen K, Hyrynkangs K, Soini Y, Alho OP, et al. Prognostic factors in tongue cancer - relative importance of demographic, clinical and histopathological factors. Br J Cancer. 2000;83:614–9.
24. Pulte D, Brenner H. Changes in survival in head and neck cancers in the late 20th and early 21st century: a period analysis. Oncologist. 2010 Jan;15:994–1001.
25. Kajja I, Sibinga CTS. Delayed elective surgery in a major teaching hospital in Uganda. Int J Clin Transfus Med. 2014;2:1–6.
26. Kigula MJB, Wegoye P. Pattern and experience with cancers treated with the chinese GWGP80 cobalt unit at Mulago hospital, Kampala. East Afr Med J. 2000;77:523–5.

Permissions

All chapters in this book were first published in CTH&N, by BioMed Central; hereby published with permission under the Creative Commons Attribution License or equivalent. Every chapter published in this book has been scrutinized by our experts. Their significance has been extensively debated. The topics covered herein carry significant findings which will fuel the growth of the discipline. They may even be implemented as practical applications or may be referred to as a beginning point for another development.

The contributors of this book come from diverse backgrounds, making this book a truly international effort. This book will bring forth new frontiers with its revolutionizing research information and detailed analysis of the nascent developments around the world.

We would like to thank all the contributing authors for lending their expertise to make the book truly unique. They have played a crucial role in the development of this book. Without their invaluable contributions this book wouldn't have been possible. They have made vital efforts to compile up to date information on the varied aspects of this subject to make this book a valuable addition to the collection of many professionals and students.

This book was conceptualized with the vision of imparting up-to-date information and advanced data in this field. To ensure the same, a matchless editorial board was set up. Every individual on the board went through rigorous rounds of assessment to prove their worth. After which they invested a large part of their time researching and compiling the most relevant data for our readers.

The editorial board has been involved in producing this book since its inception. They have spent rigorous hours researching and exploring the diverse topics which have resulted in the successful publishing of this book. They have passed on their knowledge of decades through this book. To expedite this challenging task, the publisher supported the team at every step. A small team of assistant editors was also appointed to further simplify the editing procedure and attain best results for the readers.

Apart from the editorial board, the designing team has also invested a significant amount of their time in understanding the subject and creating the most relevant covers. They scrutinized every image to scout for the most suitable representation of the subject and create an appropriate cover for the book.

The publishing team has been an ardent support to the editorial, designing and production team. Their endless efforts to recruit the best for this project, has resulted in the accomplishment of this book. They are a veteran in the field of academics and their pool of knowledge is as vast as their experience in printing. Their expertise and guidance has proved useful at every step. Their uncompromising quality standards have made this book an exceptional effort. Their encouragement from time to time has been an inspiration for everyone.

The publisher and the editorial board hope that this book will prove to be a valuable piece of knowledge for researchers, students, practitioners and scholars across the globe.

List of Contributors

Tim N. Beck and Erica A. Golemis
Program in Molecular Therapeutics, Fox Chase Cancer Center, 333 Cottman Ave, Philadelphia, PA 19111, USA
Program in Molecular and Cell Biology and Genetics, Drexel University College of Medicine, Philadelphia, PA 19129,USA

Nnamdi Eze
Section of Medical Oncology, Department of Internal Medicine, Yale University School of Medicine and Yale Cancer Center, 333 Cedar Street, Room WWW-221, New Haven, CT 06520, USA

Ying-Chun Lo
Department of Pathology, Yale University School of Medicine, New Haven, CT, USA

Barbara Burtness
Section of Medical Oncology, Department of Internal Medicine, Yale University School of Medicine and Yale Cancer Center, New Haven, CT, USA

Krista Roberta Verhoeft
Department of Clinical Oncology, Li-Ka Shing Faculty of Medicine, the University of Hong Kong, Hongkong, SAR, Hong Kong

Hoi Lam Ngan
School of Biomedical Sciences, Li-Ka Shing Faculty of Medicine, the University of Hong Kong, Hongkong, SAR, Hong Kong

Vivian Wai Yan Lui
School of Biomedical Sciences, Faculty of Medicine, the Chinese University of Hong Kong, Hongkong, SAR, Hong Kong

Firoozeh Samim
Department of Oral Medicine Oral Pathology, University of British Columbia, Vancouver, BC, Canada

Joel B. Epstein
Samuel Oschin Comprehensive Cancer Institute, Cedars-Sinai Medical Center, Los Angeles, CA, USA

Zachary S. Zumsteg
Radiation Oncology,Samuel Oschin Comprehensive Cancer Institute, Cedars-Sinai Medical Center, Los Angeles, CA, USA

Allen S. Ho
Department of Surgery, Samuel Oschin Comprehensive Cancer Institute, Cedars-Sinai Medical Center, Los Angeles, CA, USA

Andrei Barasch
Department of Medicine, Weill Cornell Medical College, New York, NY, USA

Marcelo Bonomi, Tamjeed Ahmed, Mercedes Porosnicu, Katharine Batt and Jimmy Ruiz
Section on Hematology and Oncology, Wake Forest School of Medicine, Winston-Salem, NC 27157, USA

David Warner
Internal Medicine, Wake Forest School of Medicine, Winston-Salem, NC 27157, USA

Joshua Waltonen and Christopher Sullivan
Department of Otolaryngology,Wake Forest School of Medicine, Winston-Salem, NC 27157, USA

James Cappellari
Department of Pathology, Wake Forest School of Medicine, Winston-Salem, NC 27157, USA

Henry S. Park and Roy H. Decker
Department of Therapeutic Radiology, Yale University School of Medicine, 15 York St, New Haven, CT 06519, USA

Matthew E. Witek, Randy J. Kimple, Craig R. Hullett and Paul M. Harari
Department of Human Oncology, University of Wisconsin, 600 Highland Avenue, K4/B100-0600, Madison, WI, Madison, WI 53792, USA

Aaron M. Wieland and Gregory K. Hartig
Department of Surgery, Division of Otolaryngology and Head and Neck Surgery, University of Wisconsin, Madison, WI, USA

Shuai Chen
Department of Biostatistics and Medical Informatics, University of Wisconsin, Madison, WI, USA

Tabassum A. Kennedy
Department of Radiology, University of Wisconsin, Madison, WI, USA

Evan Liang
University of Wisconsin School of Medicine and Public Health University of Wisconsin, Madison, WI, USA

Carolyn Y. Fang and Carolyn J. Heckman
Cancer Prevention and Control Program, Fox Chase Cancer Center, 333 Cottman Ave, Philadelphia, PA 19111, USA

Ting Martin Ma and Ana P. Kiess
Department of Radiation Oncology and Molecular Radiation Sciences, The Johns Hopkins University School of Medicine, Baltimore, MD 21231, USA

Hyunseok Kang
Department of Oncology, The Johns Hopkins University School of Medicine, Baltimore, MD 21287, USA

Steven P. Rowe
The Russell H. Morgan Department of Radiology and Radiological Science, The Johns Hopkins University School of Medicine, Baltimore, MD 21287, USA

Ruth J. Davis
Tumor Biology Section, Head and Neck Surgery Branch, National Institute on Deafness and Other Communication Disorders, National Institutes of Health, 10 Center Drive, Room 5B-39, Bethesda, MD 20892, USA

Nicole C. Schmitt
Tumor Biology Section, Head and Neck Surgery Branch, National Institute on Deafness and Other Communication Disorders, National Institutes of Health, 10 Center Drive, Room 5B-39, Bethesda, MD 20892, USA
Department of Otolaryngology-Head and Neck Surgery, Johns Hopkins School of Medicine, 6420 Rockledge Drive, Suite 4920, Bethesda, MD 20817, USA

Robert L. Ferris
Department of Otolaryngology, Hillman Cancer Center Research Pavilion, University of Pittsburgh, 5117 Centre Avenue, Room 2.26b, Pittsburgh, PA 15213-1863, USA
Department of Immunology, Hillman Cancer Center Research Pavilion, University of Pittsburgh, 5117 Centre Avenue, Room 2.26b, Pittsburgh, PA 15213-1863, USA
Cancer Immunology Programm, Hillman Cancer Center Research Pavilion, University of Pittsburgh Cancer Institute, 5117 Centre Avenue, Room 2.26b, Pittsburgh, PA 15213-1863, USA

Kyaw L. Aung and Lillian L. Siu
Drug Development Program, Princess Margaret Cancer Centre, University Health Network, 610 University Avenue, Suite 5-718, Toronto, ON M5G 2M9, Canada

Sylvine Carrondo Cottin, Stéphane Turcotte, Pierre Douville, François Meyer and Isabelle Bairati
Centre de recherche sur le cancer, Université Laval, 6, rue McMahon, 1899-2, Quebec City, QC G1R 2J6, Canada
Centre de recherche du CHU de Québec - Université Laval, Quebec City, QC, Canada

Faisal I. Ahmad and Daniel R. Clayburgh
Department of Otolaryngology- Head & Neck Surgery, Oregon Health and Science University, 3181 SW Sam Jackson Park Road, PV01, Portland, OR 97239, USA

Ingeborg Tinhofer and Volker Budach
Department of Radiooncology and Radiotherapy, Translational Radiation Oncology Research Laboratory, Charite University Hospital Berlin, Charitéplatz 1, 10117 Berlin, Germany
German Cancer Research Center (DKFZ), Heidelberg, and German Cancer Consortium (DKTK) partner site Berlin, Berlin, Germany

Korinna Jöhrens
Institute of Pathology, Charite University Hospital, Berlin, Germany

Ulrich Keilholz
Comprehensive Cancer Center, Charité University Hospital, Berlin, Germany

Naa A. Aryeetey and Charles Aidoo
National Center for Radiotherapy and NuclearMedicine Korle bu Teaching, Hospital, Accra, Ghana

Joel Yarney
National Center for Radiotherapy and NuclearMedicine Korle bu Teaching, Hospital Accra, Ghana
School of Medicine and Dentistry, Accra, Ghana

Verna Vanderpuye
National Center for Radiotherapy and Nuclear Medicine Korle bu Teaching, Hospital Accra, Ghana
School of Biomedical and Allied Health Science University of Ghana, Accra, Ghana

Emmanuel D. Kitcher and Kenneth Baidoo
School of Medicine and Dentistry, Accra, Ghana
Ear Nose and Throat Unit, Department of Surgery, Accra, Ghana

Alice Mensah
Department of Mathematics and Statistics, Accra Technical University, Accra, Ghana

Shrujal S. Baxi
Head and Neck Oncology Service, Department of Medicine, Memorial Sloan Kettering Cancer Center, 300 East 66th Street, Rm 1459, New York, NY 10065, USA

Emily Schwitzer and Lee W. Jones
Department of Medicine, Memorial Sloan Kettering Cancer Center, 1275 York Ave, New York, NY 10065, USA

Kyungsuk Jung
Department of Medicine, Fox Chase Cancer Center, 333 Cottman Ave, Philadelphia, PA, USA

Hyunseok Kang and Ranee Mehra
Department of Oncology, The Sidney Kimmel Comprehensive Cancer Center at Johns Hopkins, 201 N Broadway, Baltimore, MD, USA

Cassie Pan
Department of Surgery, Division of Otolaryngology, Yale University, New Haven, CT, USA

Natalia Issaeva and Wendell G. Yarbrough
Department of Otolaryngology/Head and Neck Surgery; Lineberger Cancer Center, University of North Carolina at Chapel Hill, 170 Manning Drive, Campus Chapel Hill, NC 27599, USA

Hong Li
Yale School of Medicine, New Haven, CT, USA

Henry S. Park
Yale School of Medicine, New Haven, CT, USA
Department of Therapeutic Radiology, Yale New Haven Hospital, New Haven, CT, USA
Yale Cancer Center, 330 Cedar Street, New Haven, CT 06520-8062, USA

Heather A. Osborn and Benjamin L. Judson
Yale School of Medicine, New Haven, CT, USA
Department of Surgery (Section of Otolaryngology), Yale New Haven Hospital, New Haven, CT, USA
Yale Cancer Center, 330 Cedar Street, New Haven, CT 06520-8062, USA

Sophie Hofto and Elisabeth Isenring
Faculty of Health Sciences and Medicine, Bond University, 2 Promethean Way, Robina, QLD 4226, Australia

James E. Jackson
Faculty of Health Sciences and Medicine, Bond University, 2 Promethean Way, Robina, QLD 4226, Australia
Radiation Oncology Centres, Gold Coast University Hospital, Southport, QLD, Australia.

Jessica Abbott
Gold Coast University Hospital, Southport, QLD, Australia

Juliet Asio
HIV Reference Laboratory, Uganda Virus Research Institute, Entebbe, Uganda

Adriane Kamulegeya
Department of Dentistry, College of Health Sciences, Makerere University, Kampala, Uganda

Cecily Banura
Child Health and Development Centre, College of Health Sciences, Makerere University, Kampala, Uganda

Index